Advances in Drug Delivery

Contents

AMERICAN
MEDICAL PUBLISHERS
www.americanmedicalpublishers.com

Cataloging-in-Publication Data

Advances in drug delivery / edited by Laurence Denton.
p. cm.
Includes bibliographical references and index.
ISBN 978-1-63927-856-5
1. Drug delivery systems. 2. Pharmaceutical technology. 3. Pharmacy. I. Denton, Laurence.
RS199.5 .A38 2023
615.6--dc23

American Medical Publishers,
41 Flatbush Avenue,
1st Floor, New York,
NY 11217, USA

ISBN 978-1-63927-856-5 (Hardback)

Advances in Drug Delivery

Editor: Laurence Denton

AMERICAN
MEDICAL PUBLISHERS
www.americanmedicalpublishers.com

Preface

Drug delivery system refers to the creation of a device which enables a therapeutic substance to reach a selected location in the human body without targeting the healthy tissues, cells and organs. It is a wide area of research which is related to the development of various new carrier systems and materials to be used in the delivery of drugs for efficient treatment. The novel systems of drug delivery are focused on providing sustained drug delivery with better body distribution, avoidance of drug clearance, and drug protection from harsh external environment. Furthermore, it comprises of polymeric, lipidic and proteic technologies. The evolution of nanomaterials for drug delivery known as nano-drug delivery systems (NDDSs), provides the opportunity to avoid the side effects of systemic drug administration and injury caused by the removal of tumors. This book on advances in drug delivery is a collective contribution of a renowned group of international experts. It traces significant advances in drug delivery systems. The book is an invaluable source of reference for medical practitioners, students, scientists, and researchers.

This book is a comprehensive compilation of works of different researchers from varied parts of the world. It includes valuable experiences of the researchers with the sole objective of providing the readers (learners) with a proper knowledge of the concerned field. This book will be beneficial in evoking inspiration and enhancing the knowledge of the interested readers.

In the end, I would like to extend my heartiest thanks to the authors who worked with great determination on their chapters. I also appreciate the publisher's support in the course of the book. I would also like to deeply acknowledge my family who stood by me as a source of inspiration during the project.

Editor

1

The Role of Combined Penetration Enhancers in Nasal Microspheres on In Vivo Drug Bioavailability

Giovanna Rassu [1], Luca Ferraro [2], Barbara Pavan [3], Paolo Giunchedi [1], Elisabetta Gavini [1,*] and Alessandro Dalpiaz [4]

1 Department of Chemistry and Pharmacy, University of Sassari, via Muroni 23/a, 07100 Sassari, Italy; grassu@uniss.it (G.R.); pgiunc@uniss.it (P.G.)
2 Department of Life Sciences and Biotechnology, University of Ferrara, via Borsari 46, 44121 Ferrara, Italy; frl@unife.it
3 Department of Biomedical and Specialist Surgical Sciences, University of Ferrara, via Borsari 46, 44121 Ferrara, Italy; pvnbbr@unife.it
4 Department of Chemical and Pharmaceutical Sciences, University of Ferrara, via Fossato di Mortara 19, 44121 Ferrara, Italy; dla@unife.it
* Correspondence: eligav@uniss.it

Abstract: Microspheres based on both methyl-β-cyclodextrins and chitosan were prepared by spray-drying as nasal formulations of a model polar drug to analyze, firstly, how the composition of the carrier affects drug permeation across synthetic membranes and, secondly, how it induces systemic or brain delivery of the drug. Microparticles with different weight ratios of the two penetration enhancers (10–90, 50–50, 90–10) were characterized with respect to morphology, size, structural composition, water uptake, and the in vitro drug permeation profile. The leader formulation (weight ratio of 50–50) was then nasally administered to rats; systemic and cerebrospinal fluid (CSF) drug concentrations were analyzed by high performance liquid chromatography (HPLC) over time. Microspheres obtained with a single enhancer, methyl-β-cyclodextrins or chitosan, were administered in vivo as a comparison. The in vitro properties of combined microspheres appeared modified with regard to the polymeric matrix ratio. In vivo results suggest that the optimal drug distribution between CSF and bloodstream can be easily obtained by varying the amount of these two penetration enhancers studied in the matrix of nasal microspheres.

Keywords: combined microsphere; chitosan; cyclodextrin; nasal delivery; nose to brain transport; penetration enhancer; nasal formulation; in vivo studies

1. Introduction

Absorption enhancers are agents included in formulations whose function is to increase absorption of a pharmacologically active drug by enhancing membrane permeation [1]. They are frequently employed in nasal formulations [2–5] in order to improve drug flux through nasal epithelia [6]. The main mechanisms involved in enhanced permeability of nasal membranes include (i) the transient opening of the tight junction between adjacent cells that favor paracellular diffusion through the intercellular space, and/or (ii) perturbation of lipid bilayer integrity and increased membrane fluidity promoting the transcellular permeation of drugs [1]. Permeation-enhancing excipients are investigated to develop formulations for hydrophilic drugs that have poor nasal membrane permeability [7]; among these, cyclodextrins (CDs) and chitosan are characterized by high biocompatibility, since they are able to induce their enhancing effects without causing damage to nasal mucosa [7].

Cyclodextrins, especially methylated-β-cyclodextrins, have proven to be excellent solubilizers and absorption enhancers in nasal drug delivery [2,8–10]. Owing to their ability to remove cholesterol and phospholipids from the outer half of the membrane bilayer, CDs can increase membrane fluidity [11]. Furthermore, methylated-β-cyclodextrins cause an increase in the paracellular permeability of epithelial cell layers because the cholesterol depletion influences the distribution of specific tight junction proteins (claudin 3, claudin 4, and occludin) [12]. Recently, Fenyvesi and co-workers [13] have shown that fluid-phase endocytosis of CDs can contribute to overcoming the mucosal barrier for poorly absorbed drugs.

Chitosan is one of the most-used penetration enhancers in nasal formulations [14–17]. A combination of mucoadhesion and transient opening of the tight junctions in the cell membrane allows polar drugs to pass by a paracellular pathway [2]. There are a number of chitosan salts that have better characteristics than chitosan itself; these include solubility, mucoadhesiveness, and penetration enhancement ability. The chitosan chloride salt form is the only kind of chitosan that has a specific monograph in the European Pharmacopoeia 8.0 [18].

In addition to high stability, powder formulations can also have an absorption promoting effect [2,17] by exerting a direct effect on the mucosa. Microspheres absorb water from mucus causing dehydration of the epithelial cells which leads to the opening of the tight junctions [19]. For these reasons, the formulation of solid microparticles in the presence of promotion enhancers appears advantageous for nose to brain delivery of drugs.

Traditionally cyclodextrin and chitosan have been used separately in nasal powder formulation [15,16,20] and no combination has been evaluated. Bshara and co-workers [21] formulated hydroxylpropyl-β-CD and chitosan aspartate in microemulsion and observed that the highest C_{max} and AUC values among all the formulations they tested (formulation without hydroxylpropyl-β-CD and chitosan aspartate and with chitosan aspartate alone) were most likely due to a synergistic effect of both materials on the intranasal permeation of drug.

Therefore, the aim of this work was to formulate methyl-β-cyclodextrins and chitosan in combination in spray-dried microspheres for nasal administration of a polar drug. In particular, the effects of the microparticles' composition on drug permeation across synthetic membranes were analyzed, and, then, related to systemic or brain delivery of the drug after intranasal administration.

Indeed, when administered nasally, a drug can be deposited on the respiratory or olfactory epithelia. In the first case, it may cross the respiratory mucosa by paracellular or transcellular transport, reaching the lamina propria and then blood vessel (systemic circulation) or peripheral trigeminal nerve (brainstem). If, on the other hand, the drug is deposited on the olfactory epithelium, transport to the central nervous system may be either paracellular through olfactory neurones, or transcellular through olfactory epithelial cells [7,22].

N^6-cyclopentyladenosine was selected as a model polar drug with low molecular weight.

2. Materials and Methods

2.1. Materials

Methyl-β-cyclodextrin, Cavasol® W7MPharma (Mw: 1300 g/mol; molecular substitution: 1.7) was purchased from Wacker-Chemie GmbH (München, Germany). Chitosan chloride, Protasan UP CL 113 (Mw: 160,000 g/mol; deacetylation degree, 86%) were purchased from NovaMatrix/FMC Biopolymer (Sandvika, Norway). Tegiloxan3™ silicon oil was kindly gift from Goldschmidth (Essen, Germany). N6-cyclopentyladenosine (CPA) (Mw: 335.36), N6-cyclohexyladenosine CHA, sodium acetate and acetic acid glacial were obtained from Sigma-Aldrich (Milan, Italy). Dimethylsulfoxide (DMSO) was obtained from Merck (Darmstadt, Germany). Methanol, acetonitrile, ethyl acetate, and water high performance liquid chromatography (HPLC) grade were purchased from Sigma-Aldrich (Milan, Italy). Male Wistar rats were purchased from Charles-River, Milan, Italy.

2.2. Preparation of Microspheres

Formulations of microspheres were prepared by spray drying technique with a Mini Büchi B-191 spray dryer (Büchi Laboratoriums-Technik AG, Flawil, Switzerland) using methyl-β-cyclodextrin and chitosan as excipients in different percentage ratios chosen on the basis of preliminary studies. Drug to polymer ratio 1/20 was chosen which guarantees an optimal dose for in vivo test and administration of powder amount suitable for rat nasal cavity [23]. The feed solution concentration was 0.5% (w/v). The microparticles containing both excipients in different weight ratio (10–90, 50–50, and 90–10) were prepared dissolving separately methyl-β-cyclodextrin and chitosan in water, under magnetic stirring, and solutions were mixed before the addition of CPA. The following operating conditions were utilized during spray drying: inlet and outlet temperature, 110 °C and 77 ± 2 °C, respectively; spray flow rate, 500 L/h; pump setting, 5% (1.74 ± 0.09 mL/min); and aspirator setting, 98% regardless solutions composition. The dry particles were put in a desiccator for at least 24 h. Unloaded microspheres based on methyl-β-cyclodextrin (MCb) and loaded microspheres based on chitosan (CH100) or methyl-β-cyclodextrin (MC100) were prepared as comparison.

The codes and composition of the microspheres are presented in Table 1.

Table 1. The polymer composition (% w/w), drug content (DC) and encapsulation efficiency (EE) of loaded microspheres.

Microsphere Codes	Methyl-β-Cyclodextrin	Chitosan	DC (%)	EE (%)	d_{vs} (μm)	SPAN
MC100	100	-	4.25 ± 0.05 ^{a}	88.78 ± 0.98 ^{a}	3.49 ± 0.10	2.20
MC90	90	10	4.25 ± 0.01 ^{a}	88.66 ± 0.22 ^{a}	2.74 ± 0.09	1.85
MC50	50	50	4.20 ± 0.07 ^{a}	87.87 ± 1.53 ^{a}	6.79 ± 1.84 ^{b,c}	2.24
MC10	10	90	3.81 ± 0.05	80.91 ± 1.13	6.55 ± 1.04 ^{b,c}	2.09
CH100 #	-	100	4.75 ± 0.06	95.0 ± 1.20	6.14 ± 0.84 ^{b,c}	1.66

Prepared as reference for in vivo studies [23]. ^{a} $p < 0.05$ MC10 versus MC100; versus MC90; versus MC50. ^{b} $p < 0.05$ MC100 versus CH100; versus MC50; versus MC10. ^{c} $p < 0.05$ MC90 versus CH100; versus MC50; versus MC10.

The yields of production were calculated as the weight percentage of the final product after drying, with respect to initial total amounts of drug and excipients used for the preparation.

2.3. Microsphere Characterization

2.3.1. Determination of Drug Content and Encapsulation Efficiency

To determine the real amount of CPA loaded in microspheres, 0.5 mL of water was added to an exact amount of combined formulations (containing about 0.5 mg of drug); then, 45.5 mL of methanol were added and stirred until solution was obtained. Finally, spectrophotometric analysis (UV-160A UV–Visible Recording Spectrophotometer, Shimadzu, Tokyo, Japan) was performed at 270 nm and the drug in solutions was quantified by using the calibration curve obtained in concentrations range from 2.8 to 22.4 mg/L ($y = 0.067x + 0.027$, $R^2 = 0.9997$). Analyses were carried out in triplicate.

Furthermore, an exact amount of MC100 (corresponding to 0.5 mg of CPA) was dissolved in 50 mL of methanol and solution spectrophotometrically analyzed.

The drug loaded in microspheres (DC) was calculated as the experimentally detected amount of CPA in microspheres and expressed as percentage; encapsulation efficiency (EE), as percentage, was also calculated. The following equations were applied:

$$\text{DC}\ (\%) = \left(\frac{\text{rCPA}}{\text{tCPA}}\right) \times \text{tDC}$$

$$\text{EE}\ (\%) = \left(\frac{\text{DC}}{\text{tDC}}\right) \times 100$$

where rCPA is the detected amount of CPA in microspheres, tCPA is the drug amount solubilized in feed solution and tDC the percentage of the expected theoretical value.

2.3.2. Morphological Analysis

The morphology of the microspheres was determined by observation on a scanning electron microscope (VP-SEM; Zeiss EVO40XVP, Arese, Milan, Italy). The samples were placed on double-sided tape that had previously been secured to aluminum stubs and then analyzed under an argon atmosphere at an 18 kV acceleration voltage after gold sputtering.

2.3.3. Particle Size Analysis

The particle size and particle size distribution of the microspheres were determined by laser diffraction using a Coulter Laser Sizer LS100Q (Coulter LS 100Q Laser sizer, Beckman Coulter, Miami, FL, USA). All analyses were performed at room temperature. Two mg of microspheres were suspended in 1 mL of Tegiloxan by sonication (about 4–6 s) and then analyzed. The results reported are the averages of triplicate averages. The average particle size of the microspheres was reported as the mean volume-surface diameter, d_{vs} (μm). To quantify distribution width, SPAN was calculated as previously reported [24].

2.3.4. Powder X-ray Diffraction

Powder diffraction spectra were recorded, at room temperature, on a Bruker D-8 Advance diffractometer (Brucker, Karlsruhe, Germany) with graphite monochromatized Cu Kα radiation (λ = 1.5406 Å). The data were recorded at 2θ steps of 0.02° from 3° to 50° with 2 s/step.

2.3.5. Water Uptake

The investigation of water uptake capability was carried out by the modified Enslin apparatus as previously described [25]. Microspheres (10 mg) were uniformly dispersed on a cellulose filter disk saturated with MilliQ water, lying on the top of a fritted glass support, connected with a graduated capillary. The volume of water absorbed (μL) along the time (from 0.25 up to 60 min) was measured. The result obtained is the average of three determinations (n = 3; ±SD).

2.3.6. In Vitro Permeation Test of Microspheres

The in vitro drug permeation across synthetic membrane was performed using a modified Franz diffusion system incorporating three in-line flow-through diffusion cells [26]. Regenerated cellulose membranes (pore size 0.45 μm, 47 mm diameter, Sartorius, Goettingen, Germany) saturated with octanol were chosen as lipophilic layer [20]. An amount of microspheres containing about 1.0 mg of CPA was uniformly spread out above the membrane. Acceptor compartment was filled with 100 mL of pH 6.5 phosphate buffer at 37 ± 0.5 °C, to guarantee sink condition. The flux of the medium was 6 mL/min. Permeation system was automatically coupled to UV-spectrophotometer (UV-1800, UV–Visible Recording Spectrophotometer, Shimadzu, Tokyo, Japan) and the fluid was analyzed at 270 nm at predetermined times (from 30 up to 120 min). The permeated drug was quantified by using the calibration curve obtained in concentrations range from 2.8 to 22.4 mg/L ($y = 0.0559x + 0.051$ $R^2 = 1$). All experiments were performed in triplicate. As comparison, in vitro permeation test of raw CPA was carried out.

From the values obtained, the curves of accumulated amounts (mg/cm^2) versus permeation time (min) were drawn; then, the flux (J) was determined from the slope of the steady state portion as well as the lag time (T lag) values from the x-intercept of the slope at a steady state [27].

2.4. *In Vivo Studies*

2.4.1. In Vivo CPA Administration and Quantification

Male Wistar rats (200−250 g) anesthetized during the experimental period received a femoral intravenous infusion of 0.1 mg/mL CPA dissolved in a medium constituted by 20% (*v*/*v*) DMSO and 80% (*v*/*v*) physiologic solution, with a rate of 0.2 mL/min for 10 min. At the end of infusion and at fixed time points, blood samples (100 μL) were collected and cerebrospinal fluid (CSF) samples (50 μL) were withdrawn by the cysternal puncture method described by van den Berg and co-workers [28], which requires a single needle stick and allows the collection of serial (40–50 μL) CSF samples that are virtually blood-free [29]. Four rats were employed for femoral intravenous infusions. CSF samples (10 μL) were immediately injected into high performance liquid chromatography (HPLC) system for CPA detection.

The blood samples were hemolyzed immediately after their collection with 500 μL of ice-cold water, then 50 μL of 3N NaOH and 100 μL of internal standard (10 μM CHA) were added. The samples were extracted twice with 1 mL of water-saturated ethyl acetate, and, after centrifugation, the organic layer was reduced to dryness under a nitrogen stream. One hundred and fifty microliters of a mobile phase (see below) was added, and, after centrifugation, 10 μL was injected into the HPLC system for CPA detection.

The in vivo half-life of CPA in the blood was calculated by nonlinear regression (exponential decay) of concentration values in the time range within 90 min after infusion.

Nasal administration of CPA was performed to anaesthetized rats laid on their backs, following two procedures. The first way consisted on the introduction in each nostril of rats 20 μL of an aqueous suspension of CPA (5 mg/mL) using a semiautomatic pipette which was attached to a short polyethylene tubing [29]. After the administration, blood (100 μL) and CSF samples (50 μL) were collected at fixed time points, and they were analyzed with the same procedures described above. Four rats were employed for nasal administration of CPA suspension. The second way consisted on the insufflation of loaded CPA microparticles to each nostril of the anaesthetized rats by means of single dose Monopowder P1 insufflators [30]. The insufflators were loaded with about 2.4 mg of CH100, MC100 and MC50 and their content was administered to each nostril of rats. After the administration, blood (100 μL) and CSF samples (50 μL) were collected at fixed time points, then analyzed. Four rats were employed for nasal administration of each type of microparticulate powders.

All in vivo experiments were performed in accordance with the European Communities Council Directive of September 2010 (2010/63/EU) a revision of the Directive 86/609/EEC and were approved by the Italian Ministry of Health and by the Ethical Committee of the University of Ferrara. Any effort has been done to reduce the number of the animals and their suffering.

The area under concentration curves of CPA in the blood and CSF (AUC, μg mL^{-1} min) were calculated by the trapezoidal method. All the calculations were performed by using the computer program Graph Pad Prism (GraphPad Software Incorporated, La Jolla, CA, USA).

2.4.2. HPLC Analysis

The quantification of CPA in all samples generated from the experimental procedures was performed by HPLC. The chromatographic apparatus consisted of a modular system (model LC-10 AD VD pump and model SPD-10A VP variable wavelength UV−vis detector; Shimadzu, Kyoto, Japan) and an injection valve with 20 μL sample loop (model 7725; Rheodyne, IDEX, Torrance, CA, USA). Separations were performed at room temperature on a 5 μm Hypersil BDS C-18 column (150 mm × 4.6 mm i.d.; Alltech Italia Srl, Milan, Italy), equipped with a guard column packed with the same Hypersil material. Data acquisition and processing were accomplished with a personal computer using CLASS-VP Software, version 6.12 SP5 (Shimadzu Italia, Milan, Italy). The detector was set at 269 nm. The mobile phase consisted of a ternary mixture of acetonitrile, methanol and 10 mM acetate buffer (pH 4) with a ratio of 4/40/56 ($v/v/v$). The flow rate was 0.8 mL/min and the retention time of CPA and CHA were 4.1 and 5.8 min, respectively.

The chromatographic precision, represented by relative standard deviations (RSD), was evaluated by repeated analysis ($n = 6$) of the same sample solution containing each of the examined compounds at a concentration of 10 μM. The solutes were diluted in water by 10^{-2} M stock solutions in DMSO. The RSD values ranged between 0.81% and 0.83% for the analyzed compounds. The calibration curve of peak areas versus concentration was generated in the range 0.1 to 20 μM of CPA and resulted linear ($n = 9$, $r = 0.998$, $p < 0.0001$). For CSF simulation, standard aliquots of balanced solution (PBS Dulbecco's without calcium and magnesium) in the presence of 0.45 mg/mL BSA were employed [31,32]. In this case, the chromatographic precision was evaluated by repeated analysis ($n = 6$) of the same sample solution containing 1.0 μM CPA whose RSD value was 0.92% and calibration curve of peak areas versus concentration was generated in the range 0.08 to 10 μM (corresponding to 26.8 to 3353 ng/mL), resulting linear ($n = 8$, $r = 0.994$, $p < 0.0001$). The LOD and LOQ values of CPA determination in the blood were 8.12 ng/mL (0.0002 nmoles/injection, signal-to-nose ratio of 3:1) and 26.8 ng/mL (0.0008 nmoles/injection, signal-to-noise ratio of 10:1), respectively. The accuracy of the analytical method for CPA extracted from rat whole blood was determined by comparing the peak areas of 10 μM CPA (corresponding to 3353 ng/mL) extracted at 4 °C ($n = 3$) with those obtained by injection of an equivalent concentration of the analyte dissolved in the mobile phase for HPLC analysis. The average recovery from rat whole blood ± S.E. was 86 ± 3%. The concentrations of CPA were therefore referred to as peak area ratio with respect to the internal standard CHA. The precision of this peak area ratio-based method is demonstrated by the RSD values of 1.03% for 10 μM CPA extracted from rat blood at 4 °C, whose calibration curve was linear over the range 0.15—30 μM (corresponding to 50.4 to 10,059 ng/mL; $n = 9$, $r > 0.992$, $p < 0.0001$). The LOD and LOQ values of CPA determination in the blood were 15.3 ng/mL (0.0005 nmoles/injection, signal-to-nose ratio of 3:1) and 50.4 ng/mL (0.0015 nmoles/injection, signal-to-noise ratio of 10:1), respectively.

2.5. Statistical Analysis

Data were analyzed using one-way ANOVA followed by Tukey or Bonferroni test (GraphPad Prism, version 6.02; GraphPad Software Incorporated). Difference was considered statistically significant at P values less than 0.05.

3. Results and Discussion

3.1. Preparation and Characterization of Microspheres

Spray drying appears to be a suitable method for the preparation of CPA-loaded microspheres containing methyl-β-cyclodextrin and chitosan chloride. The technique is simple and rapid as it only requires the preparation of a feed solution. Production yields were good (range from 63–72% (w/w)) with no significant differences between the formulations produced.

3.1.1. Determination of Drug Content and Encapsulation Efficiency

CPA content of the formulations and encapsulation efficiency are listed in Table 1. The drug contents of the formulations were relatively close to the theoretical values, and the encapsulation efficiency values ranged between 80% and 88%. The higher chitosan content of MC10 determined a significant decrease in drug encapsulation capacity compared to the other formulations ($p < 0.05$).

3.1.2. Morphological Analysis

Figure 1 illustrates that by increasing the percentage of methyl-β-cyclodextrin in the microspheres, the transition from a smooth to corrugated surface was gradual. In fact, CH100 and MC100 evidenced distinct morphologies. In particular, as reported in Figure 2, CH100 showed a spherical shape and smooth surface, whereas the surface of MC100 particles appeared corrugated in the presence of multiple invaginations.

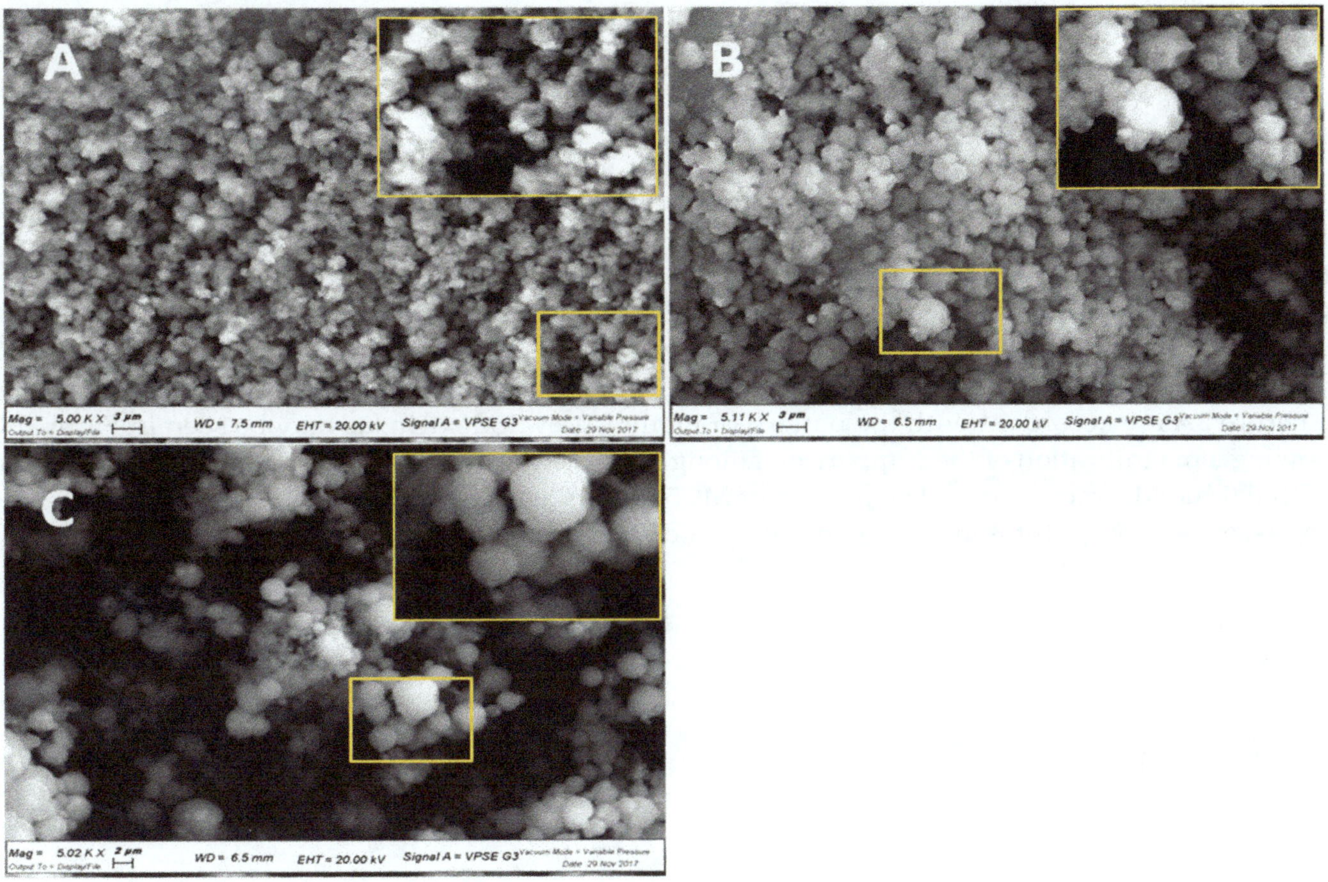

Figure 1. SEM micrographs with magnifications of 5000 times of: (**A**) MC90; (**B**) MC50; (**C**) MC10.

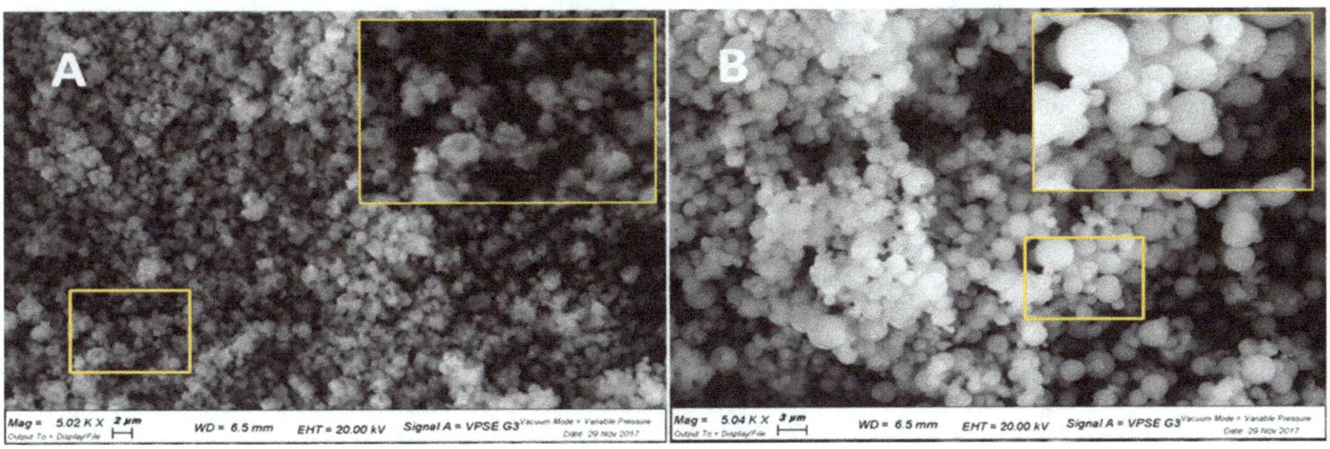

Figure 2. SEM micrographs with magnifications of 5000 times of: (**A**) MC100; (**B**) CH100.

3.1.3. Particle Size Analysis

The d_{vs} values of the formulations are reported in Table 1. The size of the microspheres, generated by spraying feed solutions with the same concentration, depends on the kind and ratio of excipients used. In fact, the weight ratio between two polymers affected the d_{vs}, which increased significantly from MC90 to MC50 and 10–90 ($p < 0.05$), but not particle size distribution ($p > 0.05$). In fact, SPAN index values were comparable, ranging between 1.85 and 2.24, indicating an almost narrow size distribution in all cases. Drug encapsulation did not significantly affect the particle size of methyl-β-cyclodextrin microspheres (MCb 4.52 ± 0.09). On the contrary, chitosan unloaded microparticles generally appeared bigger than the corresponding loaded particles. These last data would appear to be in accordance with those obtained in previous studies: indeed, size modification was observed for spray-dried chitosan microparticles as a consequence of the presence of metoclopramide [33] and CPA [23].

3.1.4. Powder X-ray Diffraction

Additional information on the solid state of the microparticles was obtained by powder X-ray diffraction. As illustrated in Figure 3A, pure CPA (black) exhibited distinct diffraction peaks. The diffractogram of the loaded microparticles did not exhibit any CPA diffraction peaks, indicating the absence of its crystalline state in the loaded form. In particular, the patterns of CH100 (red) and MC10 (blue) samples reported in Figure 3A are accordant with the pattern of chitosan, as shown in Figure 3B, showing a magnification of the comparison between pure chitosan (black) and the sample CH100 (red) diffractograms. Moreover, the patterns of MC100 (fuchsia) and MC90 (brown) samples reported in Figure 3A are accordant with the pattern of methyl-β-cyclodextrin, as may be seen in Figure 3C, showing a magnification of the comparison among pure methyl-β-cyclodextrin (red), MCb (black) and MC100 (blue) diffractograms. The pattern of MC50 sample (green) reported in Figure 3A evidenced the presence of both chitosan and methyl-β-cyclodextrin in the same sample.

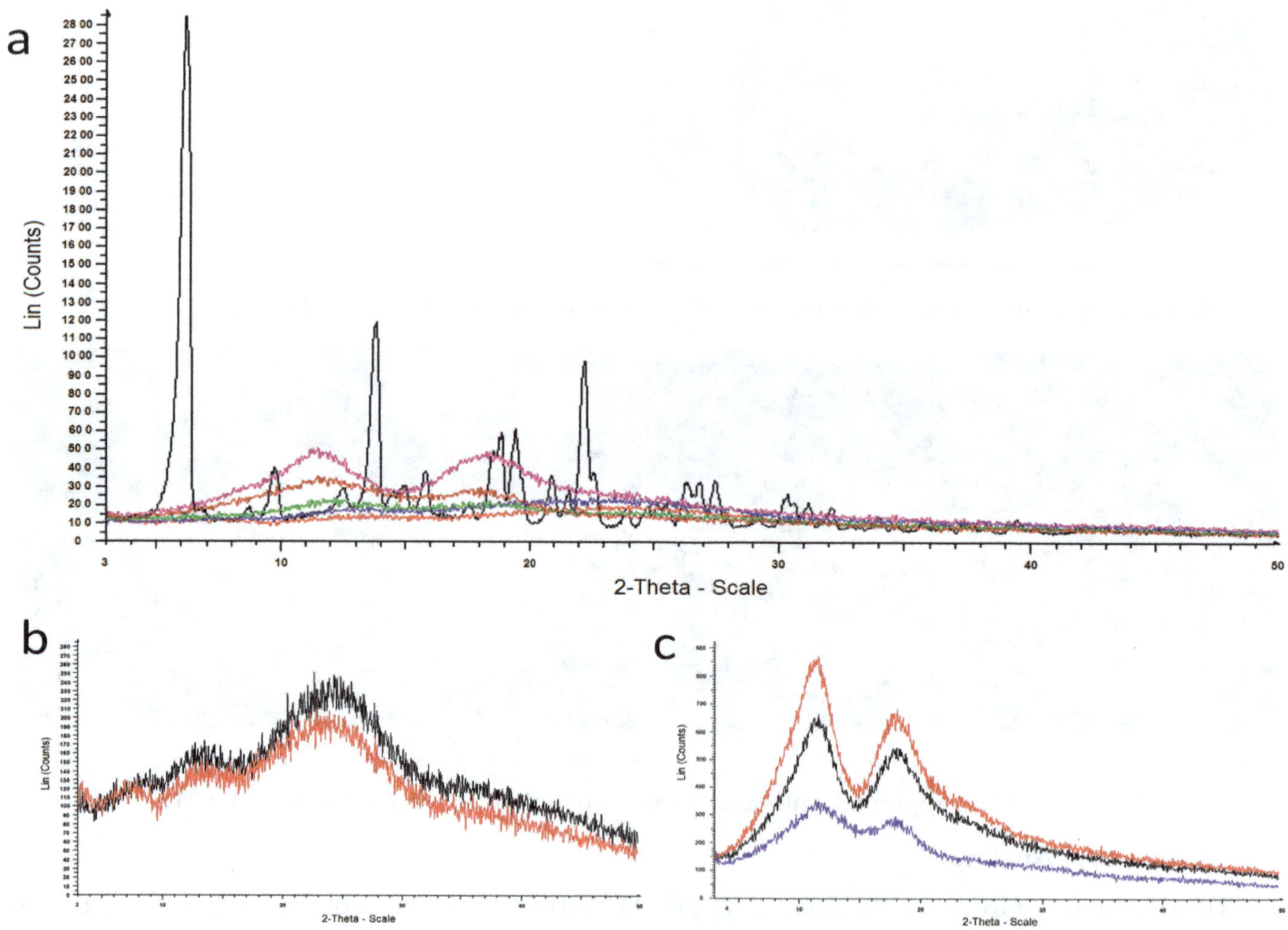

Figure 3. Powder X-ray diffraction patterns of: (**a**) CPA (black), MC90 (brown), MC50 (green) MC10 (blue), MC100 (fuchsia) and CH100 (red); (**b**) chitosan (black) and CH100 (red); (**c**) methyl-β-cyclodextrin (red), MCb (black) and MC100 (blue).

3.1.5. Water Uptake

The water uptake of formulations containing both excipients was affected by their weight ratio (Figure 4). It is well-known that methyl-β-cyclodextrin is a water soluble excipient that absorbs very little water and is then rapidly solubilized; on the contrary, chitosan salts are able to absorb water allowing them to swell and gel [20]. Consequently, the amount of water absorbed per milligram of microspheres markedly increased when the amount of chitosan was raised in the particle matrix.

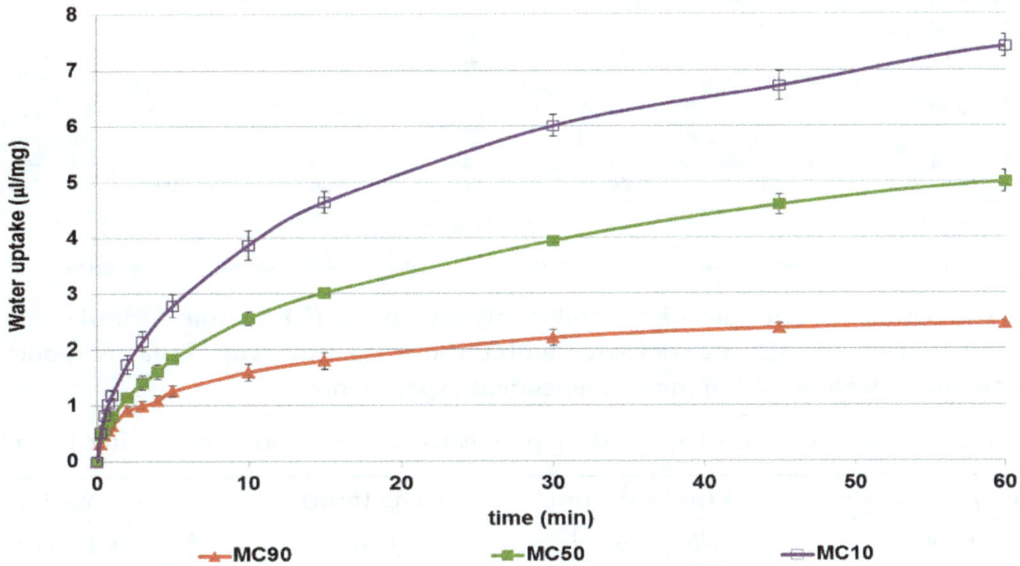

Figure 4. The water uptake capacity (µL/mg) of the microspheres. Data are reported as the mean value of three independent experiments. SD values were ≤0.17 of their corresponding means.

3.1.6. In Vitro Permeation Test of Microspheres

The in vitro permeation profiles of CPA released from microspheres, compared with those of the pure drug, are shown in Figure 5. CPA, as a hydrophilic drug, was able to permeate synthetic membrane with linear kinetic (n= 11, r = 0.984, p < 0.0001), reaching 80% of the amount tested in acceptor medium within 120 min. When encapsulated in microspheres the CPA permeation ability was modified in relation to the polymer and ratio employed as the polymeric matrix. In particular, cyclodextrin increased the flux and total amount of drug permeated when used alone (MC100), or at 90% (w/w) (MC90) (Table 2).

On the contrary, chitosan reduced the permeation of the loaded drug through lipophilic membranes (CH100: 30% of CPA permeated after 120 min). When the concentration of chitosan was 50% (MC50) and 90% (MC10) MC50, the CPA permeation flux and drug total amount significantly decreased (Table 2), reaching the zero values for MC10 sample at all time points tested (Figure 5). CPA's inability to permeate when encapsulated in MC10 could be due to the need of the elevated amount of water for its hydration (as demonstrated by the water uptake results), which was not available in the experimental conditions. Worthy of note is, firstly, chitosan's ability to reduce the permeation, and, secondly, methyl-β-cyclodextrin's ability to increase the passage of the loaded drug through lipophilic membranes regardless of the kind of drug encapsulated [20]. Among the combined formulations tested, of interest is the linear kinetic of CPA release from MC50 in the range from 20 min to 120 min (R^2 = 0.9987).

Lag time is the time required for the diffusion flow to become stable. During our experiments, it varied from 1.44 to 20.11 min (Table 2), and was affected by the hydration time of the matrix. These lag times could be considered appropriate for nasal formulations, taking into account that the half-life of clearance in nasal cavity is in the order of 15–20 min [7].

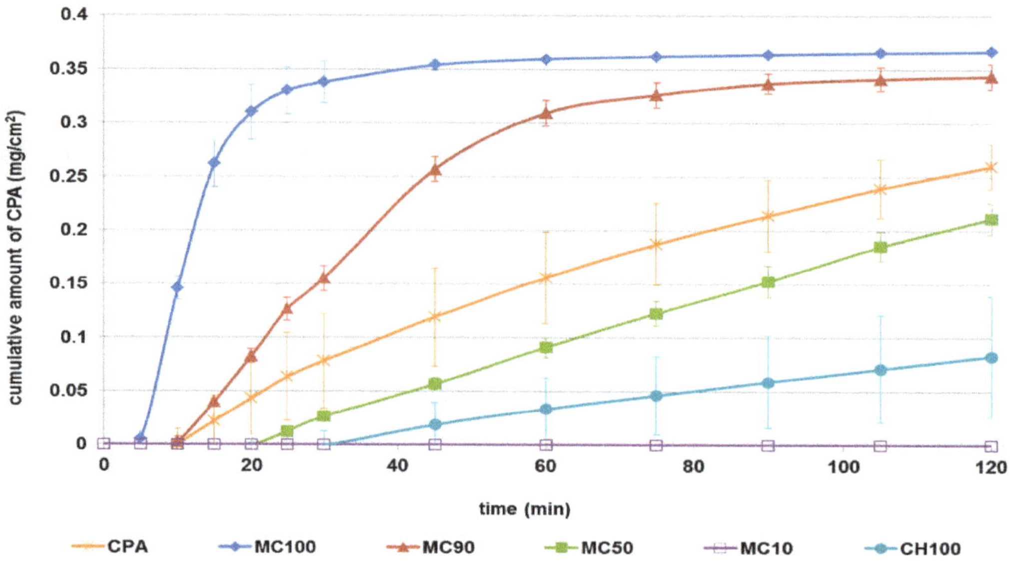

Figure 5. The permeation profiles of N6-cyclopentyladenosine (CPA) from formulations through lipophilic membranes. Profiles are compared with those of the raw drug. Data are reported as the mean ± standard deviation (SD) of three independent experiments.

Table 2. Values of flux (J), T lag and drug permeated for each formulation after 120 min.

Microsphere Codes	J (μg/cm² min)	T Lag (min)	Drug Permeated (%)
CPA	2.48 ± 0.65 [a,b,c]	1.44	83.55 ± 10.85 [d,e,g]
MC100	25.64 ± 2.14 [a]	4.64	112.56 ± 1.24 [d]
MC90	7.27 ± 0.18 [a,b]	8.96	105.87 ± 2.26 [e]
MC50	2.09 ± 0.14 [a,b]	17.62	65.46 ± 3.66 [d,e,f]
MC10	0.00 [a,b,c]	-	0.00
CH100	0.86 ± 0.53 [a,b]	20.11	22.26 ± 15.33 [d,e,f,g]

[a] $p < 0.01$ MC100 versus MC90; versus MC50; versus MC10; versus CH100 and CPA. [b] $p < 0.01$ MC90 versus MC50; versus MC10; versus CH100; versus CPA. [c] $p < 0.05$ MC10 versus CPA. [d] $p < 0.05$ MC100 versus MC50; versus CH100; versus CPA. [e] $p < 0.05$ MC90 versus MC50; versus CH100; CPA. [f] $p < 0.05$ MC50 versus CH100. [g] $p < 0.05$ CH100 versus CPA.

On the basis of the in vitro properties of microspheres made by combined penetration enhancers, MC50 was elected as the leader formulation to be in vivo tested. MC50 possessed good EE% as well as size and morphology, comparable to the other formulation containing a high amount of chitosan (MC10). Nevertheless, MC50 needed lower amounts of water to hydrate and showed a better drug release profile than MC10. On the other hand, MC90 had very similar in vitro properties to MC100, but as it is a formulation made by cyclodextrin alone, it would not be possible to evaluate the in vivo effect of the co-presence of the two penetration enhancers.

3.2. *In Vivo CPA Administration and Quantification*

The analysis of rat blood samples following the intravenous infusion of 0.2 mg of CPA indicated that the drug concentration in the blood stream was 6.11 ± 0.41 μg/mL at the end of infusion, and decreased with a terminal half-life of 6.8 ± 0.9 min. The AUC value of this profile was 37687 ± 1118 ng mL^{-1} min (Table 3). These data are in good agreement with those obtained in previous in vivo studies on CPA pharmacokinetics in rats [23,34]. On the other hand, no CPA was detected in the CSF of rats within 120 min after the end of the intravenous infusion. These results confirm that CPA is unable to reach the CNS from the bloodstream, as previously reported [23,35–37]. The microparticles (CH100, MC100 and MC50) were tested for nasal administration of CPA in order to verify its potential uptake into the CNS. Nasal administration of an aqueous suspension of CPA was also tested as control. Indeed, the nasal administration of pure CPA as powder was not performed, owing to the very low dose (200 μg in rats). Therefore, as control we employed a water suspension of the raw drug. No significant amounts of CPA were observed either in blood or in in the CSF of rats within 120 of the treatment (data not shown). A similar behavior was registered after the nasal administrations of rokitamicin [15], deferoxamine [20], and a zidovudine prodrug [16,29], as water suspensions, confirming that appropriate nasal formulations are needed in order to promote the drug uptake in the central nervous system.

Table 3. Area under concentration curves (AUC) obtained after CPA administration in rats for blood and CSF compartments.

	Blood		CSF	
Administration Way	**AUC (ng mL^{-1} min)**	**Absolute Bioavailability**	**AUC (ng mL^{-1} min)**	**Relative Bioavailability**
Intravenous	37,687 ± 1118	100	n.d.	0
Nasal (suspension)	n.d.	0	n.d.	0
Nasal (CH100)	699 ± 257	1.85%	32,910 ± 1199	100%
Nasal (MC50)	4830 ± 827 [a]	12.8%	39,900 ± 1520	121% [b]
Nasal (MC100)	13,590 ± 1451 [c]	36.0%	55,140 ± 1016	170% [c]

Data are reported as mean ± standard deviation, $n = 4$. Absolute bioavailability values are referred to AUC obtained by intravenous administration (100%); relative bioavailability values are referred to AUC obtained by nasal administration of CH100 microparticles (100%). n.d., not detectable. [a] $p > 0.05$ versus CH100; [b] $p < 0.05$ versus CH100; [c] $p < 0.001$ versus CH100.

On the contrary, nasal administration of the powder constituted by the loaded CH100, MC100 and MC50 microparticles (4.8 mg, about 200 μg of CPA) produced detectable levels of the drug in both blood and CSF, as reported in Figures 6 and 7, respectively. CH100 microparticles were previously described [23], but they were chosen as reference formulation in order to evaluate the effects induced by MC100 presence in the formulations. After nasal administration of CH100 particles, the peak concentration in the blood was detected at 60 min, with values just above the LOD of the analytical method (22 ± 12 ng/mL), indicating relatively poor CPA permeation from the nose to the bloodstream, as previously reported for this type of formulation [23]. Indeed, a comparison of the AUC values (Table 3) obtained after intravenous administration (37687 ± 1118 ng mL^{-1} min) and nasal administration (699 ± 257 ng mL^{-1} min) indicated an absolute bioavailability value of 1.85% for the microparticulate powders based on chitosan.

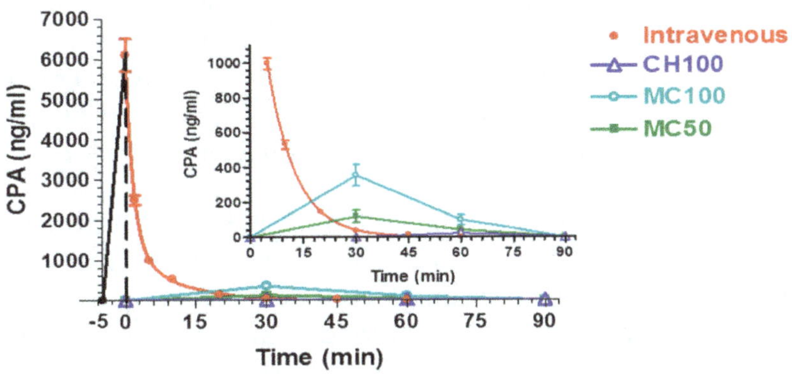

Figure 6. Blood CPA concentrations (ng/mL) after infusion or nasal administration of a 200-μg dose. The time ranging from −5 to 0 min refers to CPA IV infusion. In the inset: zoom of the same plot with expanded Y-scale (CPA blood concentration) from 0 to 1000 ng/mL. The inset highlights the concentration values obtained after administration of CH100, MC100 and MC50. Data are expressed as the mean ± standard deviation, $n = 4$.

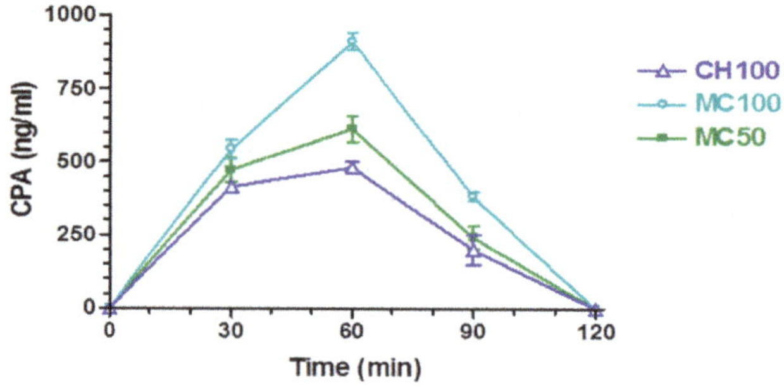

Figure 7. CPA concentrations (ng/mL) detected in the cerebrospinal fluid (CSF) after nasal administration of CH100, MC100 and MC50. Data are expressed as the mean ± standard deviation, $n = 4$.

The presence of cyclodextrins in the microparticulate nasal formulation induced an increase in CPA permeation in the bloodstream after nasal administration. Indeed, as evidenced in the inset of Figure 6, following the nasal administration of MC50 or MC100 particles, the peak plasma concentrations of CPA were detected at 30 min, with values of 118 ± 36 ng/mL or 354 ± 62 ng/mL, respectively. In this case the AUC values of MC50 or MC100 formulations were 4830 ± 827 or 13,590 ± 1451 ng mL^{-1} min, respectively, but only the MC100 value appeared significantly different from the AUC of CH100 (Table 3). The absolute bioavailability values were 12.8% and 36.0% for MC50 and MC100 samples, respectively. Table 3 summarizes the AUC and bioavailability values for the different administration routes of CPA. These data indicate that the progressive modifications of the morphology and structural composition of CH100 particles induced by the enhancement of the CDs in their composition reflects a progressive increase in systemic delivery of CPA, following their nasal administration.

Relevant amounts of CPA were detected in the CNS of rats after nasal administration of the solid microparticulate formulations. In particular, Figure 7 shows the CPA concentrations detected in the CSF: drug loaded chitosan microparticles (CH100 sample) may be seen to lead to an increase in CPA concentration values up to 481 ± 21 ng/mL within 60 min. Then, at 90 min the CPA concentration in CSF was significantly decreased (201 ± 50 ng/mL) and became undetectable at 120 min. The AUC value of this profile was found to be 32,910 ± 1199 ng mL^{-1} min. These data are in good agreement with those obtained in previous in vivo studies for this type of microparticles [23]. As registered in the bloodstream, the presence of cyclodextrins in the nasal formulations induced an increase in CPA amounts permeating in the CSF. Indeed, after nasal administration of the samples MC50 or MC100, the CPA concentrations in the CSF of rats increased up to 614 ± 44 and 911 ± 29 ng/mL, respectively, within 60 min after the nasal administration, then the values decreased to 243 ± 39 ng/mL for MC50 and 382 ± 16 ng/mL for MC100 at 90 min and became undetectable at 120 min. The AUC value of the MC50 and MC100 profiles were found to be 39,900 ± 1520 and 55,140 ± 1016 ng mL^{-1} min, respectively, with relative bioavailability values of 121% for MC50 and 170% for MC100, with respect to the CH100 formulation. These data seem to confirm that the presence of cyclodextrins in microparticulate nasal formulations can enhance drug permeation across nasal mucosa, with respect to formulations based on chitosan [20].

On the other hand, CH100 microparticles allowed us to obtain a CPA distribution between CSF and bloodstream resulting in a significantly higher ratio of concentrations than the ratios obtained by the nasal administration of the microparticles containing cyclodextrins. This aspect is evidenced in Figure 8, where the AUC ratios of CPA between CSF and bloodstream, obtained after nasal administration of the CH100, MC50 and MC100 microparticles, are reported. In particular, CH100 microparticles induced an AUC ratio of 47 ± 18, significantly higher ($p < 0.001$) than the AUC ratios obtained by nasal administration of MC50 (8.2 ± 1.6) and MC100 (3.9 ± 0.5) samples. A high AUC value can be very useful when a selective therapeutic activity of the drug is required in the central nervous system with respect to the bloodstream where the drug activity can induce severe side-effects. To the best of our knowledge, this is the first time that a modulation between the optimal uptake of a drug and its optimal distribution between CSF and bloodstream has been shown to be easily obtainable simply by varying the amount of cyclodextrins and chitosan in the microparticles.

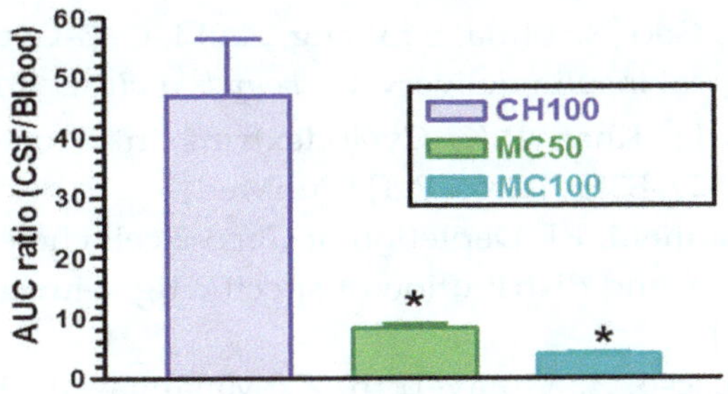

Figure 8. Ratios between CPA area under concentration curves (AUC) values between CSF and bloodstream obtained after nasal administration of the loaded microparticles CH100, MC50 and MC100. Data are expressed as the mean ± standard deviation, $n = 4$. * $p < 0.001$ versus CH100.

4. Conclusions

This study has demonstrated that the choice of penetration enhancer in nasal microspheres significantly affects the in vivo bioavailability of the encapsulated drug. In particular, methyl-β-cyclodextrin is more effective in enhancing drug permeation through respiratory and olfactory epithelia; this could be due to the changes in both paracellular and transcellular transports. On the contrary, chitosan has proven to be a selective excipient able to increase, above all, the paracellular transport of a drug through olfactory epithelia. This is, moreover, the first time that optimal drug distribution between CSF and bloodstream has been shown to be easily obtainable by varying the amount of these two penetration enhancers studied in the matrix of powder formulations.

Author Contributions: Conceptualization, E.G., P.G.; Investigation, G.R.; HPLC acquisition, analysis, validation and interpretation of data, A.D. and B.P.; Experiments on rats, L.F.; Project Administration, E.G.; Resources, P.G., A.D., L.F.; Writing—Original Draft Preparation, G.R., A.D., L.F.; Writing—Review & Editing, E.G., G.R., A.D.

Acknowledgments: The authors thank Gabriele Bertocchi (Department of Chemical and Pharmaceutical Sciences, University of Ferrara, Italy) for powder X-ray diffraction measurements.

References

1. Aungst, B.J. Absorption Enhancers: Applications and Advances. *AAPS J.* **2012**, *14*, 10–18. [CrossRef] [PubMed]
2. Davis, S.S.; Illum, L. Absorption Enhancers for Nasal Drug Delivery. *Clin. Pharmacokinet.* **2003**, *42*, 1107–1128. [CrossRef] [PubMed]
3. Gavini, E.; Rassu, G.; Haukvik, T.; Lanni, C.; Racchi, M.; Giunchedi, P. Mucoadhesive microspheres for nasal administration of cyclodextrins. *J. Drug Target.* **2009**, *17*, 168–179. [CrossRef] [PubMed]
4. Gavini, E.; Rassu, G.; Ferraro, L.; Beggiato, S.; Alhalaweh, A.; Velaga, S.; Marchetti, N.; Bandiera, P.; Giunchedi, P.; Dalpiaz, A. Influence of polymeric microcarriers on the in vivo intranasal uptake of an anti-migraine drug for brain targeting. *Eur. J. Pharm. Biopharm.* **2013**, *83*, 174–183. [CrossRef] [PubMed]
5. Yalcin, A.; Soddu, E.; Turunc Bayrakdar, E.; Uyanikgil, Y.; Kanit, L.; Armagan, G.; Rassu, G.; Gavini, E.; Giunchedi, P. Neuroprotective Effects of Engineered Polymeric Nasal Microspheres Containing Hydroxypropyl-β-cyclodextrin on β-Amyloid (1-42)-Induced Toxicity. *J. Pharm. Sci.* **2016**, *105*, 2372–2380. [CrossRef] [PubMed]
6. Williams, A.C.; Barry, B.W. Penetration enhancers. *Adv. Drug Deliv. Rev.* **2012**, *64*, 128–137. [CrossRef]
7. Illum, L. Nasal drug delivery-possibilities, problems and solutions. *J. Control. Release* **2003**, *87*, 187–198. [CrossRef]
8. Merkus, F.W.H.M.; Verhoef, J.C.; Marttin, E.; Romeijn, S.G.; van der Kuy, P.H.M.; Hermens, W.A.J.; Schipper, N.G.M. Cyclodextrins in nasal drug delivery. *Adv. Drug Deliv. Rev.* **1999**, *36*, 41–57. [CrossRef]

9. Yang, T.; Hussain, A.; Paulson, J.; Abbruscato, T.J.; Ahsan, F. Cyclodextrins in nasal delivery of low-molecular-weight heparins: In vivo and in vitro studies. *Pharm. Res.* **2004**, *21*, 1127–1136. [CrossRef] [PubMed]
10. Zhang, X.; Zhang, X.; Wu, Z.; Gao, X.; Shua, S.; Wang, Z.; Li, C. β-Cyclodextrin grafting hyperbranched polyglycerols as carriers for nasal insulin delivery. *Carbohydr. Polym.* **2011**, *84*, 1419–1425. [CrossRef]
11. Challa, R.; Ahuja, A.; Ali, J.; Khar, R.K. Cyclodextrins in Drug Delivery: An Updated Review. *AAPS PharmSciTech* **2005**, *6*, E329–E357. [CrossRef] [PubMed]
12. Lambert, D.; O'Neill, C.A.; Padfield, P.J. Depletion of Caco-2 cell cholesterol disrupts barrier function by altering the detergent solubility and distribution of specific tight-junction proteins. *Biochem. J.* **2005**, *387*, 553–560. [CrossRef] [PubMed]
13. Fenyvesi, F.; Réti-Nagy, K.; Bacsó, Z.; Gutay-Tóth, Z.; Malanga, M.; Fenyvesi, É.; Szente, L.; Váradi, J.; Ujhelyi, Z.; Fehér, P.; et al. Fluorescently labeled methyl-beta-cyclodextrin enters intestinal epithelial Caco-2 cells by fluid-phase endocytosis. *PLoS ONE* **2014**, *9*, e84856. [CrossRef] [PubMed]
14. Casettari, L.; Illum, L. Chitosan in nasal delivery systems for therapeutic drugs. *J. Control. Release* **2014**, *190*, 189–200. [CrossRef] [PubMed]
15. Gavini, E.; Rassu, G.; Ferraro, L.; Generosi, A.; Rau, J.V.; Brunetti, A.; Giunchedi, P.; Dalpiaz, A. Influence of chitosan glutamate on the in vivo intranasal absorption of rokitamycin from microspheres. *J. Pharm. Sci.* **2011**, *100*, 1488–1502. [CrossRef] [PubMed]
16. Dalpiaz, A.; Fogagnolo, M.; Ferraro, L.; Capuzzo, A.; Pavan, B.; Rassu, G.; Salis, A.; Giunchedi, P.; Gavini, E. Nasal chitosan microparticles target a zidovudine prodrug to brain HIV sanctuaries. *Antiviral Res.* **2015**, *123*, 146–157. [CrossRef] [PubMed]
17. Rassu, G.; Soddu, E.; Cossu, M.; Gavini, E.; Giunchedi, P.; Dalpiaz, A. Particulate formulations based on chitosan for nose-to-brain delivery of drugs. A review. *J. Drug Deliv. Sci. Technol.* **2016**, *32*, 77–87. [CrossRef]
18. Council of Europe. *European Pharmacopoeia Chitosan Hydrochloride*, 8th ed.; Council of Europe: Strasbourg, France, 2014; p. 1841.
19. Türker, S.; Onur, E.; Ozer, Y. Nasal route and drug delivery systems. *Pharm. World Sci.* **2004**, *26*, 137–142. [CrossRef] [PubMed]
20. Rassu, G.; Soddu, E.; Cossu, M.; Brundu, A.; Cerri, G.; Marchetti, N.; Ferraro, L.; Regan, R.F.; Giunchedi, P.; Gavini, E.; et al. Solid microparticles based on chitosan or methyl-β-cyclodextrin: A first formulative approach to increase the nose-to-brain transport of deferoxamine mesylate. *J. Control. Release* **2015**, *201*, 68–77. [CrossRef] [PubMed]
21. Bshara, H.; Osman, R.; Mansour, S.; El-Shamy, A.E.A. Chitosan and cyclodextrin in intranasal microemulsion for improved brain buspirone hydrochloride pharmacokinetics in rats. *Carbohydr. Polym.* **2014**, *99*, 297–305. [CrossRef] [PubMed]
22. Lochhead, J.J.; Thorne, R.G. Intranasal delivery of biologics to the central nervous system. *Adv. Drug Deliv. Rev.* **2012**, *64*, 614–628. [CrossRef] [PubMed]
23. Dalpiaz, A.; Gavini, E.; Colombo, G.; Russo, P.; Bortolotti, F.; Ferraro, L.; Tanganelli, S.; Scatturin, A.; Menegatti, E.; Giunchedi, P. Brain uptake of an anti-ischemic agent by nasal administration of microparticles. *J. Pharm. Sci.* **2008**, *97*, 4889–4903. [CrossRef] [PubMed]
24. Gavini, E.; Rassu, G.; Ciarnelli, V.; Spada, G.; Cossu, M.; Giunchedi, P. Mucoadhesive drug delivery systems for nose-to-brain targeting of dopamine. *J. Nanoneurosci.* **2012**, *2*, 1–9. [CrossRef]
25. Rassu, G.; Gavini, E.; Jonassen, H.; Zambito, Y.; Fogli, S.; Breschi, M.C.; Giunchedi, P. New chitosan derivatives for the preparation of rokitamycin loaded microspheres designed for ocular or nasal administration. *J. Pharm. Sci.* **2009**, *98*, 4852–4865. [CrossRef] [PubMed]
26. Gavini, E.; Spada, G.; Rassu, G.; Cerri, G.; Brundu, A.; Cossu, M.; Sorrenti, M.; Giunchedi, P. Development of solid nanoparticles based on hydroxypropyl-β-cyclodextrin aimed for the colonic transmucosal delivery of diclofenac sodium. *J. Pharm. Pharmacol.* **2011**, *63*, 472–482. [CrossRef] [PubMed]
27. Kouchak, M.; Handali, S.; Boroujeni, B.N. Evaluation of the mechanical properties and drug permeability of chitosan/Eudragit RL composite film. *Osong Public Health Res. Perspect.* **2015**, *6*, 14–19. [CrossRef] [PubMed]
28. Van den Berg, M.P.; Romeijn, S.G.; Verhoef, J.C.; Merkus, F.W. Serial cerebrospinal fluid sampling in a rat model to study drug uptake from the nasal cavity. *J. Neurosci. Methods* **2002**, *116*, 99–107. [CrossRef]

29. Dalpiaz, A.; Ferraro, L.; Perrone, D.; Leo, E.; Iannuccelli, V.; Pavan, B.; Paganetto, G.; Beggiato, S.; Scalia, S. Brain uptake of a Zidovudine prodrug after nasal administration of solid lipid microparticles. *Mol. Pharm.* **2014**, *11*, 1550–1561. [CrossRef] [PubMed]
30. Sacchetti, C.; Artusi, M.; Santi, P.; Colombo, P. Caffeine microparticles for nasal administration obtained by spray drying. *Int. J. Pharm.* **2002**, *242*, 335–339. [CrossRef]
31. Felgenhauer, K. Protein Size and CSF Composition. *Klinische Wochensch.* **1974**, *52*, 1158–1164. [CrossRef]
32. Madu, A.; Cioffe, C.; Mian, U.; Burroughs, M.; Tuomanen, E.; Mayers, M.; Schwartz, E.; Miller, M. Pharmacokinetics of Fluconazole in Cerebrospinal Fluid and Serum of Rabbits: Validation of an Animal Model used to Measure Drug Concentrations in Cerebrospinal Fluid. *Antimicrob. Agents Chemother.* **1994**, *38*, 2111–2115. [CrossRef] [PubMed]
33. Gavini, E.; Rassu, G.; Sanna, V.; Cossu, M.; Giunchedi, P. Mucoadhesive microspheres for nasal administration of an antiemetic drug, metoclopramide: In-vitro/ex-vivo studies. *J. Pharm. Pharmacol.* **2005**, *57*, 287–294. [CrossRef] [PubMed]
34. Mathot, R.A.; Appel, S.; van Schaick, E.A.; Soudijn, W.; Ijzerman, A.P.; Danhof, M. High-performance liquid chromatography of the adenosine A1 agonist N6-cyclopentyladenosine and the A1 antagonist 8-cyclopentyltheophylline and its application in a pharmacokinetic study in rats. *J. Chromatogr.* **1993**, *620*, 113–120. [CrossRef]
35. Brodie, M.S.; Lee, K.; Fredholm, B.B.; Stahle, L.; Dunwiddie, T.V. Central versus peripheral mediation of responses to adenosine receptor agonists: Evidence against a central mode of action. *Brain Res.* **1987**, *415*, 323–330. [CrossRef]
36. Tamai, I.; Tsuji, A. Transporter-mediated permeation of drugs across the blood-brain barrier. *J. Pharm. Sci.* **2000**, *89*, 1371–1388. [CrossRef]
37. Schaddelee, M.P.; Read, K.D.; Cleypool, C.G.J.; Ijzerman, A.P.; Danhof, M.; de Boer, A.G. Brain penetration of synthetic A1 receptor agonists in situ: Role of the rENT1 nucleoside transporter and binding to blood constituents. *Eur. J. Pharm. Sci.* **2005**, *24*, 59–66. [CrossRef] [PubMed]

A Mixed Thermosensitive Hydrogel System for Sustained Delivery of Tacrolimus for Immunosuppressive Therapy

Hsiu-Chao Lin [1,†], Madonna Rica Anggelia [2,3,†], Chih-Chi Cheng [1], Kuan-Lin Ku [1], Hui-Yun Cheng [2], Chih-Jen Wen [2], Aline Yen Ling Wang [2], Cheng-Hung Lin [2,3,*] and I-Ming Chu [1,*]

1 Department of Chemical Engineering, National Tsing Hua University, Hsinchu 300, Taiwan
2 Center for Vascularized Composite Allotransplantation, Department of Plastic and Reconstructive Surgery, Chang Gung Memorial Hospital, Chang Gung Medical College and Chang Gung University, Taoyuan 333, Taiwan
3 Graduate Institute of Biomedical Sciences, College of Medicine, Chang Gung University, Taoyuan 333, Taiwan
* Correspondence: lukechlin@gmail.com (C.-H.L.); imchu@che.nthu.edu.tw (I.-M.C.);

† These authors contributed equally to this work.

Abstract: Tacrolimus is an immunosuppressive agent for acute rejection after allotransplantation. However, the low aqueous solubility of tacrolimus poses difficulties in formulating an injection dosage. Polypeptide thermosensitive hydrogels can maintain a sustained release depot to deliver tacrolimus. The copolymers, which consist of poloxamer and poly(L-alanine) with L-lysine segments at both ends (P–Lys–Ala–PLX), are able to carry tacrolimus in an in situ gelled form with acceptable biocompatibility, biodegradability, and low gelling concentrations from 3 to 7 wt %. By adding Pluronic F-127 to formulate a mixed hydrogel system, the drug release rate can be adjusted to maintain suitable drug levels in animals with transplants. Under this formulation, the in vitro release of tacrolimus was stable for more than 100 days, while in vivo release of tacrolimus in mouse model showed that rejection from skin allotransplantation was prevented for at least three weeks with one single administration. Using these mixed hydrogel systems for sustaining delivery of tacrolimus demonstrates advancement in immunosuppressive therapy.

Keywords: allotransplantation; hydrogels; sustained delivery; tacrolimus

---

1. Introduction

Hydrogels are composed of crosslinked polymeric networks that can form highly hydrated semisolid materials. Because their diverse capacity to carry therapeutic agents in a depot-like form allows sustained release, hydrogels have been utilized in many applications, including drug delivery, cell therapy, and tissue engineering [1–4].

Among various types of hydrogels, thermosensitive poly(ethylene glycol)-*co*-poly(amino acids) hydrogels are capable of in situ gelling upon injection to appropriate sites in the body. They can deliver drugs or cells to specific sites with minimum invasiveness while serving as a depot for extended delivery [5–9]. These polymers belong to LCST-type materials; thus, when above a certain temperature, their aqueous solution undergoes a phase transition to the gel state, depending on the concentration. The gelling process involves a reduced hydrogen bond interaction between the hydrophilic segments of polymers and water as the temperature rises [10,11]. Different types of hydrophilic polymers are used in this gelling process, including various hydrogels, poly(ethylene glycol) (PEG) [12], methoxy poly(ethylene glycol) (mPEG) [13], and PEO–PPO–PEO copolymers (mainly the Pluronic® or poloxamer (PLX) series) [14]. Several types of polypeptides have been used in the hydrophobic portion of the polymer [12,15,16]. The fact that peptides have secondary interactions between or within themselves complicates the gelling process of these amino acid-based hydrogels, creating different types of self-assembled morphology [17–20]. Additionally, because peptide bonds possess low hydrolytic rates, compared with ester bonds, for example, hydrogels degrade at extremely slow rates. Therefore, side effects caused by long-term foreign body reactions may be a concern, or the release rates of some drugs might be too slow for intended applications.

In this study, a suitable formulation of a hydrogel carrier was sought for tacrolimus, an immunosuppressive, antirejection drug. Tacrolimus is a hydrophobic substance with low aqueous solubility. Controlled delivery of tacrolimus would avoid the low bioavailability problem and improve patient compliance statistics by reducing the administration frequency. Several delivery systems for tacrolimus have been reported, including mPEG-poly(lactic acid) nanoparticles [21], poly(lactide-*co*-glycolide) microspheres [22], and triglycerol monostearate hydrogels [23]. The in situ gelation property of the system studied here has several advantages over particulate systems or conventional hydrogel systems, including longer release time, higher encapsulation efficiency, easy administration, and applicability to various types of drugs. In particular, by combining two types of hydrogel components, the possibility of increasing the flexibility of carriers to suit distinct pharmaceutical entities and modifying release rates for better clinical outcomes is explored.

2. Materials and Methods

2.1. Materials

O,O′-Bis(2-aminopropyl) polypropylene glycol-block-polyethylene glycol-block-polypropylene glycol (Poloxamer, PLX, PPG–PEG–PPG, Mn = 900), L-alanine, hydrogen bromide (HBr/acetic acid), and a LIVE/DEAD staining kit were purchased from Sigma-Aldrich (St. Louis, MO, USA). Tacrolimus (FK506) was obtained from LC Labs (Woburn, MA, USA). Trifluoroacetic acid-d (TFA-d) and trifluoroacetic acid (TFA) were purchased from Alfa Aesar (Wall Hill, MA, USA). L-lysine-(Z) was commercially obtained from ACROS (Morris Plains, NJ, USA). Diethyl ether, hexane, and ethanol (95%) were purchased from Echo Chemicals (Toufen, Miaoli, Taiwan). Dimethyl sulfoxide (DMSO) was obtained from J.T. Baker. Dulbecco's modified eagle's medium (DMEM), fetal bovine serum (FBS), and antimycotics–antibiotics were purchased from Gibco (Grand Island, NY, USA). Toluene and tetrahydrofuran (THF) were obtained from TEDIA (Fairfield, OH, USA), and chloroform, dichloromethane (DCM), and *N,N*-dimethylformaide (DMF) were purchased from AVANTOR (Center Valley, PA, USA). All solvents were dried over CaH_2 before used.

2.2. Synthesis of L-alanine N-Carboxyanhydride (Ala-NCA), L-Lysine-(Z) N-Carboxyanhydride (Lys-(Z)-NCA), and P–Lys–Ala–PLX Block Copolymer

The copolymer synthesis was similar to that in our previous study conducted in 2016 [14] in which L-alanine (5.0 g and 56.1 mmol) and triphosgene (16.65 g, 56.3 mmol) were dissolved in anhydrous THF (150 mL) and gently stirred at 45 °C under nitrogen flux. After the reaction period of approximately 12 h, the mixture turned clear and the solution was condensed to a final volume of 15 mL through rotary evaporation. The product was precipitated in excess *n*-hexane. A similar preparation method was employed in this study: L-lysine-(Z) (5.0 g, 17.8 mmol) using 3.2 g of triphosgene (10.7 mmol) was dissolved in 60 mL of anhydrous THF. The reaction was completed within 4 h, and the mixture was then condensed and finally precipitated.

The block copolymer P–Lys–Ala–PLX was prepared through a two-step ring-opening polymerization of Ala–NCA and Lys–(Z)–NCA with PLX as the macroinitiator. Briefly, PLX (4.0 g, 5 mmol) was dissolved in 15 mL of toluene and azeotropically distilled to a final volume of approximately

5 mL to remove residual water. Ala-NCA (5.198 g) was added to the reaction flask and dissolved in 20-fold of anhydrous chloroform/DMF (2:1). The mixture was stirred at 40 °C for 24 h until the reaction was complete and then precipitated with diethyl ether. Next, pre-weighed Lys–(Z)–NCA (3.063 g) was added into the reaction flask, and the reaction was carried out at 40 °C for 24 h again. The final product was precipitated with diethyl ether.

The copolymer (Z)–Lys–Ala–PLX–Ala–Lys–(Z) was dissolved in TFA (1 g/10 mL), and a solution of 33 wt % HBr/acetic acid (0.3 mL/mol L-lysine) was added and stirred at 0 °C for 1 h. After precipitation with diethyl ether, the product was dialyzed (MWCO 1000) using a spectrum dialysis bag, lyophilized, and stored in a vacuum atmosphere for future use.

2.3. *^{1}H Nuclear Magnetic Resonanc (NMR) Spectroscopy*

A ^{1}H NMR spectrum of the 0.5 wt % copolymer solution in TFA-d was obtained using a Varian UNITY INOVA 500 MHz spectrometer (Palo Alto, CA, USA) to verify the chemical structure of the product.

2.4. *Fourier-Transformed Infrared Spectroscopy (FT-IR)*

Fourier-transformed infrared spectroscopy (FT-IR) was performed using an FTIR spectrometer (Nicolet™ iS50, Thermo Fisher Scientific, Waltham, MA, USA) equipped with an attenuated total reflectance (ATR) module. The copolymer solution prepared at 5 wt % in deionized water was injected into the test chamber. Spectra were collected at a temperature ranging from 10 to 50 °C at increments of 10 °C. The sample was equilibrated for 20 min at each temperature. The amide I band region of 1600–1700 cm^{-1} was used to collect information on secondary structures and conducted for chemical structure verification.

2.5. *Sol-to-gel Phase Transition*

The sol-to-gel transition behavior of copolymers prepared at various concentrations was investigated using the test tube inversion method. Samples were prepared in test tubes at 3 to 7 wt % in deionized water and placed in a tube rotator overnight at 4 °C until the solutes were completely dissolved. The inverted test tube test was performed at a temperature range of 10–50 °C, at increments of 1 °C. At each temperature, the sample was allowed to equilibrate for 10 min. The gelation point was designated when the solution stopped flowing while inverted and gently agitated.

2.6. *Scanning Electron Microscope (SEM)*

The copolymer mixed gel solution was prepared at 5 wt % in P–Lys–Ala–PLX and 1 wt % in Pluronic F-127 that allowed full equilibration at 4 °C overnight for future use. The hydrogel microstructure was examined using a JEOL JSM-7001F SEM system (Peabody, MA, USA). Briefly, hydrogels were gelled at 37 °C and then submerged in liquid nitrogen prior to lyophilization. To investigate the cross section, lyophilized hydrogels were carefully cut open using a scalpel blade.

2.7. *Degradation Test*

The in vitro degradation of hydrogels (100 μL) in phosphate-buffered saline (PBS) and PBS containing elastase (5 U/mL) was analyzed. Briefly, copolymer solutions were gelled in 1.5 mL tubes at 37 °C for 30 min prior to adding 1 mL of the respective degradation mediums. The medium was replaced at each time point, and the residual was weighted after washing and lyophilization.

2.8. *Biocompatibility*

The cell compatibility of the prepared mixed hydrogel was assessed. Briefly, human embryonic kidney cells (293T) were loaded onto a 24-well transwell plate at 6×10^3 cells per well and grown in DMEM media, supplemented with 10% FBS and 1% antimycotics–antibiotics. Exactly 100 μL of the copolymer solution was gelled at 37 °C in the transwell insert overlaid with 1 mL of culture media. LIVE/DEAD staining with fluorescence microscopy observation was performed on the third and seventh days to quantitate the viability of the cells, and a 3-(4,5-dimethylthiazol-2-yl)-2,5-diphenyltetrazolium bromide (MTT) assay was simultaneously performed to detect cell proliferation. Briefly, cells were treated with 3-(4,5-dimethylthiazol-2-yl)-2,5-diphenyltetrazolium bromide (10% *v/v* in medium) in each well for 3 hours before 200 μL of DMSO was added. The solution was collected and analyzed.

2.9. Drug Release In Vitro

The hydrogels P–Lys–Ala–PLX 5 wt % and Pluronic F-127 1 wt % were combined, solubilized in deionized water, and then mixed with tacrolimus in tubes to afford 1 mL solutions of the final drug concentration with 10 or 20 mg/mL. A negative control of the mixed hydrogel without tacrolimus was used. 100 μL copolymer solutions were loaded into a 1.5 mL tube and kept at 37 °C for 10 min before adding 1 mL of PBS with 2% tween 20 as the conditional medium. At each time point, aliquots were collected using HPLC analysis to ascertain the tacrolimus concentration. A linear calibration curve over the concentration range of 1000 μg/mL to 1 μg/mL was constructed, and the tacrolimus concentration was interpolated accordingly.

2.10. Drug Release In Vivo

Male Lewis (LEW) rats, weighing 300 to 350 g, were obtained from the National Laboratory Animal Center and were housed under pathogen-free conditions at the Animal Center of Linkou Chang Gung Memorial Hospital according to protocols approved by Institutional Animal Care and Use Committee of Chang Gung Memorial Hospital (IACUC No. 2017121807, approved date, 14 May 2018). Those rats ($n = 3$) were injected subcutaneously with 1 mL mixed hydrogels loaded with tacrolimus at 10 mg/mL. To analyze the in vivo release rate of tacrolimus, whole blood was drawn from the tail vein of those rats on days 7, 14, and 28 and put into the VACUETTE® EDTA tubes. Whole blood concentration of tacrolimus was quantitated by liquid chromatography-tandem mass spectrometry (LC-MS/MS) (Waters, Milford, MA, USA) at the Department of Laboratory Medicine, Linkou Chang Gung Memorial Hospital. The performance characteristics and assay method has been described previously. [24] The method for tacrolimus assay showed linearity over the calibrator range, $r > 0.999$, with the range measurement: 1.1–38.5 ng/mL and accuracy 108%. For intra-day and inter-day precision, the CV was <6.6%. This method showed no carryover or ion suppressant. The calibration solution (6PLUS1® RMultilevel Calibrator Immunosuppressants in Whole Blood) was purchased from Chromsystems (Munich, Germany) and contained tacrolimus and a blank calibration fluid (blank calibrator)). Further, 100 μL of calibration solution, quality control solution, and sample were loaded into a 1.5 mL centrifuge tube, and 300 μL of 0.1 M zinc sulfate containing internal standards (FK-506) were added. The mixtures were then vigorously vortexed for 30 s then centrifuged at 12,000 rpm for 15 min to completely precipitate the protein. The 300 μL supernatant was removed, placed in a 96-well collection tray, and put into the autosampler.

3. Results and Discussion

3.1. The Synthesis and Characterization of P–Lys–Ala–PLX and Pluronic F-127

Thermosensitive hydrogels composed of amphiphilic block copolymers were used in this study, specifically PLX-poly(L-alanine-lysine) (P–Lys–Ala–PLX). The ^{1}H-NMR spectra of the triblock copolymer are illustrated in Figure 1A, where peaks corresponding to copolymers are observed and successful synthesis of copolymers is confirmed. The molecular weights, as measured by Gel Permeation Chromatography (GPC) and ^{1}H NMR, are displayed in Table 1. Briefly, the molar mass polydispersity of the triblock copolymer is 1.51, and the weight average molecular weight (Mw) is 3817 Da.

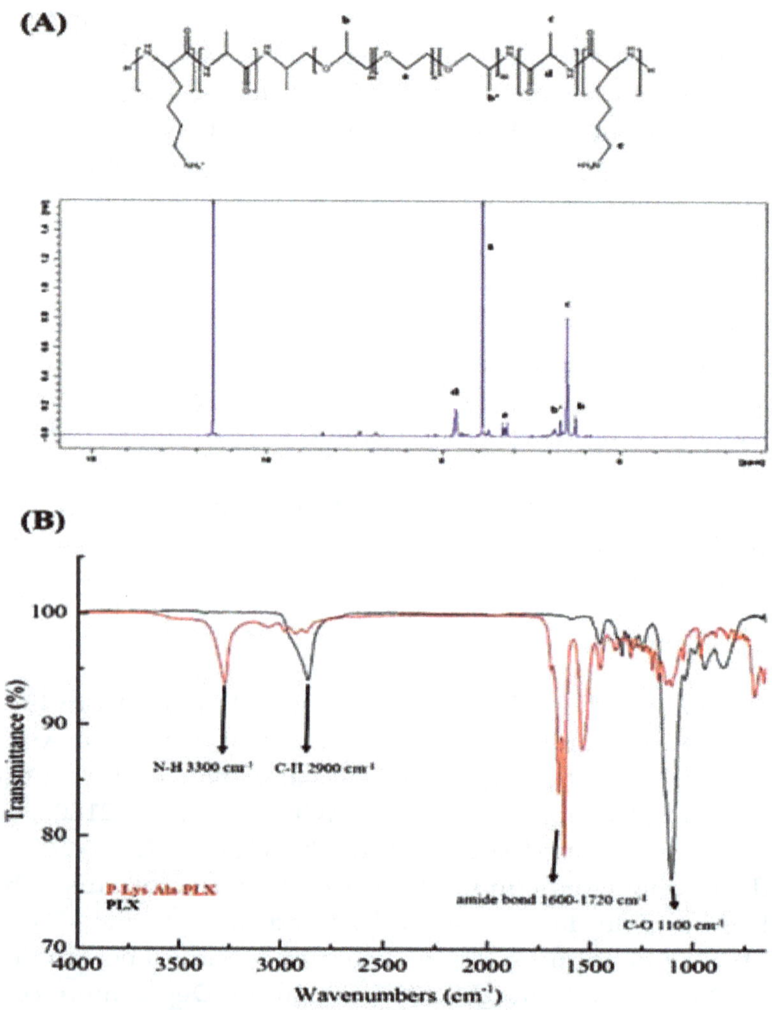

Figure 1. (**A**) ^{1}H-NMR of poloxamer (PLX)-poly(L-alanine-lysine) (P–Lys–Ala–PLX) copolymer in trifluoroacetic acid-d (TFA-d). (**B**) FT-IR spectra of P–Lys–Ala–PLX (red line) and PLX (black line) samples obtained via an attenuated total reflectance (ATR) module (2900 cm^{-1}, alkane of Pluronic F-127; 3345 cm^{-1}, amide of poly(L-alanine) and poly(L-lysine); 1637 cm^{-1} and 1540 cm^{-1}, amide I and II of poly(L-alanine) and poly(L-lysine); 1100 cm^{-1}, carbon-oxygen bond of PLX.

Table 1. The molecular weight and polydispersity as determined by GPC and ^{1}H NMR.

	Ala	Lys	Mn ^{a}	Mw ^{b}	PDI ^{b}
P–Lys–Ala–PLX	19.4	1.8	2528	3817	1.51

^{a}. Determined by ^{1}H NMR. ^{b}. Determined by GPC.

ATR-FTIR was used to verify the synthesis of the copolymer P–Lys–Ala–PLX and compared with that of *O,O′*-Bis(2-aminopropyl) polypropylene glycol-block-polyethylene glycol-block-polypropylene glycol (Poloxamer, PLX), which has the same characteristic peaks as the PLX segment of P–Lys–Ala–PLX. As in Figure 1B, peaks at 3300 cm^{-1} (N–H bond) and 1600–1720 cm^{-1} (amide bond) are from polypeptides, while those found at 2900 cm^{-1} (C–H) and 1100 cm^{-1}(C–O) are from the PLX segment. The characterization and structure of the triblock copolymer P–Lys–Ala–PLX is explained in our 2016 study [14].

The sol–gel transition phase diagram is represented in Figure 2. In the room to body temperature range, P–Lys–Ala–PLX underwent a sol-to-gel transition in the concentration range from 3% to 7%. The gelation temperature decreased as the concentration of copolymers increased. For solutions with a copolymer concentration lower than 3 wt %, hydrogels were unable to form stable gels under the inverted test tube test despite significant increases in viscosity at higher temperatures. Consequently, copolymer concentrations of 4 to 5 wt % were chosen for further formulation studies.

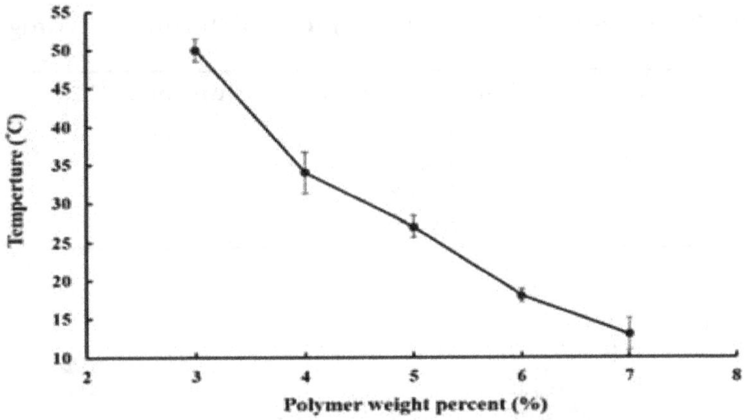

Figure 2. Sol–gel transition profile of aqueous solutions of P–Lys–Ala–PLX.

The internal structure of the P–Lys–Ala–PLX hydrogel was examined through scanning electronic microscopy, as portrayed in Figure 3. A plate-like structure was dominant with some fibrous features within. This type of morphology is typical for PLX-poly(alanine) hydrogels.

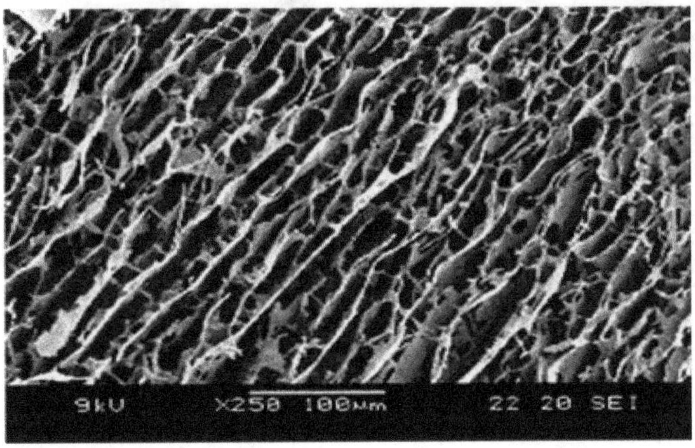

Figure 3. SEM image of P–Lys–Ala–PLX hydrogels.

3.2. Development of Mixed Hydrogel Formulation

After the preliminary in vivo drug release tests with the P–Lys–Ala–PLX hydrogel, extremely slow tacrolimus release rates and a considerably low plasma concentration of tacrolimus were observed. Unexpected transplant rejection resulted from these tests (data not shown) because drug concentrations were low. The slow in vivo release rate of the drug may be caused by the slow degradation rate of the hydrogel in vivo. Therefore, the hydrogel formulation should be modified to accelerate drug release at effective concentrations and sustain the release for more than 30 days. Pluronic F-127 has been mentioned to modulate the drug release rate [25]. The addition of Pluronic F-127, an approved fast-degrading hydrogel, to the P–Lys–Ala–PLX hydrogel system may provide a solution to accelerate the release rate.

A series of hydrogel formulations of 1 to 3 wt % Pluronic F-127 powder mixed into 4 or 5 wt % P–Lys–Ala–PLX were studied, as shown in Table 2. Sol-to-gel transition properties, cytotoxicity, drug encapsulation efficiency, and the release rate were measured. The formulation of 5 wt % P–Lys–Ala–PLX with 1 wt % Pluronic F-127 (sample 5:1) had a lower transition temperature than the other three groups, as demonstrated in Figure 4A. Additionally, the sample 5:1 had the highest drug encapsulation efficiency (Figure 4B). Consequently, the formulation of the sample 5:1 was chosen for further studies.

Table 2. The series formulation test group of the mixed hydrogels.

Group	P–Lys–Ala–PLX	Pluronic F-127
1	4 wt %	2 wt %
2	5 wt %	1 wt %
3	5 wt %	2 wt %
4	5 wt %	3 wt %

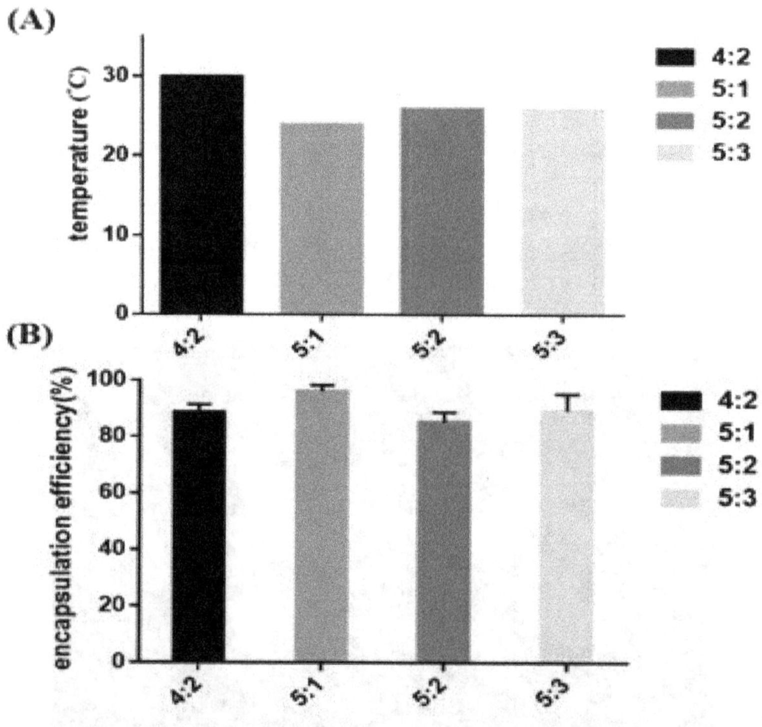

Figure 4. (**A**) The sol-to-gel transition temperature of mixed hydrogels without tacrolimus; (**B**) the encapsulation efficiency of tacrolimus in mixed hydrogels.

3.3. Biodegradability

Degradation behavior of hydrogels in a buffer solution with and without the enzyme elastase at 37 °C was observed. P–Lys–Ala–PLX gels (5 wt %) incubated with elastase (5 U/mL) resulted in a mass loss of 40% after 14 days, as displayed in Figure 5, whereas gels incubated with the buffer solution lost only 10% of the original mass. The sample 5:1 incubated with elastase had a mass loss of 50% after 14 days, whereas those without the enzyme lost only 15% of the original mass. The mass loss of mixed hydrogels was higher than that of the P–Lys–Ala–PLX hydrogel because Pluronic F-127 was more prone to dissolve back to an aqueous solution. In short, hydrogels were stable when proteinases were absent, and Pluronic F-127 accelerated degradation rates.

SEM micrographs of lyophilized P–Lys–Ala–PLX and a sample 5:1 mixed hydrogel are shown in Figure 6. The mixed hydrogels exhibited more porous structures and space resulting from the incorporation of Pluronic F-127. After the 14-day degradation, samples of mixed hydrogels revealed larger pores and looser structure resulting from the faster dissolution or disintegration of Pluronic F-127.

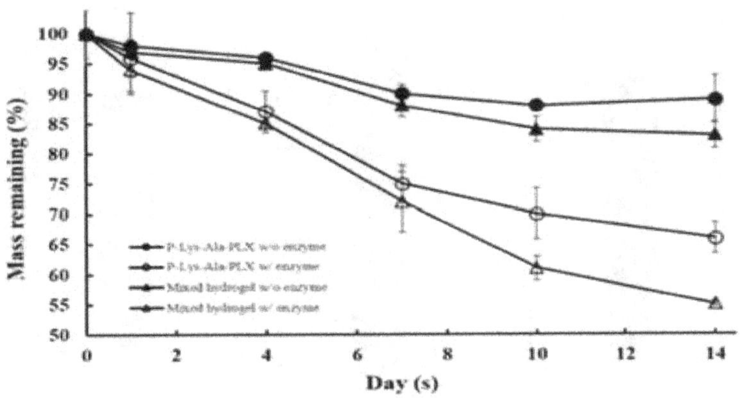

Figure 5. Degradation profiles of P–Lys–Ala–PLX and sample 5:1 mixed hydrogel in phosphate-buffered saline (PBS) with or without 5 U/mL elastase (n = 6).

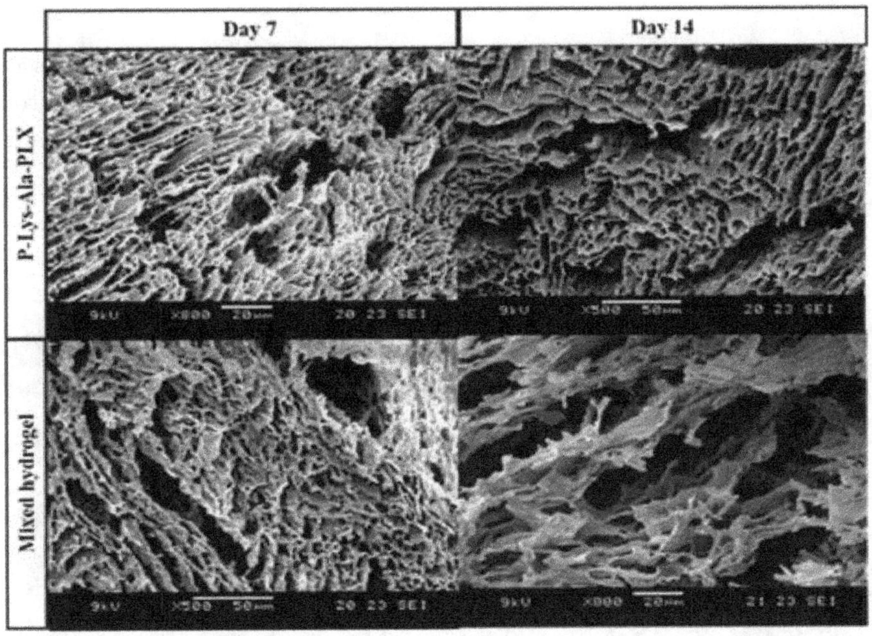

Figure 6. SEM microphotographs of P–Lys–Ala–PLX hydrogel and sample 5:1 mixed hydrogel after degradation in PBS with 5 U/mL elastase at 37 °C for 7 and 14 days.

3.4. *Biocompatibility*

The dispersion of insoluble tacrolimus particles in the hydrogel solution was rather challenging [21,22]. Certain solvents must be used to dissolve tacrolimus during the encapsulation process to assure an even distribution of the drug. Acceptable solvents should be nontoxic to cells and not interfere in the sol–gel transition of the polymeric system.

Several solvents that can dissolve tacrolimus were chosen, including DMSO, ethanol, and transcutol P. Ethanol had the least toxicity and highest dissolving power when water was present (data not shown). To reduce the toxicity of ethanol to the cells, tacrolimus was dissolved in ethanol as 100 mg/mL or 200 mg/mL stock solutions, which were then used to prepare the 10 mg/mL and 20 mg/mL drug-carrying hydrogels, respectively. Tacrolimus encapsulated in the gel gradually precipitated out as small evenly dispersed solid particles when ethanol diffused into the surrounding aqueous environment. When the gel pellet was placed in a 10-time volume of medium and the residual ethanol concentration was below 1 wt %, its conditioned medium exerted little effect on the cells in the in vitro toxicity test (see Figure 7).

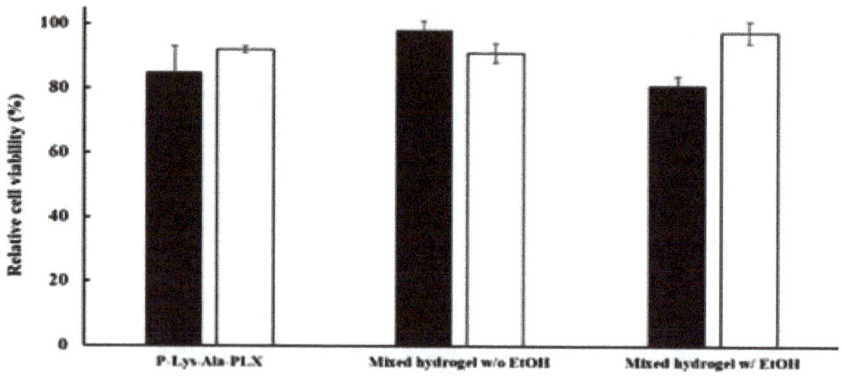

Figure 7. Cytotoxicity of conditioned mediums of various formulations by the MTT assay. Mixed hydrogels: 5:1 P–Lys–Ala–PLX to Pluronic F-127. Ethanol was added to the gel as in the 10 mg/mL formulation but without the drug. The black bar was on day 3 (black) and the white bar was on day 7.

Cellular compatibility under encapsulation of prepared hydrogels was evaluated using LIVE/DEAD staining, in which live cells stained green and dead cells were red. To evaluate the cytotoxicity of materials, in the medium, cells were cultivated in contact with hydrogels in transwells. The cells showed acceptable viability in culture for 3 to 7 days with both P–Lys–Ala–PLX and mixed hydrogels, as related in Figure 8.

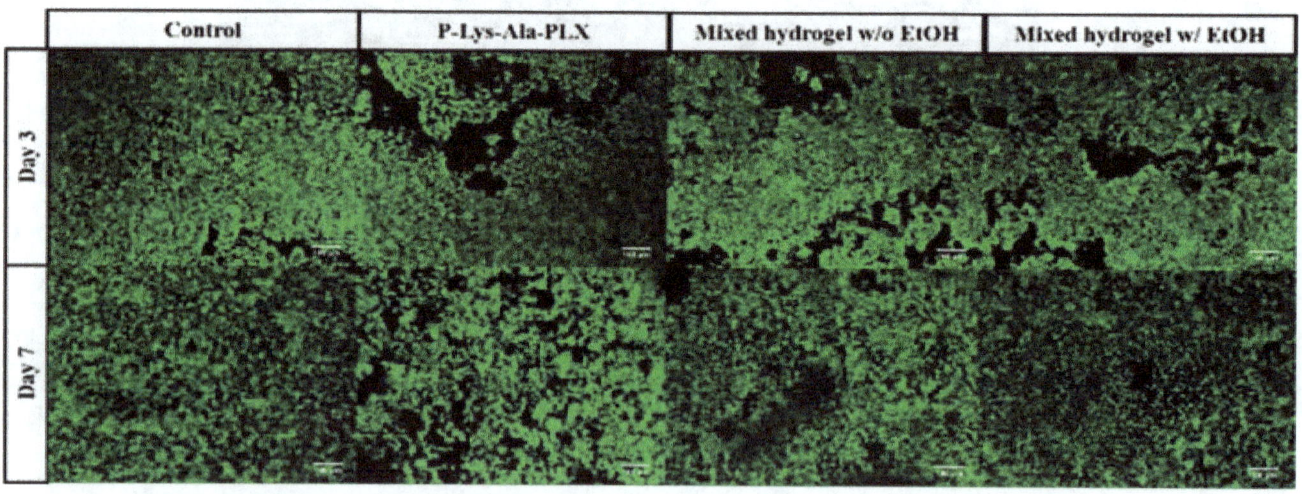

Figure 8. The LIVE/DEAD staining of 293T cells was co-cultured with various hydrogels without the drug.

3.5. Tacrolimus Encapsulation and Release

The feasibility of hydrogels as an efficient local drug delivery system for tacrolimus was studied first under in vitro conditions. The encapsulation efficiency and release of tacrolimus in mixed hydrogel were measured. The values of encapsulation efficiency (EE) of the sample 5:1 mixed hydrogel were measured at two levels of drug content, where EE = (experimental drug loading)/(theoretical drug loading) × 100%. The results are presented in Table 3. The data indicated the hydrogel encapsulated tacrolimus rather well, with the EE at approximately 96%–98% in triplicate samples. Drug release rates in P–Lys–Ala–PLX or the sample 5:1 mixed hydrogel was measured for a one-month period. The release rates were stable and higher in the mixed hydrogel at both drug content levels, as illustrated in Figure 9. No burst release was observed, and the sustained release of tacrolimus was achieved. Release rates correlated with hydrogel degradation (e.g., see Figure 5) and thereby suggest that the enhanced disintegration of mixed hydrogels was responsible for higher drug release rates in mixed hydrogels. These results demonstrate the ability to modify the release rate by using mixed hydrogels.

Table 3. The encapsulation efficiency of 5:1 mixed hydrogel for tacrolimus.

Group	Encapsulation Efficiency (%)
10 mg/mL	96.13 ± 1.56
20 mg/mL	98.5 ± 0.97

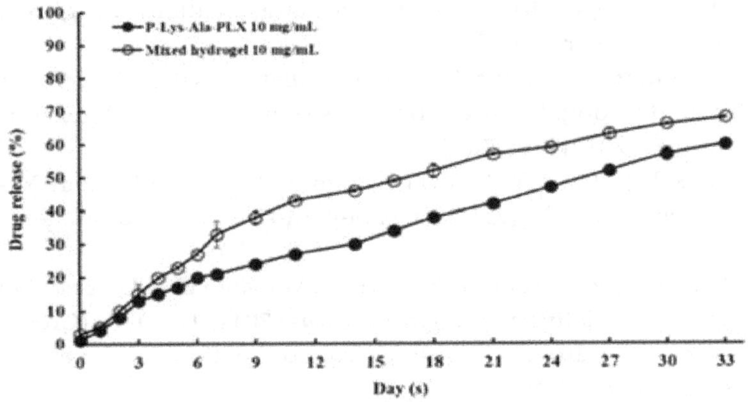

Figure 9. In vitro tacrolimus release as a fraction of total encapsulated drug.

For the mixed hydrogel with 10 mg/mL tacrolimus group, preliminary in vivo drug release tests were conducted. The aim was to establish a correlation between our in vitro release data and the corresponding data in a plasma concentration when 1 mL of the formulation was injected subcutaneously in a mouse. More comprehensive pharmacokinetic work, together with allotransplantation animal study, is currently underway, and results will be presented in a separate paper. As exhibited in Table 4, plasma concentrations of tacrolimus during a 28-day period after administration were stable at approximately 10 ng/mL, a level generally considered clinically relevant [23,26]. Therefore, the linear in vitro release rates reflected consistent in vivo plasma concentrations.

Table 4. Whole blood concentrations of tacrolimus: In vivo drug release results from mixed hydrogels containing 10 mg/mL tacrolimus.

Tacrolimus (ng/mL)	Time (Days)		
	7 (n = 3)	14 (n = 3)	28 (n = 3)
	8.5 ± 1.5	12.2 ± 2.1	10.1 ± 1.6

4. Conclusions

Tacrolimus is a potent immunosuppressive age that can be used for patients who receive allotransplantation. The current daily or twice-daily oral dosage forms may encounter patient compliance problems. Encapsulation of tacrolimus by in situ gelling hydrogels is a feasible way to deliver this drug. Using the mixed hydrogel system developed in this study, steady and extended delivery was achieved. The use of toxic solvents was avoided and the formulation exhibited high biocompatibility with 293T cells in vitro with high encapsulation efficiency of drug and good gelling properties. Preliminary in vivo data also confirm a stable plasma concentration of the drug for an extended period of time. In summary, the newly designed formulation of mixed hydrogels is a promising delivery system for tacrolimus and, perhaps, other highly hydrophobic compounds.

Author Contributions: Conceptualization, I.-M.C. and C.-H.L.; methodology, A.Y.L.W.; software, C.-J.W.; validation, C.-C.C., H.-C.L. and M.R.A.; formal analysis, K.-L.K. and H.-Y.C.; investigation, C.-C.C.; writing—original draft preparation, H.-C.L. and M.R.A.; writing—review and editing, I.-M.C.; supervision, I.-M.C. and C.-H.L.; project administration, I.-M.C. and C.-H.L.; funding acquisition, I.-M.C. and C.-H.L.

References

1. Hoare, T.R.; Kohane, D.S. Hydrogels in drug delivery: Progress and challenges. *Polymer* **2008**, *49*, 1993–2007. [CrossRef]
2. Wichterle, O.; Lim, D. Hydrophilic Gels for Biological Use. *Nature* **1960**, *185*, 117. [CrossRef]
3. Drury, J.L.; Mooney, D.J. Hydrogels for tissue engineering: Scaffold design variables and applications. *Biomaterials* **2003**, *24*, 4337–4351. [CrossRef]
4. Kopeček, J. Hydrogel biomaterials: A smart future? *Biomaterials* **2007**, *28*, 5185–5192. [CrossRef] [PubMed]
5. Ko, D.Y.; Shinde, U.; Yeon, B.; Jeong, B. Recent progress of in situ formed gels for biomedical applications. *Prog. Polym. Sci.* **2013**, *38*, 672–701. [CrossRef]
6. Jeong, Y.; Joo, M.K.; Bahk, K.H.; Choi, Y.Y.; Kim, H.T.; Kim, W.K.; Lee, H.J.; Sohn, Y.S.; Jeong, B. Enzymatically degradable temperature-sensitive polypeptide as a new in-situ gelling biomaterial. *J. Control. Release* **2009**, *137*, 25–30. [CrossRef] [PubMed]
7. Boustta, M.; Colombo, P.-E.; Lenglet, S.; Poujol, S.; Vert, M. Versatile UCST-based thermoresponsive hydrogels for loco-regional sustained drug delivery. *J. Control. Release* **2014**, *174*, 1–6. [CrossRef] [PubMed]
8. Klouda, L. Thermoresponsive hydrogels in biomedical applications: A seven-year update. *Eur. J. Pharm. Biopharm.* **2015**, *97*, 338–349. [CrossRef]
9. Yu, L.; Ding, J. Injectable hydrogels as unique biomedical materials. *Chem. Soc. Rev.* **2008**, *37*, 1473–1481. [CrossRef]
10. Nguyen, M.K.; Lee, D.S. Injectable Biodegradable Hydrogels. *Macromol. Biosci.* **2010**, *10*, 563–579. [CrossRef]
11. Yu, L.; Chang, G.; Zhang, H.; Ding, J. Temperature-induced spontaneous sol–gel transitions of poly (D,L-lactic acid-*co*-glycolic acid)-*b*-poly (ethylene glycol)-*b*-poly (D,L-lactic acid-*co*-glycolic acid) triblock copolymers and their end-capped derivatives in water. *J. Polym. Sci. Part A Polym. Chem.* **2007**, *45*, 1122–1133. [CrossRef]
12. Yeon, B.; Park, M.H.; Moon, H.J.; Kim, S.J.; Cheon, Y.W.; Jeong, B. 3D culture of adipose-tissue-derived stem cells mainly leads to chondrogenesis in poly (ethylene glycol)-poly (L-alanine) diblock copolymer thermogel. *Biomacromolecules* **2013**, *14*, 3256–3266. [CrossRef] [PubMed]
13. Peng, S.; Lai, Z.T.; Hong, D.W.; Chu, I.M.; Lai, P.L. Controlled release of strontium through neutralization reaction within a methoxy (polyethylene glycol)-polyester hydrogel. *J. Appl. Biomater. Funct. Mater.* **2017**, *15*, e162–e169. [CrossRef] [PubMed]
14. Lin, J.-Y.; Lai, P.-L.; Lin, Y.-K.; Peng, S.; Lee, L.-Y.; Chen, C.-N.; Chu, I.M. A poloxamer-polypeptide thermosensitive hydrogel as a cell scaffold and sustained release depot. *Polym. Chem.* **2016**, *7*, 2976–2985. [CrossRef]
15. Yun, E.J.; Yon, B.; Joo, M.K.; Jeong, B. Cell therapy for skin wound using fibroblast encapsulated poly (ethylene glycol)-poly (L-alanine) thermogel. *Biomacromolecules* **2012**, *13*, 1106–1111. [CrossRef] [PubMed]
16. Chiang, P.R.; Lin, T.Y.; Tsai, H.C.; Chen, H.L.; Liu, S.Y.; Chen, F.R.; Hwang, Y.S.; Chu, I.M. Thermosensitive hydrogel from oligopeptide-containing amphiphilic block copolymer: Effect of peptide functional group on self-assembly and gelation behavior. *Langmuir* **2013**, *29*, 15981–15991. [CrossRef] [PubMed]
17. Cui, H.; Zhuang, X.; He, C.; Wei, Y.; Chen, X. High performance and reversible ionic polypeptide hydrogel based on charge-driven assembly for biomedical applications. *Acta Biomater.* **2015**, *11*, 183–190. [CrossRef] [PubMed]
18. Cheng, Y.; He, C.; Xiao, C.; Ding, J.; Zhuang, X.; Huang, Y.; Chen, X. Decisive role of hydrophobic side groups of polypeptides in thermosensitive gelation. *Biomacromolecules* **2012**, *13*, 2053–2059. [CrossRef] [PubMed]
19. Oh, H.J.; Joo, M.K.; Sohn, Y.S.; Jeong, B. Secondary Structure Effect of Polypeptide on Reverse Thermal Gelation and Degradation of l/dl-Poly (alanine)–Poloxamer–l/dl-Poly (alanine) Copolymers. *Macromolecules* **2008**, *41*, 8204–8209. [CrossRef]
20. Choi, Y.Y.; Jang, J.H.; Park, M.H.; Choi, B.G.; Chi, B.; Jeong, B. Block length affects secondary structure, nanoassembly and thermosensitivity of poly (ethylene glycol)-poly (L-alanine) block copolymers. *J. Mater. Chem.* **2010**, *20*, 3416–3421. [CrossRef]

21. Xu, W.; Ling, P.; Zhang, T. Toward immunosuppressive effects on liver transplantation in rat model: Tacrolimus loaded poly (ethylene glycol)-poly (D,L-lactide) nanoparticle with longer survival time. *Int. J. Pharm.* **2014**, *460*, 173–180. [CrossRef] [PubMed]
22. Tajdaran, K.; Shoichet, M.S.; Gordon, T.; Borschel, G.H. A novel polymeric drug delivery system for localized and sustained release of tacrolimus (FK506). *Biotechnol. Bioeng.* **2015**, *112*, 1948–1953. [CrossRef] [PubMed]
23. Gajanayake, T.; Olariu, R.; Leclere, F.M.; Dhayani, A.; Yang, Z.; Bongoni, A.K.; Banz, Y.; Constantinescu, M.A.; Karp, J.M.; Vemula, P.K.; et al. A single localized dose of enzyme-responsive hydrogel improves long-term survival of a vascularized composite allograft. *Sci. Transl. Med.* **2014**, *6*, 249ra110. [CrossRef] [PubMed]
24. Huang, Y.F.; Lai, P.C.; Huang, Y.C.; Chiang, Y.S.; You, H.L.; Lin, C.N.; Ning, H.C. Development of an ultra-performance liquid chromatography tandem mass spectrometric method for simultaneous quantitating four immunosuppressant drugs. *J. Biomed. Lab. Sci.* **2015**, *27*, 61–68.
25. Kojarunchitt, T.; Hook, S.; Rizwan, S.; Rades, T.; Baldursdottir, S. Development and characterisation of modified poloxamer 407 thermoresponsive depot systems containing cubosomes. *Int. J. Pharm.* **2011**, *408*, 20–26. [CrossRef] [PubMed]
26. Kojima, R.; Yoshida, T.; Tasaki, H.; Umejima, H.; Maeda, M.; Higashi, Y.; Watanabe, S.; Oku, N. Release mechanisms of tacrolimus-loaded PLGA and PLA microspheres and immunosuppressive effects of the microspheres in a rat heart transplantation model. *Int. J. Pharm.* **2015**, *492*, 20–27. [CrossRef] [PubMed]

3

Gold Nanocage-Incorporated Poly(ε-Caprolactone) (PCL) Fibers for Chemo-photothermal Synergistic Cancer Therapy

Ju Hyang Park [1], Hojun Seo [2], Da In Kim [1], Ji Hyun Choi [1], Jin Ho Son [1], Jongbok Kim [3], Geon Dae Moon [2,*] and Dong Choon Hyun [1,*]

1 Department of Polymer Science and Engineering, Kyungpook National University, Daegu 41566, Korea; pjh99279@naver.com (J.H.P.); dada7230@naver.com (D.I.K.); jode1532@naver.com (J.H.C.); mlbask7@naver.com (J.H.S.)

2 Dongnam Regional Division, Korea Institute of Industrial Technology, Busan 46938, Korea; dark911205@gmail.com

3 Department of Materials Science and Engineering, Kumoh National Institute of Technology, Gumi, Gyeongbuk 39177, Korea; jb1956k@gmail.com

* Correspondence: gmoon@kitech.re.kr (G.D.M.); dong.hyun@knu.ac.kr (D.C.H.)

Abstract: This paper introduces a new fibrous system for synergistic cancer therapy, which consists of gold nanocage (AuNC)-loaded poly(ε-caprolactone) (PCL) fibers with encapsulation of a chemotherapeutic anticancer drug in their core and loading of a phase-changeable fatty acid in their sheath. Under on–off switching of near-infrared (NIR) light irradiation, the excellent photothermal ability and photostability of AuNCs allows repeated, significant heating of the fibers to a temperature available to hyperthermia. Simultaneously, the NIR light-induced heat generation enables the melting out of the loaded fatty acid, leading to a rapid release of the drug molecules from the fibers. The combination of this NIR light-triggered drug release with the repeated hyperthermia treatment exhibits excellent anticancer efficacy.

Keywords: PCL; electrospinning; combination therapy; photothermal therapy; NIR-triggered drug release

1. Introduction

Over the past several decades, considerable effort has been dedicated to the fabrication of polymeric fibers. These have a large surface area and high aspect ratio, and are applicable to a broad spectrum of applications, including air filtration, catalysis, energy harvesting and conversion, electronics, sensors, and in regenerative medicine [1–7]. Among many strategies that have been developed for the production of polymeric fibers, electrospinning has been extensively explored due to its merits such as simplicity, high efficiency, low cost, and high reproducibility [3]. More importantly, it allows a variety of functional molecules to be easily loaded into polymeric fibers [8], which has expanded the applicability of the fibers to the biomedical treatment of diseases through the delivery and even the controlled release of drugs [9].

Recently, the use of electrospun polymeric fibers in biomedical application has been directed towards the therapy of cancer, an intractable health issue worldwide. Such electrospun fibres possess unique features including high drug loading efficiency, good stability as a bulk material, and ease in temporal release of drugs [10–14]. In particular, their implantability at tumor sites or in the cavities remaining after surgical removal of solid tumors enables a localized release of chemotherapeutic drugs, which can maintain a low concentration of the systematic drugs while allowing their sufficient dosage locally [12]. However, the use of chemotherapeutic drugs can bring inevitably several problems such as drug resistance and toxicity in side effects [13,15,16]. Furthermore, it is difficult to sufficiently eliminate tumors using drugs only, even though they are useful for treating many types of cancers.

In addressing these issues, combination therapy, which uses the synergistic effects of two or more treatment modalities, has been developed for higher therapeutic efficacy. Photothermal therapy (PTT), in which an incident light is converted into heat for destroying cancer cells, has been used together with chemotherapy because it can induce a selective death of cancer cells [17,18]. As the combination strategy, until recently, electrospun polymeric fibers have been incorporated with both chemotherapeutic drugs and photothermal agents. As an exemplary case, smart electrospun fibers, which can potentially realize a synergistic effect of chemotherapy and PTT, were produced by Burdick and coworkers [19]. They encapsulated gold nanorods (AuNRs), as a photothermal agent, and drug molecules into poly(*N*-isopropylacrylamide-co-polyethylene glycol acrylate) (PNPA) fibers with thermosensitivity. Near-infrared (NIR) light-triggered release of the loaded drug occurred by an interplay of the photothermal effect of AuNRs with the temperature responsiveness of PNPA. Mao and coworkers fabricated Yb^{3+}/Er^{3+} co-doped $CaTiO_3$ nanofibers [12]. Increase in local temperature at the surface of the fibers by NIR light irradiation enhanced the vibration of poly(acrylic acid) (PAA) chains functionalized on the surface of the fibers, weakening an electrostatic bonding between the fibers and preloaded doxorubicin anticancer drug molecules. As a result, NIR light-triggered release of the drug was achieved. Recently, Kim and coworkers demonstrated the use of poly(ε-caprolactone) (PCL) fibers functionalized by NIR light-responsive polypyrrole (PPy) for synergistic cancer therapy [13]. Under an on–off operation of NIR light, the fibers allowed a precisely controlled release of paclitaxel anticancer drug together with a repeated application of NIR light-triggered hyperthermia, which exhibited excellent anticancer efficacy. Nevertheless, for their practical application in cancer therapy, the systems need to stop the undesirable drug release in non-triggered state and/or the loss of activity of chemotherapeutic drugs arising from the use of multi-stage physicochemical processes [20]. Alternatively, a system, consisting of PCL hollow fibers with entrapment of indocyanine green (ICG) in their sheath, was developed for combination therapy [21]. However, the use of ICG as a photothermal agent would make the repeated hyperthermia of the system difficult due to its loss of photothermal ability by photobleaching or chemical/thermal denaturation.

In this study, we introduce a PCL fibrous system incorporated with gold nanocages (AuNCs) that can function as a NIR light-absorbing photothermal agent with excellent stability. The incorporation of AuNCs enables a significant heating of the fibers upon exposure to NIR light. This NIR light-triggered heat generation can be repeatedly achieved through an on–off switching of NIR light irradiation, leading to a significant death of cancer cells by repeated hyperthermia treatment. Additional loading of the anticancer drug doxorubicin and a phase-changeable fatty acid to the fibres will enhance the anticancer activity of the system more through NIR light-triggered release of the drug in combination with hyperthermia.

2. Materials and Methods

2.1. Materials

The following chemicals were purchased from Sigma-Aldrich (St. Louis, MO, USA): PCL (Mn $\approx$ 45,000 Da), WST-1 solution, doxorubicin hydrochloride (DOX), Span 80, silver trifluoroacetate (CF_3COOAg), sodium hydrosulfide hydrate (NaHS), poly(vinylpyrrolidone) (PVP, Mw $\approx$ 55,000 Da), lauric acid (LA), stearic acid (SA), *O*-[2-(3-mercaptopropionylamino)ethyl]-*O*′-methylpolyethylene glycol (PEG-thiol, Mw $\approx$ 5000 Da), and gold (III) chloride trihydrate ($HAuCl_4{\cdot}3H_2O$). Ethylene glycol (EG) and sodium chloride (NaCl) were obtained from J.T. Baker (Phillipsburg, NJ, USA) and Duksan

Chemical (Daegu, Korea), respectively. Human breast cancer SK-BR-3 cells and fibroblast (FB) cells were procured from Korea Cell Line Bank (KCLB, Seoul, Korea).

2.2. Preparation of Eutectic Mixture of Fatty Acids

We prepared a eutectic mixture of fatty acids with a melting point of 39 °C as previously reported [22]. Briefly, 0.8 g of LA and 0.2 g of SA were first put together in a glass vial (20 mL), followed by heating at 90 °C in nitrogen (N_2) atmosphere with magnetic stirring at 500 rpm. After 1 h, the fatty acid mixture was cooled down to 25 °C in ambient air.

2.3. Synthesis and Phase Transfer of AuNCs

First, EG (50 mL) was added to a 250 mL round bottom flask and then heated at 150 °C under magnetic stirring using a heating mantle, followed by the addition of a NaHS solution in EG (0.6 mL, 3 mM). After 4 min, 5 mL of a HCl solution in EG (3 mM) was added, followed by 12.5 mL of a PVP solution in EG (20 mg/mL). Then, 4 mL of CF_3COOAg solution in EG (282 mM) was additionally injected to synthesize silver nanocubes (AgNCs). After 30 min, the reaction was quenched in an ice-water bath, followed by centrifugation and washing with acetone and deionized (DI) water (18.2 MΩ). The resultant AgNCs were converted into AuNCs using a previously reported procedure with several minor modifications [23]. In a typical synthesis process, an aqueous solution of $HAuCl_4$ (0.75 mM) was prepared. A specific amount of the $HAuCl_4$ solution was then added dropwise into 5 mL of an aqueous solution of AgNCs (0.01 mg/mL) preheated to 90 °C. After 10–15 min, the sample was cooled down to 25 °C and a sufficient amount of NaCl was added to remove the AgCl precipitated in the synthesis. The sample was then centrifuged three times at 9000 rpm for 20 min. The collected AuNCs were re-dispersed in DI water and stored in the dark until further use.

To achieve phase transfer of the as-synthesized AuNCs from water phase to organic, their surface was modified. In order to accomplish this, 1 mg of the as-synthesized AuNCs was dispersed in 5 mL of DI water, followed by adding 1 mL of an aqueous solution of PEG-thiol (1 wt%) and 3 mL of chloroform. The solution mixture was mechanically agitated using a vortex mixer for 2 min, and thus the AuNCs were transferred from the water phase to the chloroform. The chloroform phase was then extracted, followed by centrifugation, washing with fresh chloroform, and drying in ambient air. The resultant sample was stored at 4 °C until further use.

2.4. Fabrication of Electrospun Fibers

To fabricate electrospun fibers, a water-in-oil (W/O) emulsion was first prepared. To accomplish this, a Span 80 solution in chloroform was made by dissolving 2 g of the surfactant in 38 g of the solvent. The solution was mixed with 200 μL of an aqueous solution containing DOX (3 mg) to generate a W/O emulsion using a high-speed mixer at a rotation rate of 15,000 rpm. The resultant W/O emulsion (3.5 g) was mixed with the eutectic mixture of fatty acids, the phase-transferred AuNCs, and PCL (1.5 g). The weight fraction of the eutectic mixture to PCL (f_{fatty}) was varied. Polymeric fibers loaded with AuNCs and DOX were produced by electrospinning the prepared W/O emulsion. For the electrospinning, the W/O emulsion was filled into a syringe (5 mL) with attachment to a stainless steel needle (22 gauge) and a voltage in the range of 6 and 8 kV was applied to the needle. The feed rate of the emulsion was fixed at 0.03 mL/h and an electrically grounded aluminum foil, placed 20 cm away from the needle, was used as a collector. Loading of DOX into the fibers was confirmed using a confocal laser scanning microscope (CLSM) (LSM700, Carl Zeiss, Oberkochen, Germany) and the amount of the loaded drug was quantified through UV–VIS spectral measurement (T60, PG Instrument, Leicestershire, United Kingdom), as previously reported [21].

2.5. NIR Light-Induced Heat Generation

The photothermal ability of the as-synthesized AuNCs and the phase-transferred AuNCs was characterized using a digital thermometer (Scilab Co., Daejeon, Korea). In a typical procedure, 0.5 mg of the particles was dispersed in 5 mL of dispersion medium (DI water for the former and chloroform for the latter). Each sample was exposed to 1 W/cm^2 NIR light with a wavelength of 808 nm (LASERLAB Co., Anyang, Korea) for 50 min. For checking the photothermal behavior of the AuNC-loaded fibers, a mesh made of 20 mg of the fibers with a dimension of 1 cm × 1 cm was first prepared, followed by exposing to NIR light irradiation (1 W/cm^2). The thermal infrared images and the temperature change were obtained with the use of a thermal infrared camera (G100EX, Avio, Tokyo, Japan).

2.6. Release of DOX from Fibers in Response to NIR Light Irradiation

To obtain the release profiles of DOX, we prepared 100 mg of AuNC-loaded PCL fibers encapsulating DOX, followed by immersing in 5 mL of phosphate-buffered saline (PBS) solution at pH 7.4. After incubation in a thermostat preheated to 37 °C for 4 h under mild agitation, NIR light irradiation (1 W/cm^2, 808 nm) was applied to the sample for 5 min to increase the temperature to 45 °C. After the treatment, the sample was re-incubated at 37 °C. At different time intervals, 1 mL of the solution was taken out and the concentration of DOX in it was characterized using UV–VIS spectrophotometry, as previously reported [21]. After characterization, the solution was poured back for further testing. For each time interval, three samples were tested.

2.7. Cell Viability Test

The cytotoxicity of NIR light irradiation (1 W/cm^2, 808 nm) was examined using a previously reported procedure [20]. Additionally, we investigated the cytotoxicity of phase-transferred AuNCs, which was achieved by introducing a solution of the particles (10 μL) in dimethyl sulfoxide with a certain concentration to the cells cultured through the aforementioned procedure. The sample without the treatment with the nanoparticles and NIR irradiation was used as a control. The cell viability was determined using WST-1 assay.

The biocompatibility of plain PCL fibers, AuNC-incorporated PCL fibers, AuNC-incorporated PCL fibers loaded with DOX, and AuNC-incorporated PCL fibers with loading of the fatty acid mixture and DOX was also tested using FB cells. Meshes with a dimension of 1 cm × 1 cm were first prepared from each type of fibers (20 mg) and then placed in each well of a 24-well cell culture plate. After their sterilization for 30 min under UV light irradiation, FB cells were cultured on the meshes as reported previously [20]. The anticancer activity of those fibers and PCL fibers loaded with the fatty acid mixture and DOX against SK-BR-3 cells was evaluated using a live/dead cell assay as well as a WST-1 assay. SK-BR-3 cells cultured on the meshes made of each type of fibers through the aforementioned procedure were subsequently treated with 1 W/cm^2 NIR light (5 min of exposure per treatment), followed by incubation at 37 °C for an additional 19–24 h according to the number of the exposure to conduct the WST-1 assay and the live/dead assay using a commercially available kit (Biotium, Fremont, CA, USA).

2.8. Characterization

Transmission electron microscope (TEM) analysis was performed on the fibers incorporated with AuNCs and the as-synthesized AuNCs using a HT7700 (Hitachi) operated at 75 kV. The morphology of the produced fibers was also investigated using a scanning electron microscope (SEM) (SU8220, Hitachi, Tokyo, Japan) with an accelerating voltage of 3 kV. Differential scanning calorimetry (DSC) measurement was conducted using DSC Q100 (TA Instrument, New Castle, DE, USA). Typically, samples with a weight of approximate 3 mg were used for scanning in the range of −70 and 250 °C at a scanning rate of 2 °C/min. X-ray diffraction (XRD) patterns were recorded in the range of 2θ = 10° to 90° using a Rigaku D/MAX II X-ray diffractometer with Cu K_α radiation.

2.9. Statistical Analysis

Student's *t*-test was used to examine the differences between two groups, and a one-way analysis of variance (ANOVA) with a Tukey's post hoc test was performed to examine the differences among four groups. $p < 0.01$ was considered to indicate a statistically significant difference.

3. Results and Discussion

NIR light, which has the minimum absorption by human blood and body tissues, is known to penetrate into soft tissues up to several inches in depth and to be converted into heat with a photothermal agent [24], which makes it advantageous for PTT. To achieve NIR light-induced cancer therapy, a NIR light-sensitive system was made of biocompatible/ biodegradable PCL fibers incorporated with AuNCs. The unique plasmonic property of AuNCs due to an interaction of light with their conduction band electrons allows photon energy to be efficiently converted into thermal energy [25]. When the generated heat increases the temperature of the system to a window available for hyperthermia (ca. 40–45 °C) [26], inactivation and eventual death of cancer cells will occur. Since AuNCs are non-susceptible to photobleaching and chemical/thermal denaturation [27], the hyperthermia can be repeatedly achieved.

AuNCs were synthesized using a galvanic replacement reaction between AgNCs (Figure S1, Supplementary Materials) and $HAuCl_4$. When a very small amount of $HAuCl_4$ solution was added to an aqueous solution of AgNCs, the replacement reaction was activated at a specific site on the surface of each AgNC, generating a hole (Figure 1A). As the reaction proceeded, the hole worked as an anode, oxidizing Ag atoms. Consequently, the released electrons moved to the surface of the AgNCs for reducing $HAuCl_4^-$, leading to an epitaxial growth of Au atoms on the AgNCs [28]. As the Au layer formed, the holes functioned as a site for the dissolution of Ag, transforming the AgNCs into a hollow structure (Figure 1B). When the amount of the $HAuCl_4$ solution was increased, the hollow interior would be larger in size, forming Au-Ag nanoboxes with a uniform wall (Figure 1C). The Ag atoms in the nanoboxes would be selectively removed with the further addition of $HAuCl_4$, eventually leading to the formation of AuNCs with a porous structure (Figure 1D).

Figure 1E shows UV-VIS–NIR extinction spectra for the samples of Figure 1A–D dispersed in DI water, indicating that their surface plasmon resonance (SPR) band was dependent on the amount of $HAuCl_4$ used. When a larger amount of $HAuCl_4$ was used, the extinction peak appeared at a longer wavelength. For example, the sample of Figure 1B exhibited an extinction peak at 575 nm, while the SPR peak for the solution of AuNCs (Figure 1D) was red-shifted to 790 nm in the NIR region. This shift in SPR band had a direct impact on the photothermal ability of the samples. Figure 1F shows the change in temperature of each sample during exposure to 1 W/cm^2 NIR light irradiation with a wavelength of 808 nm, indicating that the temperature of all the samples was increased by NIR light irradiation. However, the exact profiles differed. The sample of Figure 1A exhibited a temperature increase to 35 °C, while the increase in temperature up to 37 °C was seen in the sample of Figure 1B. The largest temperature rise was observed for the sample of Figure 1D because the SPR peak of this sample well matched the central wavelength of the laser source [29]. This result indicates that AuNCs could be a photothermal agent responding to NIR light.

For the fabrication of NIR light-sensitive fibrous system, loading of AuNCs into polymeric fibers is required. To accomplish this, the particles should be dispersed in organic media without aggregation. We phase-transferred the as-synthesized AuNCs from the aqueous phase to the organic using thiolated PEG as a transfer agent. PEG-thiol was first introduced to an aqueous solution containing the as-synthesized AuNCs, followed by chloroform. As shown in Figure 2A, the organic phase and the aqueous phase containing the particles were phase-separated because of their immiscibility. After vigorous agitation, most of the particles transferred from the water phase to the chloroform in 30 min (Figure 2B) [30]. This successful phase transfer was due to the surface modification caused by the strong affinity between the surface of AuNCs and the thiol group [30,31]. After extraction, centrifugation, and washing, the particles were re-dispersed in fresh chloroform to make a W/O emulsion for electrospinning (Figure 2C).

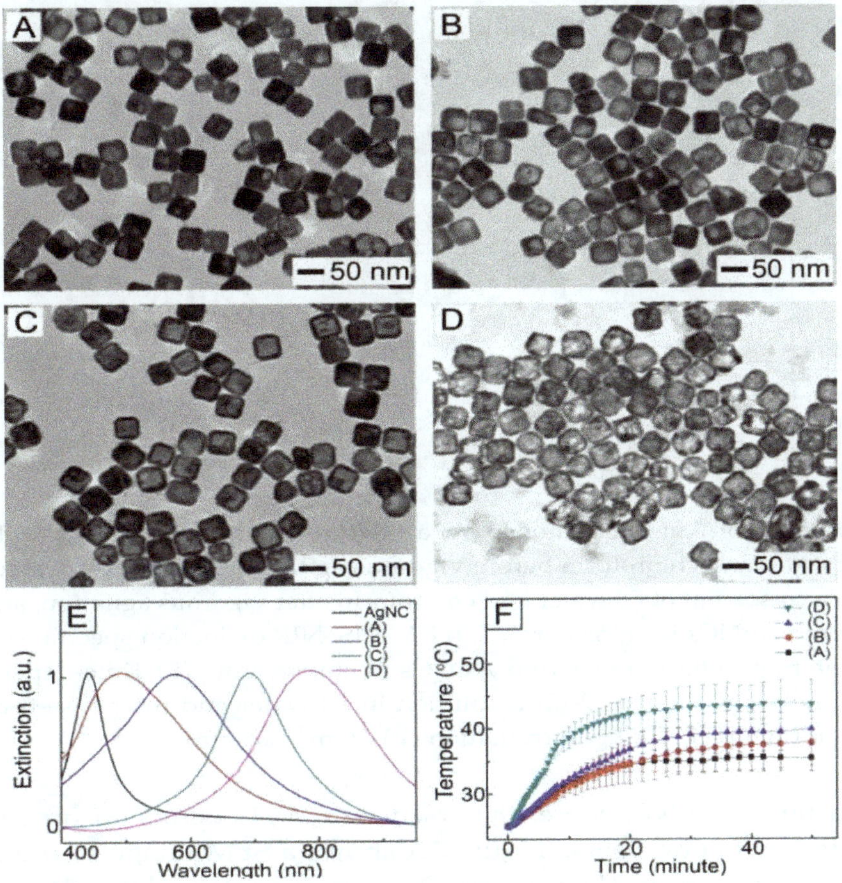

Figure 1. (**A–D**) TEM images of the particles obtained after the reaction of AgNCs with different amounts of $HAuCl_4$ solution: (**A**) 0.06, (**B**) 0.08, (**C**) 0.15 and (**D**) 0.2 mL. (**E**) UV–VIS–NIR extinction spectra for the particles of (**A–D**) in DI water. (**E**) UV–VIS–NIR extinction spectra for the particles of (**A–D**) and AgNCs in DI water. (**F**) Change in temperature for the particles of (**A–D**) in DI water with a concentration of 0.1 mg/mL under NIR light irradiation (1 W/cm^2, 808 nm).

Figure 2D shows UV–VIS–NIR extinction spectra for the as-synthesized AuNCs dispersed in DI water and the phase-transferred AuNCs dispersed in chloroform. No broadening of the SPR band was observed for the latter as compared with the former, which implies that aggregation among the AuNCs and change in their morphology did not happen during the phase transfer process. On the other hand, the phase transfer caused a red-shift in SPR band and the extinction peak moved to 815 nm in the NIR region, which was a result of change in the refractive index of the local environment surrounding the AuNCs [32].

We tested the photothermal conversion property of the phase-transferred AuNCs by exposing a solution of the phase-transferred particles in chloroform to NIR light irradiation. As shown in Figure 2E, the temperature of the sample increased in response to NIR light irradiation and its time-dependent temperature profile was similar to that of the aqueous solution of the as-synthesized AuNCs, which suggest that the photothermal ability of AuNCs was still kept after the phase transfer process. We also measured the optical property of the phase-transferred AuNCs after NIR light treatment. No change in the SPR band was observed after the treatment (Figure S2, Supplementary Materials), implying that the particles maintained their morphology without aggregation after NIR light irradiation. These results reveal that the phase-transferred AuNCs had excellent photostability.

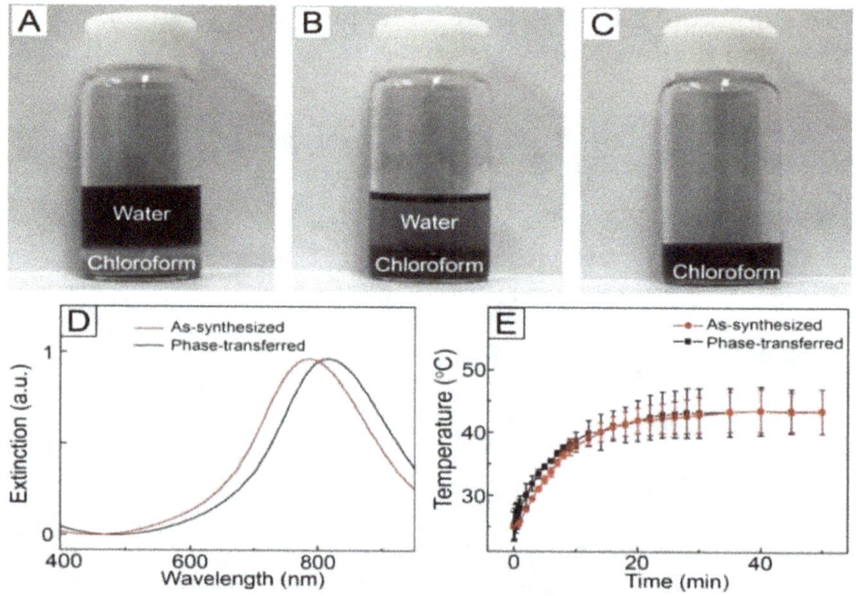

Figure 2. Photographs of AuNC solutions: (**A**) a mixture solution of AuNCs and PEG-thiol in a co-solvent of DI water and chloroform before vigorous agitation, (**B**) a mixture solution of AuNCs and PEG-thiol in a co-solvent of DI water and chloroform after vigorous agitation, and (**C**) a solution of phase-transferred AuNCs in chloroform. (**D**) UV–VIS–NIR extinction spectra for as-synthesized AuNCs in DI water and phase-transferred AuNCs in chloroform. (**E**) Time-dependent change in temperature for the as-synthesized AuNC solution in DI water and the phase-transferred AuNC solution in chloroform under NIR light irradiation (1 W/cm^2, 808 nm).

The phase-transferred AuNCs were dispersed in a W/O emulsion prepared for fabrication of NIR light-sensitive polymeric fibers. Figure 3A shows a SEM image of the fibers produced by electrospinning the W/O emulsion. The used W/O emulsion contained the phase-transferred AuNCs of 0.1 wt% without any inclusion of drug. The produced fibers had a smooth surface and their average diameter was 2.84 $\pm$ 0.12 µm. Figure 3B shows a TEM image of a single fiber of Figure 3A. It was found that a hollow interior, which can be a reservoir of hydrophilic drug, was formed in the core of the fiber, which was a result of a big difference in the surface energy between water droplet phase and chloroform one that were present within the W/O emulsion [21]. A magnified image of the region, marked by a black box, is shown in the inset, demonstrating that the phase-transferred AuNCs were well distributed within the fiber. Figure 3C shows XRD patterns for the phase-transferred AuNCs, plain PCL fibers, and the fibers of Figure 3A. The XRD pattern from the sample of Figure 3A contained the peaks generated by the AuNCs as well as those corresponding to the plain PCL fibers. This result also confirms that the nanoparticles were successfully loaded into the fibers.

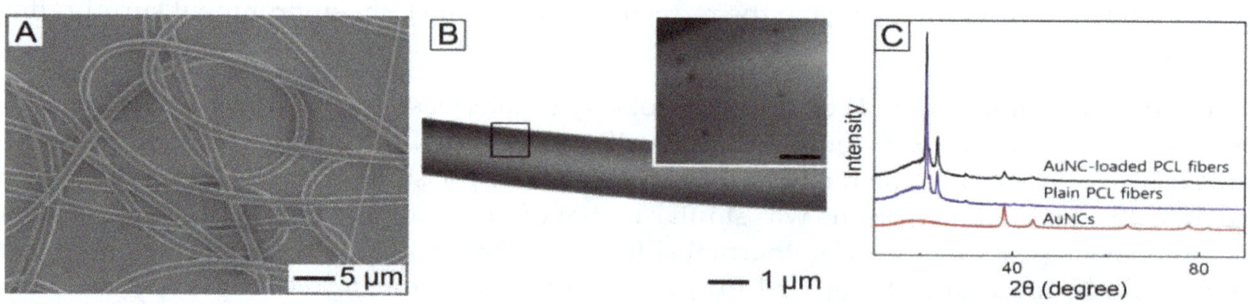

Figure 3. (**A**) SEM and (**B**) TEM images of PCL fibers loaded with AuNCs. The scale bar in the inset is 300 nm. (**C**) XRD patterns for AuNCs, plain PCL fibers, and AuNC-loaded PCL fibers.

To investigate a NIR light sensitivity of the fibers loaded with AuNCs, the fibres were exposed to NIR light irradiation and then their change in temperature observed. Figure 4A shows the time-lapse thermal infrared photographs of the fibers of Figure 3A under NIR light with a power density of 1 W/cm^2. When the fibers were exposed to NIR irradiation, a drastic change in color from blue to red was observed at the center of the images (marked with a white box) where the fibers were placed. This change in color implies that the temperature of the sample increased due to the loading of AuNCs with photothermal conversion capability. Change in the concentration of AuNCs in the W/O emulsion had an influence on the heat generation property of the fibers. As shown in Figure 4B, the sample without the inclusion of AuNCs exhibited no significant change in temperature under NIR light irradiation, whereas the use of the W/O emulsion with 0.01 wt% AuNCs allowed the temperature rise to 33 °C. When the concentration increased to 0.1 wt%, the temperature reached 45 °C. This result was because the higher concentration of AuNCs would lead to loading of the more amount of the particles into the fibers, which resulted in stronger heat generation.

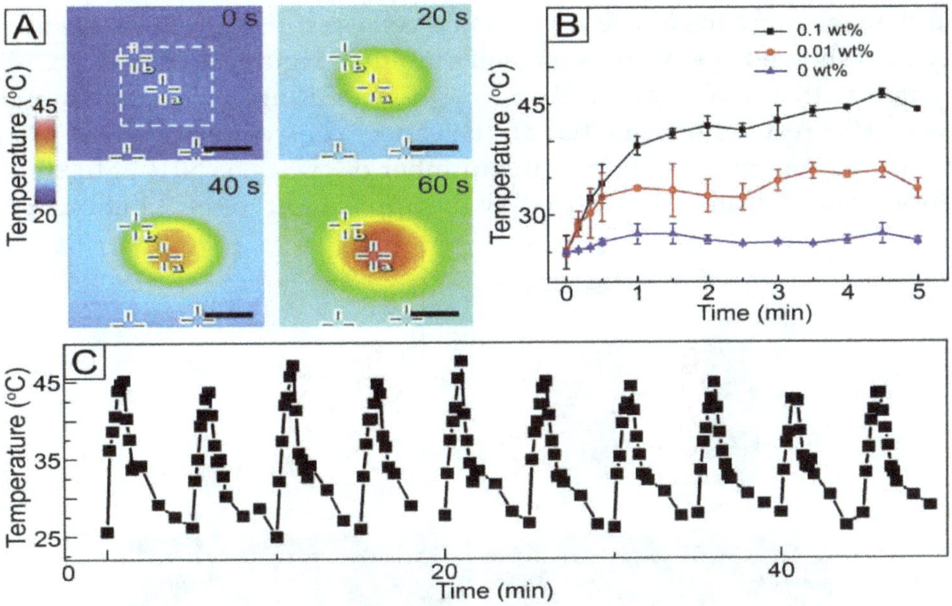

Figure 4. (**A**) Time-lapse thermal infrared images of AuNC-loaded fibers under NIR light irradiation (1 W/cm^2, 808 nm). The scale bar is 0.5 cm. (**B**) Change in temperature for the fibers, which were produced from the W/O emulsions with different concentration of AuNCs, under NIR light (1 W/cm^2, 808 nm). (**C**) Time-dependent temperature curve for AuNC-loaded fibers under on–off switching of NIR light (1 W/cm^2, 808 nm).

The NIR light-triggered heat generation could reversibly happen when NIR light irradiation was applied in an on–off manner, as shown in Figure 4C. The treatment with NIR light for 1 min changed the temperature of the sample of Figure 3A from 26 to 45 °C, and the temperature returned to 26 °C after the light remained off for 4 min. This NIR light-sensitive manner in temperature change was still kept when the light was switched on and off ten times under the same condition, which indicates that the fibers would be useful for repeated hyperthermia treatment.

We evaluated the anticancer ability of the fibers against SK-BR-3 cells. Before the evaluation, we checked the cytotoxicity of NIR light to the cells. Figure S3A (Supplementary Materials) shows the viability of SK-BR-3 cells after exposure to 1 W/cm^2 NIR light, determined using a WST-1 assay. The viability of the cells was >90% for all the conditions compared with the control without the treatment of NIR light. In addition, we tested the cytotoxicity of the phase-transferred AuNCs and the result reveals that the particles were biocompatible (Figure S3B, Supplementary Materials). These results suggest that their effects on the anticancer ability of the fibers were negligible.

Figure 5A shows the viabilities of SK-BR-3 cells treated with plain PCL fibers and AuNC-loaded PCL fibers of Figure 3A. Under no exposure to NIR light, both the samples exhibited cell viabilities >90%. A similar result was also observed with FB cells (Figure S4, Supplementary Materials). The high viabilities indicate that the fibers are biocompatible. On the other hand, when irradiated with NIR light, only the fibers loaded with AuNCs had a lower cell viability (78%). This decrease in cell viability was because the photothermal conversion generated by the loaded particles increased the temperature of the sample to 45 °C for hyperthermia, and consequently damaged the cells. However, many cells were still alive, even though they might be weakened.

This hyperthermia effect could be strengthened by increasing the number of cycles of NIR light irradiation. Figure 5B shows the cell viability with respect to the number of NIR light treatments, demonstrating that the value of viability decreased as the number of the treatments increased. Two cycles of NIR light treatment yielded a cell viability of 44%, while four cycles of the treatment reduced the value to 16%. This decrease in viability can be explained by the shock effect [33]. The repeated, rapid temperature change due to multiple cycles of on–off operation of NIR light irradiation could damage more the already weakened cells, resulting in more destruction of the cells. Live/dead assay also showed the decrease in cell viability. Figure 5C shows a CLS micrograph of SK-BR-3 cells treated with AuNC-loaded fibers under no NIR light, which exhibited only a bright green fluorescence. This result suggests that all the cancer cells were still alive. On the other hand, the red fluorescence became more visible as the number of cycles of NIR light treatment increased (Figure 5D–F), implying cell death was induced by the applications of NIR light-driven hyperthermia.

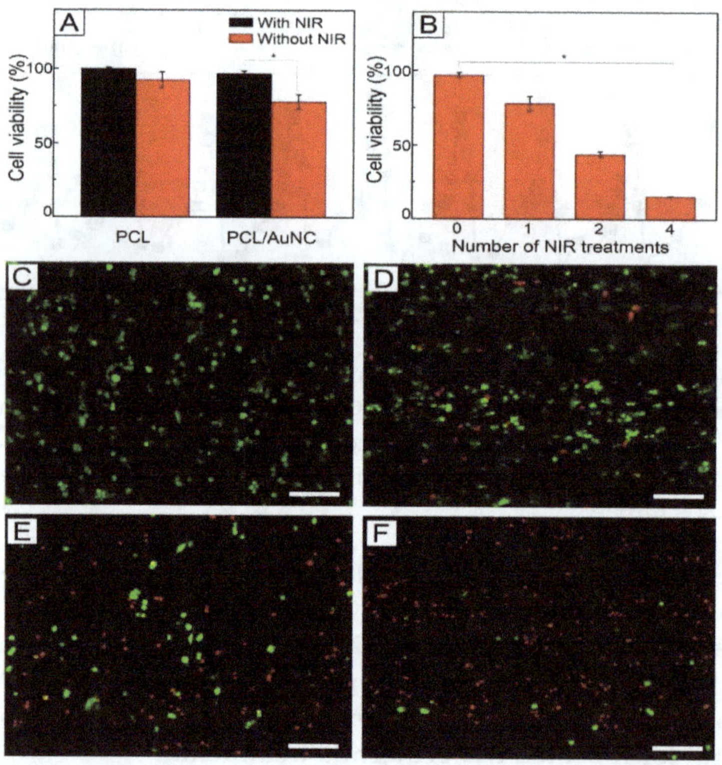

Figure 5. (**A**) Viability of SK-BR-3 cells treated with plain PCL and AuNC-loaded PCL fibers without and with NIR irradiation (1 W/cm^2, 808 nm). (**B**) Viability of SK-BR-3 cells treated with AuNC-loaded PCL fibers under on–off switching of NIR light irradiation (1 W/cm^2, 808 nm). * indicates $p < 0.01$. (**C–F**) CLS micrographs showing live (green) and dead (red) SK-BR-3 cells treated with AuNC-loaded PCL fibers under different numbers of cycles of 1 W/cm^2 NIR light irradiation: (**C**) Zero, (**D**) one, (**E**) two, and (**F**) four cycles. The scale bars are 100 μm.

However, the use of only NIR light-induced hyperthermia cannot achieve a satisfactory therapeutic efficacy because of the non-uniform distribution of heat generated within a tumor [13]. Furthermore, residual cancer cell survival after the treatment can cause metastasis or recurrence [20]. To improve the anticancer activity of the AuNC-loaded fibers, we additionally loaded a chemotherapeutic drug, DOX, into the fibers together with a biocompatible, phase-changeable fatty acid that could induce a NIR-light triggered release of the drug [21,22,26]. Figure 6A shows a SEM image of AuNC-loaded PCL fibers with the inclusion of the drug and the fatty acid mixture of LA and SA, which were produced by electrospinning a W/O emulsion containing DOX in the water phase and the fatty acid mixture (f_{fatty} = 0.05) in the oil phase. The average diameter of the fibers was 2.88 ± 0.14 μm, which was similar to that for the sample of Figure 3A. A cross-sectional SEM image is shown in the inset, demonstrating that the fibers had a hollow interior and a smooth surface. These results indicate that the addition of the fatty acid mixture and the drug did not affect the formation of fibers or their structure. Figure 6B–D show CLS images of the single fiber of Figure 6A. Red fluorescence generated from DOX is observed in the fluorescence image of Figure 6B, suggesting that the drug molecules were well loaded in the fibers. The merged image (Figure 6D) with its corresponding optical image (Figure 6C) clearly demonstrates that DOX was placed in the central region of the fiber. Taken together with the inset of Figure 6A, this result indicates that the drug molecules were encapsulated in the hollow core of the fibers.

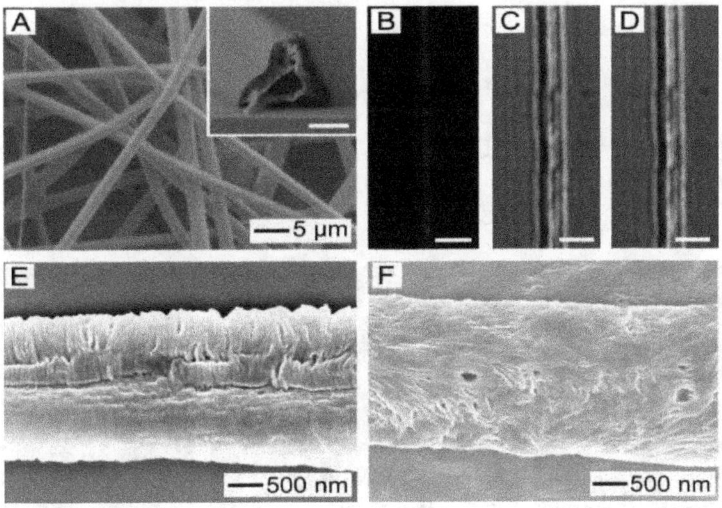

Figure 6. (**A**) SEM image of AuNC-loaded fibers containing the fatty acid mixture and DOX, which were produced using a W/O emulsion of f_{fatty} = 0.05. The inset scale is 1 μm. (**B–D**) CLS micrographs showing the fluorescence from DOX loaded in the as-spun fiber. The scales are 3 μm. (**E,F**) SEM images of AuNC-loaded fibers after exposure to 1 W/cm^2 NIR light. The fibers were made using W/O emulsions of: (**E**) f_{fatty} = 0.05 and (**F**) f_{fatty} = 0.1.

To check the inclusion of the fatty acid mixture into the fibers, DSC measurement was conducted. The fibers of Figure 6A exhibited two sharp peaks at 39 and 59 °C (Figure S5, Supplementary Materials), which corresponded to the melting points of the fatty acid mixture and PCL, respectively [22]. This result reveals the successful loading of the fatty acid mixture into the fibers. After introduction of 1 W/cm^2 NIR light irradiation to increase the temperature of the fibers to 45 °C, the peak at 39 °C given by the fatty acid mixture disappeared (Figure S5), indicating that the mixture was removed from the fibers. This removal was a result of NIR light-induced photothermal effect. Upon exposure to NIR light, a photothermal conversion was caused by the loaded AuNCs, increasing the local temperature of the sample above the melting point of the fatty acid mixture and melting out the mixture from the fibers. Consequently, small pores were generated in the sheath of the fibers, as shown in Figure 6E. The size and density of the formed pores increased with f_{fatty} (Figure 6F) because of the inclusion of the larger amount of the mixture in the fibers.

Figure 7A shows the release profiles of DOX from the fibers produced from the W/O emulsions with different values of f_{fatty}. The sample with no inclusion of the fatty acid mixture (f_{fatty} = 0) did not release the drug molecules over 4 h without NIR light treatment. A similar result was also observed for the fibers produced with the use of the W/O emulsion of f_{fatty} = 0.05 because the fatty acid mixture present in the solid state blocked the diffusion-out of the encapsulated drug molecules. When 1 W/cm^2 NIR light was irradiated for 5 min, the sample of f_{fatty} = 0 still did not release the drug molecules, whereas the fibers of f_{fatty} = 0.05 allowed the release of 33% DOX for 4 h since NIR light was irradiated. The release in the latter case resulted from the formation of the pores in response to NIR light, as visualized in Figure 6E. The formation of the pores caused by the melting out of the loaded fatty acid could increase the surface area of the fibers, allowing an easy uptake of the PBS buffer into the fibers and a generation of effective paths for the preloaded drug molecules to be released quickly [22]. This NIR light-triggered release could be controlled by varying the value of f_{fatty}. When f_{fatty} increased to 0.1, the release of 55% DOX was achieved over the same period. This difference was attributed to the larger size and density of the generated pores for the sample of f_{fatty} = 0.1 (Figure 7F), which increased surface area [21] and consequently led to the faster release of the drug.

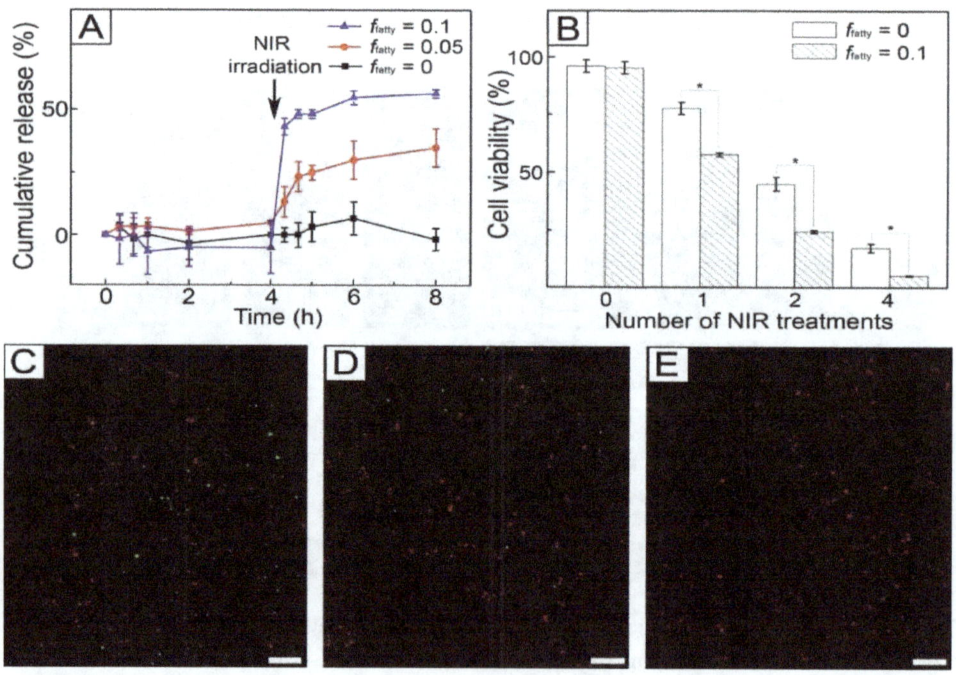

Figure 7. (**A**) Release profiles of DOX from AuNC-loaded fibers containing the fatty acid mixture and the drug. The cumulative release (%) percentage was defined as a ratio of the accumulated amount of released drug at a given time to the initial amount loaded. (**B**) Viability of SK-BR-3 cells treated with AuNC-loaded fibers containing the fatty acid mixture and DOX under different numbers of cycles of 1 W/cm^2 NIR light irradiation. The fibers were made using W/O emulsions of f_{fatty} = 0 and 0.1. * indicates $p < 0.01$. (**C–E**) CLS micrographs showing live (green) and dead (red) SK-BR-3 cells treated with the fibers of f_{fatty} = 0.1 under different numbers of cycles of 1 W/cm^2 NIR light irradiation: (**C**) one, (**D**) two, and (**E**) four cycles. The scale bars are 100 μm.

Figure 7B shows the viability of SK-BR-3 cells treated with the fibers of f_{fatty} = 0 and 0.1 in Figure 7A. When the fibers were not exposed to NIR light, the cell viabilities were above 90%. In the case of FB cells, the similar result was also observed (Figure S4). These results were because the fibers were biocompatible and the drug encapsulated in their core was not released, as indicated by the result of *in vitro* release in Figure 7A. When NIR light was irradiated, the cell viability was reduced for both the systems. However, their anticancer ability was different. The cell viability for the system with f_{fatty} = 0 was similar to that of Figure 5B because the loaded drug molecules were not released

(Figure 7A) and consequently only hyperthermia occurred. In the case of the system with $f_{fatty} = 0.1$, the cell viability decreased to 57% after one cycle of NIR light, which was lower than the value (77%) of the fibers with $f_{fatty} = 0$ with the use of only hyperthermia. This decrease in cell viability was due to the synergistic effect of the drug release and hyperthermia. The effect was much stronger with the increase of the number of cycles of NIR light treatment. Two cycles of NIR irradiation reduced the cell viability to 24%, and four cycles led to a cell viability of 4%. This cell death was also confirmed using a live/dead assay (Figure 7C–E), demonstrating that the majority of the cells were dead after four cycles of the treatment, as shown in Figure 7E.

4. Conclusions

A fibrous system for synergistic cancer therapy was successfully developed using a simple emulsion electrospinning technique. The system consisted of AuNC-incorporated PCL fibers encapsulating an anticancer drug, DOX, in their core and loading a phase-changeable fatty acid in their sheath. The excellent photothermal ability and photostability of AuNCs led to the repeated, significant heating of the fibers in response to on–off switching of NIR light irradiation. When the irradiation increased the temperature of the system to a window suitable for hyperthermia, the death of cancer cells was observed. The NIR light-induced heat generation also simultaneously allowed the release of the drug molecules through the pores in the fibers generated by the melting of the loaded fatty acid. The combination of this NIR light-triggered drug release with the repeated hyperthermia treatment exhibited excellent therapeutic efficacy in an in vitro model. Thus, the fibers have potential in synergistic cancer therapy with a combination of NIR-triggered hyperthermia and chemotherapy.

Author Contributions: G.D.M. and D.C.H. conceived and designed the experiments; J.H.P., H.S., D.I.K., J.H.C., and J.H.S. performed the experiments and analyzed the data; J.B.K. reviewed the data; J.H.P., G.D.M. and D.C.H. wrote the paper.

References

1. Kadam, V.V.; Wang, L.; Padhye, R. Electrospun nanofibre materials to filter air pollutants—A review. *J. Ind. Text.* **2018**, *47*, 2253–2280. [CrossRef]
2. Lu, P.; Qiao, B.; Lu, N.; Hyun, D.C.; Wang, J.; Kim, M.J.; Liu, J.; Xia, Y. Photochemical deposition of highly dispersed Pt nanoparticles on porous CeO_2 nanofibers for the water-gas shift reaction. *Adv. Funct. Mater.* **2015**, *25*, 4153–4162. [CrossRef]
3. Shi, X.; Zhou, W.; Ma, D.; Ma, Q.; Bridges, D.; Ma, Y.; Hu, A. Electrospinning of nanofibers and their applications for energy devices. *J. Nanomater.* **2015**. [CrossRef]
4. Lee, B.S.; Park, B.; Yang, H.S.; Han, J.W.; Choong, C.; Bae, J.; Lee, K.; Yu, W.-R.; Jeong, U.; Park, J.-J.; et al. Effects of substrate on piezoelectricity of electrospun poly(vinylidene fluoride)-nanofiber-based energy generators. *ACS Appl. Mater. Interfaces* **2014**, *6*, 3520–3527. [CrossRef] [PubMed]
5. Park, M.; Im, J.; Park, J.; Jeong, U. Micropatterned stretchable circuit and strain sensor fabricated by lithography on an electrospun nanofiber mat. *ACS Appl. Mater. Interfaces* **2013**, *5*, 8766–8771. [CrossRef] [PubMed]
6. Park, M.; Im, J.; Shin, M.; Min, Y.; Park, J.; Cho, H.; Park, S.; Shim, M.-B.; Jeon, S.; Chung, D.-Y.; et al. Highly stretchable electric circuits from a composite material of silver nanoparticles and elastomeric fibers. *Nat. Nanotechnol.* **2012**, *7*, 803–809. [CrossRef] [PubMed]
7. Braghirolli, D.I.; Steffens, D.; Pranke, P. Electrospinning for regenerative medicine: A review of the main topics. *Drug Discov. Today* **2014**, *19*, 743–753. [CrossRef]
8. Yu, D.G.; Zhu, L.M.; White, K.; Branford-White, C. Electrospun nanofiber-based drug delivery systems. *Health* **2009**, *1*, 67–75. [CrossRef]
9. Chen, M.; Li, Y.F.; Besenbacher, F. Electrospun nanofibers-mediated on-demand drug release. *Adv. Healthc. Mater.* **2014**, *3*, 1721–1732. [CrossRef]

10. Yang, G.; Wang, J.; Wang, Y.; Li, L.; Guo, X.; Zhou, S. Implantable active-targeting micelle-in-nanofiber device for efficient and safe cancer therapy. *ACS Nano* **2015**, *9*, 1161–1174. [CrossRef]
11. Zhang, J.; Wang, X.; Liu, T.; Liu, S.; Jing, X. Antitumor activity of electrospun polylactide nanofibers loaded with 5-fluorouracil and oxaliplatin against colorectal cancer. *Drug Deliv.* **2016**, *23*, 784–790. [CrossRef] [PubMed]
12. Liu, H.; Fu, Y.; Li, Y.; Ren, Z.; Li, X.; Han, G.; Mao, C. A fibrous localized drug delivery platform with NIR-triggered and optically monitored drug release. *Langmuir* **2016**, *32*, 9083–9090. [CrossRef] [PubMed]
13. Tiwari, A.P.; Hwang, T.I.; Oh, J.-M.; Maharjan, B.; Chun, S.; Kim, B.S.; Joshi, M.K.; Park, C.H.; Kim, C.S. pH/NIR-responsive polypyrrole-functionalized fibrous localized drug-delivery platform for synergistic cancer therapy. *ACS Appl. Mater. Interfaces* **2018**, *10*, 20256–20270. [CrossRef] [PubMed]
14. Chen, P.; Wu, Q.S.; Ding, Y.P.; Chu, M.; Huang, Z.M.; Hu, W. A controlled release system of titanocene dichloride by electrospun fiber and its antitumor activity in vitro. *Eur. J. Pharm. Biopharm.* **2010**, *76*, 413–420. [CrossRef] [PubMed]
15. Tran, T.H.; Nguyen, H.T.; Pham, T.T.; Choi, J.Y.; Choi, H.G.; Yong, C.S.; Kim, J.O. Development of a graphene oxide nanocarrier for dual-drug chemo-phototherapy to overcome drug resistance in cancer. *ACS Appl. Mater. Interfaces* **2015**, *7*, 28647–28655. [CrossRef] [PubMed]
16. Cheng, M.; Wang, H.; Zhang, Z.; Li, N.; Fang, X.; Xu, S. Gold nanorod-embedded electrospun fibrous membrane as a photothermal therapy platform. *ACS Appl. Mater. Interfaces* **2014**, *6*, 1569–1575. [CrossRef] [PubMed]
17. Hu, S.H.; Fang, R.H.; Chen, Y.W.; Liao, B.J.; Chen, I.W.; Chen, S.Y. Photoresponsive protein−graphene−protein hybrid capsules with dual targeted heat-triggered drug delivery approach for enhanced tumor therapy. *Adv. Funct. Mater.* **2014**, *24*, 4144–4155. [CrossRef]
18. Jian, W.H.; Yu, T.W.; Chen, C.J.; Huang, W.C.; Chiu, H.C.; Chiang, W.H. Indocyanine green-encapsulated hybrid polymeric nanomicelles for photothermal cancer therapy. *Langmuir* **2015**, *31*, 6202–6210. [CrossRef] [PubMed]
19. Ramanan, V.V.; Hribar, K.C.; Katz, J.S.; Burdick, J.A. Nanofiber–nanorod composites exhibiting light-induced reversible lower critical solution temperature transitions. *Nanotechnology* **2011**, *22*. [CrossRef]
20. Choi, J.H.; Seo, H.; Park, J.H.; Son, J.H.; Kim, D.I.; Kim, J.; Moon, G.D.; Hyun, D.C. Poly(D,L-lactic-co-glycolic acid) (PLGA) hollow fiber with segmental switchability of its chains sensitive to NIR light for synergistic cancer therapy. *Colloids Surf. B* **2019**, *173*, 258–265. [CrossRef]
21. Park, J.H.; Choi, J.H.; Son, J.H.; Hwang, S.J.; Seo, H.; Kang, I.K.; Park, M.; Kim, J.; Hyun, D.C. Poly(ε-caprolactone) (PCL) fibers incorporated with phase-changeable fatty acid and indocyanine green for NIR light-triggered, localized anti-cancer drug release. *Polymer* **2018**, *135*, 211–218. [CrossRef]
22. Park, J.H.; Ahn, H.; Kim, J.; Hyun, D.C. Phase-changeable fatty acid available for temperature-regulated drug release. *Macromol. Mater. Eng.* **2016**, *301*, 887–894. [CrossRef]
23. Skrabalak, S.E.; Au, L.; Li, X.; Xia, Y. Facile synthesis of Ag nanocubes and Au nanocages. *Nat. Protoc.* **2007**, *2*, 2182–2190. [CrossRef] [PubMed]
24. Riley, R.S.; Day, E.S. Gold nanoparticle-mediated photothermal therapy: Applications and opportunities for multimodal cancer treatment. *Wiley Interdiscip. Rev. Nanomed. Nanobiotechnol.* **2017**, *9*, e1449. [CrossRef] [PubMed]
25. Vats, M.; Mishra, S.K.; Baghini, M.S.; Chauhan, D.S.; Srivastava, R.; De, A. Near infrared fluorescence imaging in nano-therapeutics and photo-thermal evaluation. *Int. J. Mol. Sci.* **2017**, *18*, 924. [CrossRef] [PubMed]
26. Sun, T.; Zhang, Y.S.; Pang, B.; Hyun, D.C.; Yang, M.; Xia, Y. Engineered nanoparticles for drug delivery in cancer therapy. *Angew. Chem. Int. Ed.* **2014**, *53*, 12320–12364. [CrossRef] [PubMed]
27. Skrabalak, S.E.; Chen, J.; Sun, Y.; Lu, X.; Au, L.; Cobley, C.M.; Xia, Y. Gold nanocages: Synthesis, properties, and applications. *Acc. Chem. Res.* **2008**, *41*, 1587–1595. [CrossRef]
28. Sun, Y.; Xia, Y. Mechanistic study on the replacement reaction between silver nanostructures and chloroauric acid in aqueous medium. *J. Am. Chem. Soc.* **2004**, *126*, 3892–3901. [CrossRef]
29. Chen, J.; Wang, D.; Xi, J.; Au, L.; Siekkinen, A.; Warsen, A.; Li, W.-Y.; Zhang, H.; Xia, Y.; Li, X. Immuno gold nanocages with tailored optical properties for targeted photothermal destruction of cancer cells. *Nano Lett.* **2007**, *7*, 1318–1322. [CrossRef]

30. Alkilany, A.M.; Bani Yaseen, A.I.; Park, J.; Eller, J.R.; Murphy, C.J. Facile phase transfer of gold nanoparticles from aqueous solution to organic solvents with thiolated poly(ethylene glycol). *RSC Adv.* **2014**, *4*, 52676–52679. [CrossRef]
31. Liu, M.; Law, W.C.; Kopwitthaya, A.; Liu, X.; Swihart, M.T.; Prasad, P.N. Exploring the amphiphilicity of PEGylated gold nanorods: Mechanical phase transfer and self-assembly. *Chem. Commun.* **2013**, *49*, 9350–9352. [CrossRef] [PubMed]
32. Serrano-Montes, A.B.; Jimenez de Aberasturi, D.; Langer, J.; Giner-Casares, J.J.; Scarabelli, L.; Herrero, A.; Liz-Marzán, L.M. A general method for solvent exchange of plasmonic nanoparticles and self-assembly into SERS-active monolayers. *Langmuir* **2015**, *31*, 9205–9213. [CrossRef] [PubMed]
33. Huang, C.; Soenen, S.J.; Rejman, J.; Trekker, J.; Chengxun, L.; Lagae, L.; Ceelen, W.; Wilhelm, C.; Demeester, J.; De Smedt, S.C. Magnetic electrospun fibers for cancer therapy. *Adv. Funct. Mater.* **2012**, *22*, 2479–2486. [CrossRef]

4

Intestinal Drug Absorption Enhancement by *Aloe vera* Gel and Whole Leaf Extract: In Vitro Investigations into the Mechanisms of Action

Anja Haasbroek [1], Clarissa Willers [1], Matthew Glyn [2], Lissinda du Plessis [1] and Josias Hamman [1,*]

[1] Centre of Excellence for Pharmaceutical Sciences (Pharmacen™), Potchefstroom Campus, North West University, Potchefstroom 2520, South Africa; 22692592@nwu.ac.za or anjahaasbroek11@gmail.com (A.H.); 20672322@nwu.ac.za (C.W.); Lissinda.duPlessis@nwu.ac.za (L.d.P.)

[2] Preclinical Drug Development Platform (PCDDP), Potchefstroom Campus, North West University, Potchefstroom 2520, South Africa; mglynmglyn@live.co.uk

* Correspondence: sias.hamman@nwu.ac.za

Abstract: The co-administration of absorption enhancing agents with macromolecular drugs (e.g., protein and peptide drugs) has been identified as a means to improve the oral bioavailability of these drugs. Absorption-enhancing agents of natural origins have received a great deal of attention due to their sustainable production, in support of green chemistry. In previous studies, certain parts of the *Aloe vera* leaf (e.g., gel and whole leaf extract) have shown a potential to enhance drug permeation across the intestinal epithelial barrier. The mechanism of the drug-absorption-enhancement action and the capacity for absorption-enhancement of the *A. vera* gel and whole leaf, were investigated in this study. A clear decrease in transepithelial electrical resistance (TEER) of Caco-2 cell monolayers exposed to *A. vera* gel and wholeleaf extract, in various concentrations, indicated the opening of tight junctions between the epithelial cells. The transport of Fluorescein isothiocyanate (FITC)-dextran, with a molecular weight of 4 kDa (FD-4), could be enhanced across the Caco-2 cell monolayers, by the *A. vera* gel and whole-leaf extract, but not the FITC-dextran with larger molecular weights (i.e., 10, 20, and 40 kDa), which indicated a limited drug absorption enhancement capacity, in terms of the molecular size. Accumulation of FD-4 between the Caco-2 cells (and not within the cells), after treatment with the *A. vera* gel and whole-leaf extract was shown with a confocal laser scanning microscopy (CLSM) imaging, indicating that the paracellular transport of FD-4 occurred after the interaction of the *A. vera* gel and whole-leaf extract, with the epithelial cell monolayers. Furthermore, changes in the F-actin distribution in the cytoskeleton of the Caco-2 cell monolayers was observed by means of a fluorescence staining, which confirmed tight junction modulation as the mechanism of action for the absorption enhancement effect of the *A. vera* gel and whole-leaf extract.

Keywords: *Aloe vera*; gel; whole leaf; absorption enhancement; Caco-2; confocal laser scanning microscopy; F-actin; FITC-dextran; tight junctions; transepithelial electrical resistance

1. Introduction

The oral route of drug administration is associated with relatively high patient compliance and is more affordable, when compared to the injection therapies [1]. Reasons for a high patient compliance with the oral route of administration, include self-treatment, ease of use, and its non-invasive nature [2]. On the other hand, oral drug administration is challenged by the low bioavailability of certain drugs, such as macromolecular drugs [1]. The general low-membrane permeability and oral bioavailability of large compounds (molecular weight > 500 Da) can be ascribed to their unfavorable physico-chemical properties [3], as well as the harsh gastrointestinal environment where enzymatic and chemical activity cause extensive degradation, especially, of protein and peptide drugs [4].

For an orally administered drug to have its desired pharmacological effect, the drug must reach the systemic circulation via absorption, through the intestinal epithelial layer [5], which can occur via the paracellular or transcellular pathways [6,7]. The paracellular pathway is the transport of drug molecules between epithelial cells and occurs by means of size-limited passive diffusion, through the tight junctions and intercellular spaces. Hydrophilic macromolecules, such as peptide and protein drugs are mainly transported via the paracellular route, since they cannot penetrate cell membranes [7,8], however, their paracellular movement is severely restricted by the tight junctions between the adjacent epithelial cells [9]. A promising approach to improve the oral absorption of these hydrophilic macromolecules is the co-administration of absorption enhancers [7].

Tight junctions (zonula occludens) are one of three intercellular complexes, with adherence junctions (zonula adherens) and desmosomes (macula adherens), which link epithelial cells together. Tight junctions can be described as dynamic multi-protein complex structures consisting of various transmembrane proteins, with the main proteins being occludin, tricellulin, and the claudin family. These proteins are connected to the cell actin cytoskeleton, via the scaffolding protein zonula occludens-1 (ZO-1). Thus, a change in the actin distribution can be linked to a modulation of one or more tight junction proteins [10,11]. The dynamic nature of the tight junction ensures that it can be modulated by different stimuli, resulting in an increased paracellular absorption, in a reversible and potentially safe manner [12]. Tight junction modulation can be experimentally confirmed by transepithelial electrical resistance (TEER) measurements, as well as the permeability of paracellular markers. In addition, microscopic examination after staining of cell components and intercellular accumulation of fluorescent probes, can be used to indicate the opening of tight junctions as a mechanism of paracellular drug-absorption enhancement [13,14].

Oral drug-absorption enhancement of protein and peptide drugs can be defined as the process of improving the movement of the drug molecules across the intestinal epithelium, which can be accomplished by the incorporation of functional excipients, in dosage forms. This improved membrane permeation should be accomplished without damaging the cells or causing toxic effects [15,16]. Absorption enhancers are chemical adjuvants that are co-administered with peptides and proteins, to increase their bioavailability, by reversibly removing or disrupting the intestinal barrier, with minimal tissue damage [17]. The mechanisms through which this can be achieved include decreasing mucus viscosity, changing membrane fluidity, disrupting the structural integrity of the intestinal wall or modulating the tight junctions [17,18].

Many compounds have already been investigated for their potential drug-absorption enhancing abilities, including various chemicals of natural origin that are derived from plants (capsaicin, piperine, quercetin, and *Aloe vera*) and from animals (chitosan and zonula occludens toxin). Different mechanisms of absorption enhancement have been suggested for these chemical absorption-enhancing agents, such as regulation of gastrointestinal function, enzyme inhibition, P-gp efflux inhibition, mucoadhesion, and tight junction modulation [12,19–24].

Aloe vera is a succulent perennial xerophyte that displays the water-storage mechanisms in leaves, such as the formation of a viscous mucilage to survive in arid regions with little or irregular rainfall [25,26]. The innermost part of the leaf is made up of clear, moist, soft, and slippery tissue that consists of thin-walled parenchyma cells [27]. As a result, the thick fleshy leaves contain amongst other compounds, storage carbohydrates, such as acetylated mannan (acemannan or aloverose) and cell wall carbohydrates, such as cellulose and hemicellulose [28].

Aloe vera has long been used in traditional medicine, where the latex has been used for its laxative effects and the gel was mainly used for the treatment of wounds and skin ailments, such as psoriasis and genital herpes [29]. Other uses that have also been ascribed to *A. vera* components include anti-bacterial, anti-cancer, anti-diabetic, anti-fungal, anti-obesity, anti-viral effects, and gastric protection against ulcers [25,29,30].

A study was conducted to evaluate the effect of *A. vera* liquid preparations on the absorption of vitamin C and E, in human subjects, and it was found that *A. vera* markedly improved the oral bioavailability of both these vitamins [31]. It was shown in an in vitro study that the *A. vera* gel and whole-leaf extract had the ability to markedly enhance the transport of insulin across the Caco-2 cell monolayers [32]. Thereafter, several in vitro studies were conducted on the effect of the *A. vera* gel and whole-leaf extract on macromolecular and other hydrophilic compounds, across intestinal epithelial cell monolayers, excised intestinal tissues [32–35], excised skin [36,37], and across excised buccal mucosa [38]. The P-gp-modulating effects of the *A. vera* juice was investigated by Djuv and Nilsen [39], but they found that the *A. vera* juice did not inhibit the P-gp mediated transport of digoxin, in a statistically significant way in any of the concentrations that were tested.

The aim of this study was to identify the mechanism of action by which the *A. vera* gel and the whole leaf extract, enhance the gastrointestinal absorption of macromolecules, as well as to establish the capacity of these materials in terms of the size of the molecules, which can be moved across the intestinal epithelium. This was done by determining the transport of the FITC-dextran with different molecular weights across the Caco-2 cell monolayers, after treatment with the *A. vera* gel and whole-leaf extract, by TEER studies, by visualization of the accumulation of the FITC-dextran (4 kDa) between the Caco-2 cells, on the monolayers grown on membrane inserts, and by fluorescence staining and visualization of the F-actin structure of the Caco-2 cells, after incubation with the *A. vera* gel and the whole-leaf extract.

2. Materials and Methods

2.1. Materials

Dehydrated *Aloe vera* gel powder 200X (Dalton Max 700® gel) and whole leaf, decolourised, spray-dried *Aloe vera* powder 100X (whole-leaf extract) were kindly donated by Improve USA. Inc. (De Soto, TX, USA). Chitosan (ChitoClear® with a degree of deacetylation of 96% and viscosity of 8 cP for a 1% solution) was purchased from Primex (Siglufjordur, Iceland). Fluorescein isothiocyanate (FITC)-dextran with molecular weight (MW) of 4 kDa (FD-4), 10 kDa (FD-10), 20 kDa (FD-20), and 40 kDa (FD-40), as well as Lucifer Yellow, were purchased from Sigma-Aldrich/Merck (Darmstadt, Germany). CytoPainter® Phalloidin iFluor 488 and Fluoroshield® mounting medium, with propidium iodide, were purchased from Abcam (Cambridge, MA, USA).

2.2. Chemical Characterisation of the A. vera Gel and the Whole-Leaf Extract

Quantitative proton nuclear magnetic resonance (^{1}H-NMR) analysis was used to chemically characterise the *A. vera* gel and the whole-leaf extract, by determining the content of certain marker molecules, including aloverose, glucose, malic acid, and iso-citric acid (whole-leaf marker), as previously described [40].

2.3. Chemical Characterisation of N-Trimethyl Chitosan Chloride

N-trimethyl chitosan chloride (TMC) was synthesised from chitosan (ChitoClear®, degree of deacetylation of 96% and viscosity of 8 cP, for a 1% solution), as previously described [41], and characterized by the means of ^{1}H-NMR spectroscopy, using an Avance III 600 Hz NMR spectrometer (Bruker BioSpin Corporation, Rheinstetlen, Germany). A sample of the TMC (100 mg) was dissolved in 2 mL D_2O and analyzed in the NMR spectrometer, at 80 °C, with a suppression of the water peak. The degree of quaternization of the TMC was calculated from the ^{1}H-NMR spectra, by using Equation (1), as previously described [42]:

$$DQ\ (\%) = \left[\left(\frac{\int TM}{\int H}\right) \times \frac{1}{9}\right] \times 100 \quad (1)$$

where DQ (%) is the percentage of the degree of quaternization, $\int$TM is the integral of the trimethyl amino group (quaternary amino) peak at 3.7–4.0 ppm, on the ^{1}H-NMR spectra, and $\int$H is the integral of the ^{1}H peaks from 4.7–6.2 ppm, on the ^{1}H-NMR spectra.

2.4. Caco-2 Cell Culturing

The Caco-2 cells were procured from the European Collection of Authenticated Cell Cultures (ECACC). Caco-2 cells were cultured in a growth medium that consisted of high-glucose Dulbecco's Modified Eagles Medium (DMEM), supplemented with 10% *v*/*v* fetal bovine serum (FBS), 1% *v*/*v* non-essential amino-acid solution (NEAA), 1% *v*/*v* penicillin/streptomycin (10,000 U/mL penicillin and 10,000 U/mL streptomycin), 1% *v*/*v* amphotericin B (250 μg/mL), and 2 mM L-glutamine. The cells were incubated at 37 °C and exposed to 95% humidified air and 5% CO_2. The Caco-2 cells were used between passages 51–56.

2.5. Cell Monolayer Integrity

The integrity of the cell monolayers was confirmed by measuring the TEER, as well as determining the permeation of the exclusion marker, Lucifer yellow [43,44].

Prior to each permeation experiment, the TEER of the Caco-2 cell monolayers was measured to confirm the formation of a confluent cell monolayer on the insert membrane. The minimum TEER values, as indicated in Table 1, were required and considered as indicative of the presence of intact cell monolayers, in the different Transwell® plates (Corning Costar®, Corning, NY, USA) [45–47].

Table 1. Required transepithelial electrical resistance (TEER) values, as indicative of the intact Caco-2 cell monolayers, on different Transwell®plate insert membranes.

Type of Transwell® Plate	TEER Value Measured (Ω)	TEER Value Normalized for Surface Area (Ω·cm^2)
Transwell® 6-well plates (surface area = 4.67 cm^2) [45]	150	700.5
Transwell® 24-well plates (surface area = 0.33 cm^2) [46]	750	247.5
Snapwell® 6-well plates (surface area = 1.12 cm^2) [47]	179	200.0

Lucifer yellow was used as an exclusion transport marker molecule, to confirm the formation of confluent Caco-2 cell monolayers on the inserts of each Transwell® plate. The growth medium was aspirated from the basolateral chambers of the 6-well Transwell® plate and replaced with the appropriate volume of pre-heated serum-free DMEM, buffered with *N*-(2-hydroxyethyl) piperazine-*N*-(2-ethanesulfonic acid) (HEPES) (pH = 7.4), and incubated for 30 min, at 37 °C. After 30 min, the Transwell® plates were removed from the incubator, the growth medium was aspirated from the apical chambers and replaced with an appropriate volume of a pre-heated Lucifer yellow solution (i.e., 50 μg/mL in serum-free DMEM) [44]. The Transwell® plates were incubated with the Lucifer yellow solution and samples (200 μL) were withdrawn from the basolateral chamber, every 20 min, for 120 min, and replaced with equal volumes of pre-heated serum-free DMEM buffered with HEPES. The Lucifer yellow concentration in the samples was quantified by means of fluorescence spectroscopy, at excitation, and at emission wavelengths of 485 nm and 535 nm, respectively [48]. The percentage transport of Lucifer yellow across the Caco-2 cell monolayer should be less than 2% for the two-hour transport period, to indicate intact cell monolayers [48]. Furthermore, apparent permeability coefficient (P_{app}) values of the Lucifer yellow $\leq 0.2 \times 10^{-6}$ cm/s [43] or 0.66–0.75 $\times 10^{-6}$ cm/s [44], were considered indicative of the formation of intact Caco-2 cell monolayers.

2.6. *In Vitro Transepithelial Electrical Resistance (TEER) Study*

Caco-2 cells were cultured in Transwell® 24-well plates (Corning Costar®) on insert membranes, with a surface area of 0.33 cm^2 and pore size of 0.4 μm, to form confluent monolayers. The positive control consisted of 0.5% *w/v* TMC (a known tight junction modulator), while the test solutions consisted of *A. vera* gel and whole-leaf extract, each in four different concentrations ranging from 0.1 % *w/v* to 1.5% *w/v*. Serum-free DMEM alone was used as the negative control.

The TEER measurements of the Caco-2 cell monolayers on insert membranes in 24-well Transwell® plates commenced one hour prior to addition of the test solutions, to obtain the TEER values, at a baseline level. DMEM buffered with HEPES (pH = 7.4) (1 mL) was added to the basolateral chamber and incubated for 30 min, prior to the addition of the test solutions (200 μL) to the apical chamber on top of the cell monolayers, on the filter membranes. The TEER (T_0) was measured directly, after application of the test solutions to the apical chamber. TEER measurements were then taken at 20 min intervals up to 120 min, after addition of test solutions. TEER was measured with a Millicell ERS meter (Millipore, Billerica, MA, USA) that was connected to a set of chopstick electrodes.

2.7. *In Vitro Permeation Studies*

Caco-2 cells were cultured in Transwell® 6-well plates (Corning Costar®) on insert membranes, with a surface area of 4.67 cm^2 and a pore size of 0.4 μm, to form confluent monolayers. For the in vitro permeation study, four different FITC-dextran (i.e., FD-4, FD-10, FD-20 and FD-40) solutions were prepared, each in a concentration of 125 μg/mL, in serum-free DMEM. Four different concentrations of each of the *A. vera* gel and whole leaf extract (ranging from 0.1 % *w/v* to 1.5% *w/v*) were added to each of the FITC-dextran solutions, to prepare the experimental solutions. Control groups consisted of each FITC-dextran in serum-free DMEM, without *A. vera* gel and the whole-leaf extract.

The in vitro permeation of each of the FITC-dextran molecules, in the absence and presence of the different *A. vera* gel and the whole-leaf extract solutions, was determined in the apical to basolateral (AP-BL, absorptive) direction, across the Caco-2 cell monolayers. First, the growth medium was aspirated from the basolateral chamber and replaced with 2.5 mL pre-heated serum-free DMEM buffered with HEPES (pH = 7.4) and placed back in the incubator (37 °C), to equilibrate for 30 min. After 30 min, the Transwell® plates were removed from the incubator and the growth medium from the apical chamber was aspirated and replaced with 2.5 mL of each of the experimental solutions pre-heated to 37 °C. Samples (200 μL) were extracted from the basolateral chamber at 20 min intervals for a total period of 120 min and replaced with 200 μL pre-heated DMEM buffered with HEPES. The quantification of the FITC-dextran concentrations, in the samples, was done by means of fluorescence spectroscopy, at excitation and at emission wavelengths of 494 and 518 nm, respectively.

The percentage transport was calculated from the concentration of each FITC-dextran (i.e., FD-4, FD-10, FD-20, and FD-40) measured in the samples withdrawn from the basolateral chamber, at each time interval. The percentage transport was calculated with the following equation:

$$\%\text{Transport} = \frac{\text{Drug concentration at specific time interval}}{\text{Initial FITC} - \text{dextran dose}} \times 100 \tag{2}$$

The apparent permeability coefficient (P_{app}) values were calculated from the percentage transport data across the Caco-2 cell monolayers, for each of the FITC-dextran molecules. P_{app} is defined as the permeability rate that is normalized by the surface area, across which the permeation occurs, as well as the concentration, assuming the starting concentration in the acceptor (basolateral) chamber is zero [49]. The P_{app} was calculated by using the following equation [50,51]:

$$P_{app} = {}^{dc}/{}_{dt} \frac{1}{(A \cdot 60 \cdot C_0)}, \tag{3}$$

where P_{app} is the apparent permeability coefficient ($cm \cdot s^{-1}$), (dc/dt) represents the permeability rate (concentration/min, represented by the slope of the transport curve), A is the permeation surface area (cm^2), and C_0 is the starting concentration of the permeant.

From the P_{app} values, the permeation-enhancement ratio (R) values were calculated by the following equation [32]:

$$R = \frac{P_{app}\ \text{experiment}}{P_{app}\ \text{control}} \quad (4)$$

where R is the permeation-enhancement ratio, P_{app} experiment is the apparent permeability coefficient for the test solution, and P_{app} control is the apparent permeability coefficient for the control group.

2.8. Caco-2 Cell Monolayers for the Confocal Laser Scanning Microscopy (CLSM) Study

For the CLSM visualisation studies (for both the transport pathway and the F-actin filament studies), the Caco-2 cells were cultured in Snapwell® 6-well plates (Corning Costar®), with removable filter-rings, which had a surface area of 1.12 cm^2 and a pore size of 0.4 μm, to form confluent cell monolayers. Stock solutions of the FITC-dextran 4 kDa (FD-4, 1 mg/mL), the *A. vera* gel, the *A. vera* whole-leaf extract (2.0% *w*/*v*), and TMC (1.0% *w*/*v*), were each prepared, separately, in a serum-free DMEM. These stock solutions were used to prepare the experimental solutions, which consisted of combinations of the FITC-dextran and each of the permeation enhancers solutions (i.e., *A. vera* gel, *A. vera* whole leaf, and TMC) in a 1:1 ratio that were applied to the Caco-2 cell monolayers. The final concentrations of the test solutions were, therefore, 1.0% *w*/*v A. vera* gel, 1.0% *w*/*v A. vera* whole-leaf extract and 0.5% *w*/*v* TMC, while the final concentration of FITC-dextran (FD-4) in the mixture, applied to the cell monolayers, was 0.5 mg/mL. The negative control group consisted of serum-free DMEM, without any of the chemical permeation enhancers.

For the fluorescence staining, a 10× CytoPainter® Phalloidin iFluor 488 solution was prepared by diluting 5 μL of a 1000× phalloidin conjugate in dimethyl sulfoxide (DMSO) stock solution with 500 μL PBS, containing 1.1% *v*/*v* foetal bovine serum (FBS). The 0.1% *v*/*v* Triton X100 solution was prepared by diluting 3 μL of the 100× Triton X-100 solution to 300 μL with phosphate buffer saline (PBS).

2.8.1. Fluorescence Staining

Visualisation of the Transport Pathway

After 21 days of culturing, in the Snapwell® 6-well plates, and confirmation of the cell monolayer formation, the cell monolayers were incubated with the above-mentioned experimental solutions for 2 h at 37°C, 5% CO_2, and 95% air (i.e., the same conditions as for the in vitro permeation study).

After the 2 h incubation period, the cells were fixed with 4% formaldehyde for 10 min [52,53] and gently rinsed, once, with ice-cold PBS [54]. After fixation, the cell monolayers were prepared on the microscope slides, as described below in Section 2.8.2, and confocal images were taken with a Nikon Eclipse TE-3000 inverted microscope (Nikon Instruments, Melville, NY, USA), equipped with 60× and 100× ApoPlanar oil immersion objectives and a DSRi1 Nikon digital camera, for real-time imaging. The microscope was linked to a Nikon D-Eclipse C1 confocal system. The images were taken at room temperature, under light exclusion. All experiments were done in triplicates.

Visualization of the F-Actin Filaments in the Cytoskeleton

Staining of the F-actin in the cytoskeleton of the Caco-2 cells was used to identify if opening of tight junctions was the mechanism of action of the *A. vera* gel and the whole-leaf extract, in terms of drug-absorption enhancement [55,56]. The cell monolayers in the Snapwell® 6-well plates were incubated with the experimental permeation enhancer solutions (*A. vera* gel and whole-leaf extract without FD-4) for 2 h, at 37 °C, 5% CO_2, and 95% air. The cell monolayers were then fixed with 4% formaldehyde, for 10 min, and gently rinsed, once, with ice-cold PBS. Fixation was followed by permeabilization (to increase the accessibility of the F-actin to the CytoPainter® Phalloidin iFluor probe) with 0.1% Triton X-100 for, 3 min, after which the cell monolayers were gently rinsed with PBS. Thereafter, F-actin staining was done with 10X CytoPainter® Phalloidin iFluor 488 for 60 min and gently rinsed for 5 min, with PBS. The cell monolayers were prepared on the microscope slides, as described below in Section 2.8.2, and images were taken with CLSM, as described above. All experiments were done in triplicates.

2.8.2. Preparation of the Microscope Slides for the Confocal Laser Scanning Microscopy (CLSM)

The filter-ring was removed from the Snapwell® insert and placed onto a glass plate, to add support before the filter membrane was cut loose with a scalpel. The filter membrane was cut into smaller sections and a section with a size of, approximately, 1.12 cm × 0.3 cm was transferred to a microscope slide. Three to four drops of the Fluoroshield® mounting medium, containing propidium iodide [57], were added and spread-out, evenly. Care was taken not to touch the cell monolayer on the filter membrane. The propidium iodide, contained in the mounting media was used to visualize the cell nuclei. Finally, the excess Fluoroshield® mounting medium was removed by gently touching the slide with a piece of paper towel, and then a coverslip was added.

2.8.3. Imaging with Confocal Laser Scanning Microscopy

The CLSM was equipped with an Argon Ion laser (emission wavelength of 488 nm or 515 nm), a Helium Neon polarised laser (emission wavelength of 543 nm), and a blue Diode laser (emission wavelength of 409 nm). The excitation and emission wavelengths used for the imaging of the FITC-dextran, Phalloidin iFluor, and the propidium iodide are shown in Table 2.

Table 2. Excitation and emission wavelengths of the dyes and transport marker used in the confocal imaging experiments [51,54,57].

Compound	Excitation Wavelength (nm)	Emission Wavelength (nm)
FITC-dextran	494	518
Phalloidin iFluor	493	517
Propidium Iodide	535	615

2.9. Data Analysis

Data analyses on the in vitro permeation results were performed with STATISTICA Version 12 (Statsoft, Tulsa, OK, USA, 2013). All data sets were subjected to the Brown-Forsythe test to establish the normality and homogeneity of the data distribution. Normally distributed data were analyzed by analysis of variance (ANOVA) with Dunnet's post-hoc tests (two-sided). For data sets that were not normally distributed, non-parametric Kruskal-Wallis testing was applied. Statistically significant differences were accepted when $p < 0.05$.

3. Results and Discussion

3.1. Characterisation of the A. vera Gel and the Whole-Leaf Extract

The quantitative ^{1}H-NMR analysis indicated that the *A. vera* gel contained 15.2% aloverose; 9.8% glucose; 2.0% citric acid, and 20.7% malic acid, while the *A. vera* whole-leaf extract contained 4.9% aloverose; 8.6% glucose, 8.9% citric acid, 24.7% malic acid, and 14.6% iso-citric acid, or whole-leaf marker [33].

3.2. Characterization of the N-trimethyl Chitosan (TMC)

The degree of quaternization (DQ) of the TMC was calculated to be 45.995%, from the ^{1}H-NMR spectrum of the TMC (Figure 1), using Equation (1).

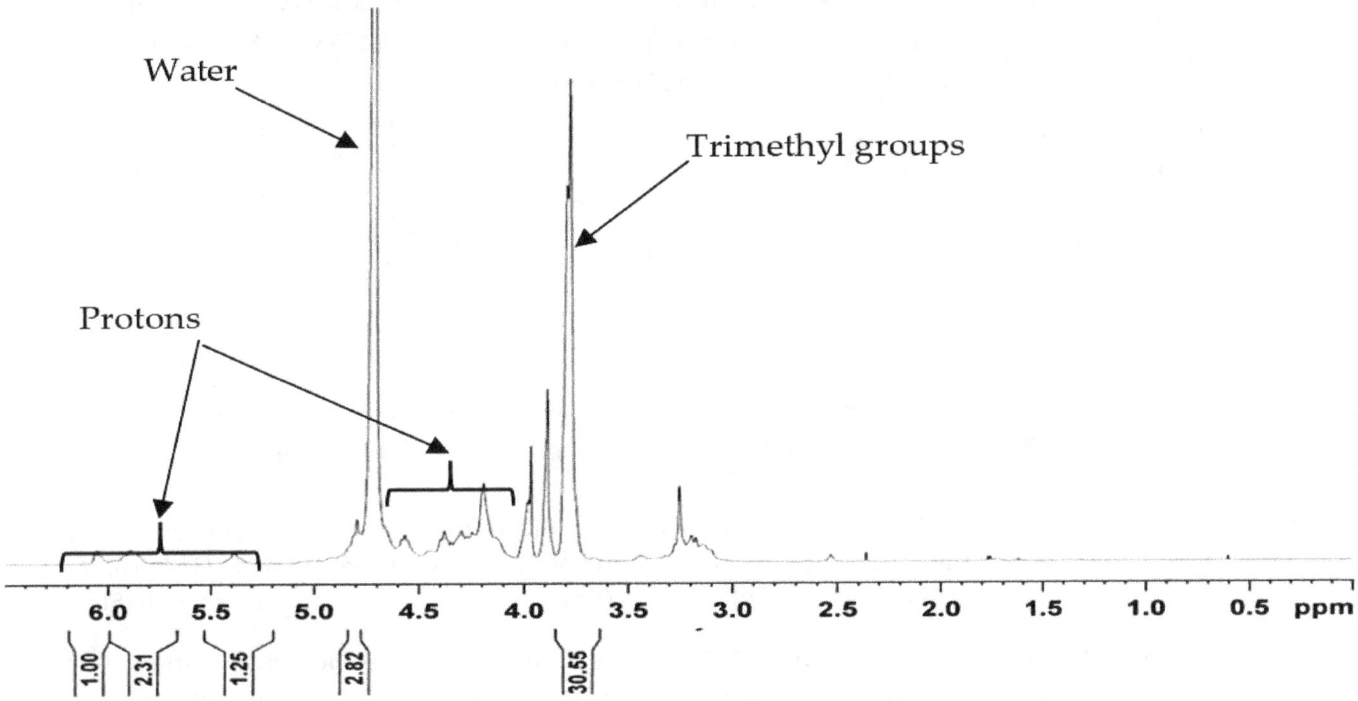

Figure 1. Proton nuclear magnetic resonance (^{1}H-NMR) spectrum for the *N*-trimethyl chitosan chloride (TMC).

3.3. Cell Monolayer Integrity Using Lucifer Yellow

The cumulative percentage transport of Lucifer yellow, across the Caco-2 cell monolayers was below 2%, over a period of 120 min, which indicated an acceptable integrity of the Caco-2 cell monolayers, as suggested by Wahlang et al. [48]. The apparent permeability coefficient (P_{app}) value for the Lucifer yellow was calculated to be 0.346×10^{-6} cm/s, from the transport curve, which was also within the range of the suggested P_{app} values for the Lucifer yellow, when transported across the Caco-2 cell monolayers, with an acceptable integrity, namely $0.2–0.75 \times 10^{-6}$ cm/s [43,44].

3.4. In Vitro Transepithelial Electrical Resistance (TEER) Study

The TEER value of a cell monolayer is indicative of the tight junction integrity and a decrease in TEER has been related to the opening of tight junctions and, therefore, also to an increase in the paracellular permeability [56]. The TEER studies were performed to indicate the capability of the *A. vera* gel and the whole-leaf extract, to open tight junctions. From the results it was clear that maximum TEER reduction was already evident at 20 min, after application of the test solutions, and the TEER started to recover over the 120 min period, towards the initial value. The percentage TEER of the Caco-2 cell monolayers, after application of the test solutions and the positive control (i.e., TMC) plotted as a function of time, are shown in Figure 2, for four different concentrations of the *A. vera* gel, and in Figure 3, for the four different concentrations of the *A. vera* whole-leaf extract.

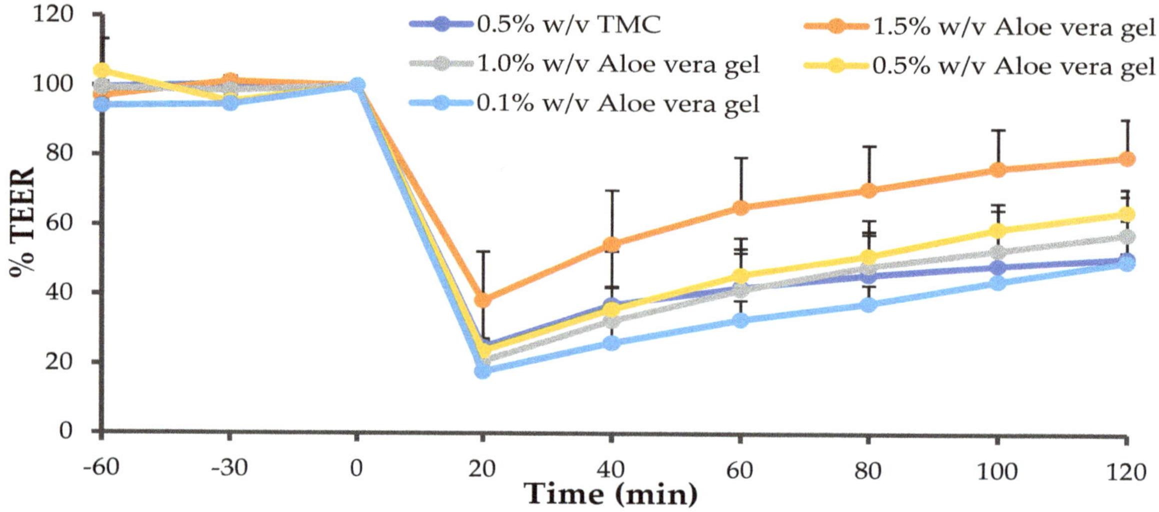

Figure 2. Percentage transepithelial electrical resistance (TEER) of the Caco-2 cell monolayers, after application of the *A. vera* gel, at different concentrations, and *N*-trimethyl chitosan chloride (TMC) (0.5% *w/v*, positive control), plotted as a function of time ($n = 3$) (Error bars represent standard deviation (SD)).

From Figure 2, it is clear that a rapid (within 20 min) and relatively large decrease in the percentage TEER of Caco-2 cell monolayers occurred after the application of the *A. vera* gel solutions, which was similar in extent to that of the positive control (TMC at 0.5% *w/v*), except for the 1.5% *w/v* *A. vera* gel solution, which exhibited a lower TEER reduction effect. The decrease in TEER caused by the *A. vera* gel on the Caco-2 cell monolayers was inversely proportional to the concentration applied. This could probably be explained by the increase in the viscosity of the *A. vera* gel solutions, with each concentration increase, which may have decreased the diffusion of ions across the Caco-2 cell monolayers.

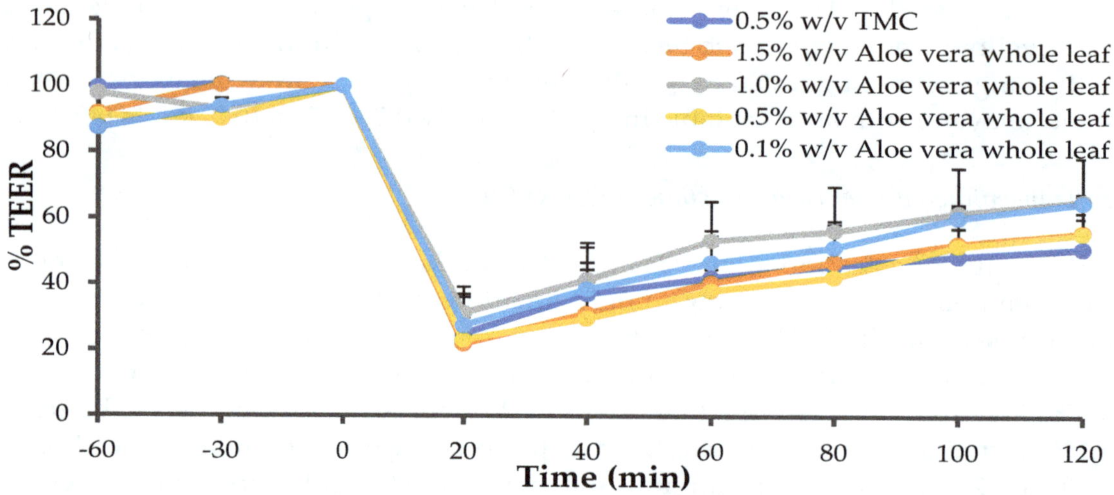

Figure 3. Percentage TEER of the Caco-2 cell monolayers after the application of the *A. vera* whole leaf, at different concentrations, and TMC (0.5% *w/v*, positive control) plotted as a function of time ($n = 3$) (Error bars represent SD).

From Figure 3, it is evident that the *A. vera* whole-leaf extract solutions caused a rapid and relatively large decrease in the TEER of the Caco-2 cell monolayers, which started to recover towards the initial value, over the period of 120 min. Furthermore, the decrease in TEER caused by some of the *A. vera* whole-leaf extract solutions, was larger than that of the positive control (0.5% *w/v* TMC). However, the reduction in TEER did not correlate, directly or inversely, with the concentration of the *A. vera* whole-leaf extract solutions.

Nonetheless, the TEER reduction results are in line with previous studies on the application of the *A. vera* gel and whole leaf extract on epithelial surfaces [32,33,35]. The TEER results indicated that the *A. vera* gel and whole-leaf extract were capable of opening tight junctions between the Caco-2 cells.

3.5. In Vitro Permeation Studies

The *A. vera* gel and whole-leaf extract showed the ability to enhance the transport of the FITC-dextran with a molecular weight of 4 kDa, across the Caco-2 cell monolayers, however, no transport could be detected for the FITC-dextran molecules, with molecular weights of 10 kDa (FD-10), 20 kDa (FD-20), and 40 kDa (FD-40), in the absence or presence of the *A. vera* gel and whole-leaf extract solutions, across the Caco-2 cell monolayers.

The transport curves and apparent permeability coefficient (P_{app}) values of the FD-4, across the Caco-2 cell monolayers, in the absence and presence of four different concentrations of the *A. vera* gel and whole-leaf extract, respectively, are shown in Figures 4–7.

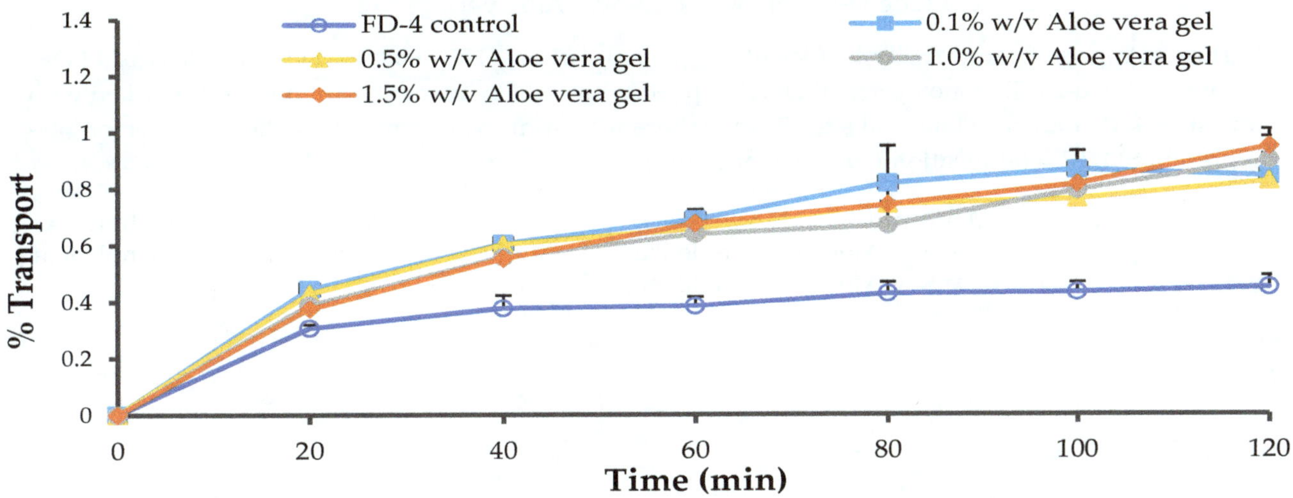

Figure 4. Percentage transport of the Fluorescein isothiocyanate (FITC)-dextran (FD) (FD-4 with MW of 4 kDa) plotted as a function of time, across the Caco-2 cell monolayers, in the absence (FD-4 control) and presence of the *Aloe vera* gel solutions, with different concentrations ($n = 3$; error bars represent SD).

From Figure 4, a clear increase in the percentage transport of FD-4, in relation to the negative control (FD-4 alone), can be seen for all concentrations of the *A. vera* gel solutions that were applied to the Caco-2 cell monolayers, with the FD-4. The transport of the FD-4, alone, showed an initial increase until 20 min, whereafter it reached a plateau, over the rest of the 120 min transport period. While in the presence of the *A. vera* gel it continued to be transported, albeit at a slower rate than the first 20 min.

A slightly higher than the two-fold increase in the transport of the FD-4 (R or permeation-enhancement ratio values indicated on Figure 5) in relation to the control group (FD-4 alone) was shown for all the concentrations of the *A. vera* gel solutions tested. The transport of the FD-4 was, statistically, significantly higher ($p < 0.05$) in the presence of all the *A. vera* gel solutions, compared to the transport of the control group (FD-4 alone). *A. vera* gel, therefore, showed the ability to significantly enhance the transport of a macromolecule (FD-4), across intestinal epithelial cell monolayers (Caco-2), which is in line with previous findings [32–34].

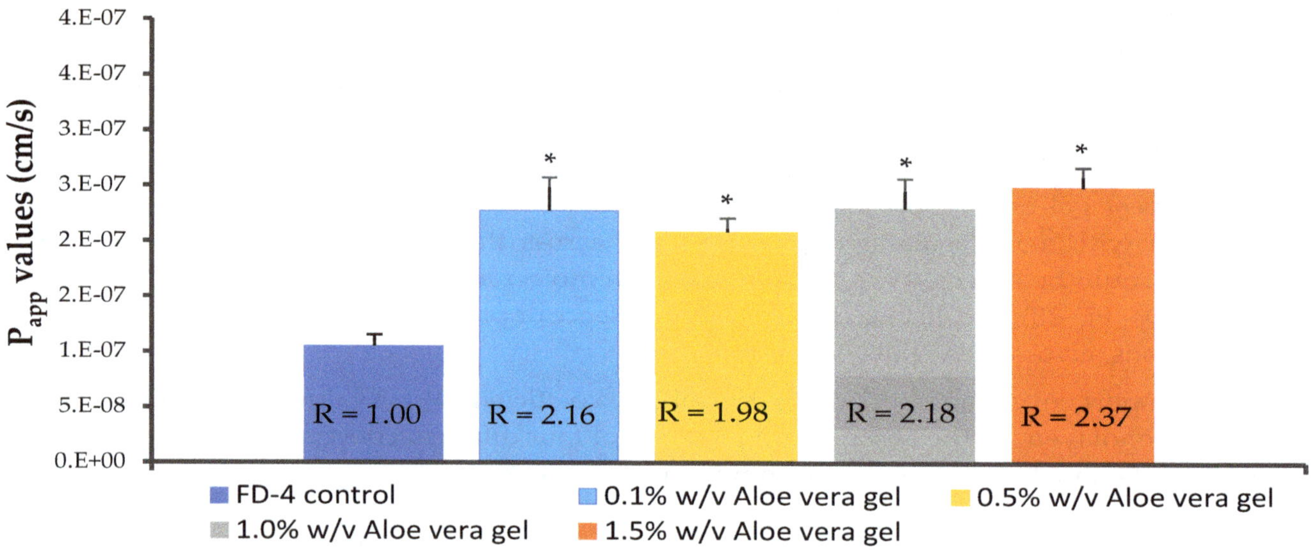

Figure 5. Apparent permeability coefficient (P_{app}) values of the FITC-dextran (FD-4 with MW of 4 kDa), across the Caco-2 cell monolayers, when co-applied with the *Aloe vera* gel solutions. Bars marked with an asterisk (*) indicate statistical significant differences from the control ($p < 0.05$) ($n = 3$; error bars represent SD) (R = permeation-enhancement ratio).

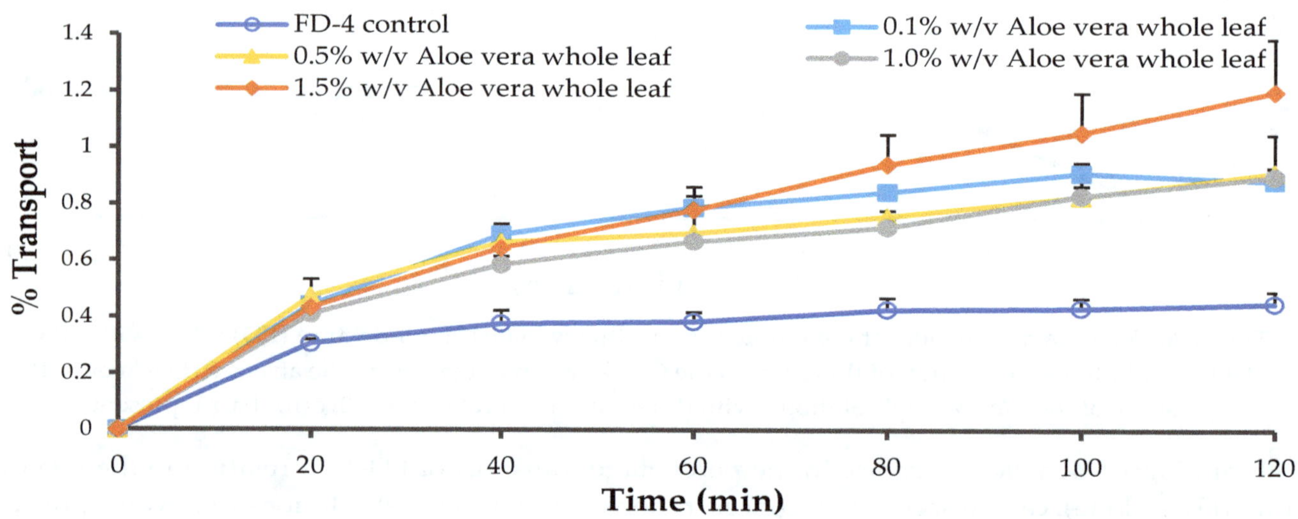

Figure 6. Percentage transport of the FITC-dextran (FD-4 with MW of 4 kDa) plotted as a function of time, across the Caco-2 cell monolayers, in the absence (FD-4 control) and presence of the *Aloe vera* whole-leaf extract solutions, with different concentrations ($n = 3$; error bars represent SD).

From Figure 6, a distinct increase in the FD-4 transport across the Caco-2 cell monolayers can be seen for all the concentrations of the *A. vera* whole-leaf extract solutions, when compared to the negative control group (FD-4 alone). The transport of the FD-4 alone (negative control) reached a plateau after 20 min, and only slightly increased, further, over the remainder of the transport period (120 min); while in the presence of the *A. vera* whole-leaf extract, it continued to be transported.

The transport of the FD-4 in the presence of all concentrations of the *A. vera* whole-leaf extract solutions, were significantly higher (Figure 7) than that of the control group (FD-4 alone) ($p < 0.05$). *A. vera* whole-leaf extract has, therefore, shown the ability to significantly enhance the transport of a macromolecular model compound (FD-4), across the intestinal epithelial cell monolayers (Caco-2), which is in line with previous findings [32–34]. The absorption-enhancing effect of the *A. vera* whole-leaf extract was in agreement with the TEER reduction results and can, therefore, most probably be attributed to its tight junction-modulating activities.

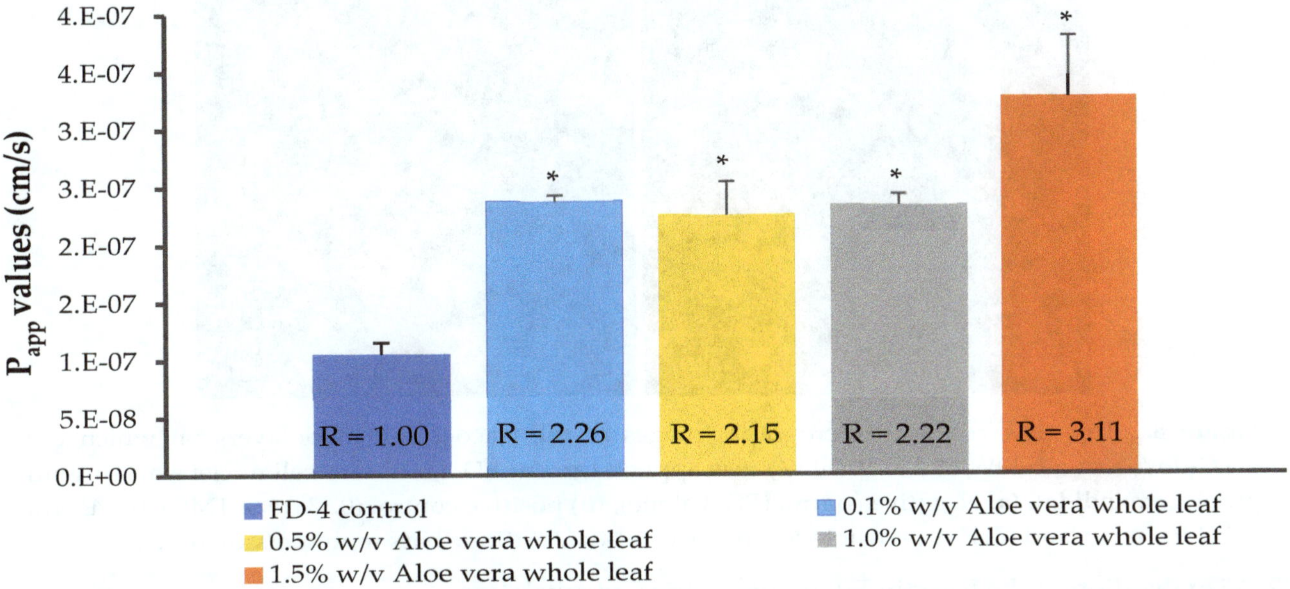

Figure 7. Apparent permeability coefficient (P_{app}) values of the FITC-dextran (FD-4 with MW of 4 kDa) across the Caco-2 cell monolayers, when co-applied with the *Aloe vera* whole-leaf extract solutions. Bars marked with an asterisk (*) indicate statistically significant differences from the negative control group ($p < 0.05$) ($n = 3$; error bars represent SD) (R = permeation-enhancement ratio).

3.6. Confocal Laser Scanning Microscopy (CLSM)

3.6.1. Visualization of the Transport Pathway

Figure 8 shows the top-view confocal micrograph images of the Caco-2 cell monolayers to which the FD-4 was applied, in the absence (negative control) and presence of the *A. vera* gel and whole-leaf extract, as well as TMC (positive control).

From the confocal micrograph images in Figure 8, the intercellular accumulation of FD-4 (green) between the Caco-2 cells can be observed, when it was applied with the absorption enhancers (Figure 8b–d), compared to no accumulation in the negative control (Figure 8a). This accumulation in the intercellular spaces between the cells indicated a movement of the FD-4 molecules, via the paracellular pathway. The CLSM image of the positive control (0.5% *w*/*v* TMC, a known tight junction modulator and paracellular absorption enhancer) is in accordance to previously published papers [58,59]. The lack of green fluorescence inside the cells, confirmed that the incubation with TMC, the *A. vera* gel, and *A. vera* whole-leaf extract, did not damage the cell membranes. The paracellular accumulation of the FD-4, in the presence of the *A. vera* gel and the whole-leaf extract, corresponded with the TEER reduction results and is most probably the result of their ability to modulate tight junctions.

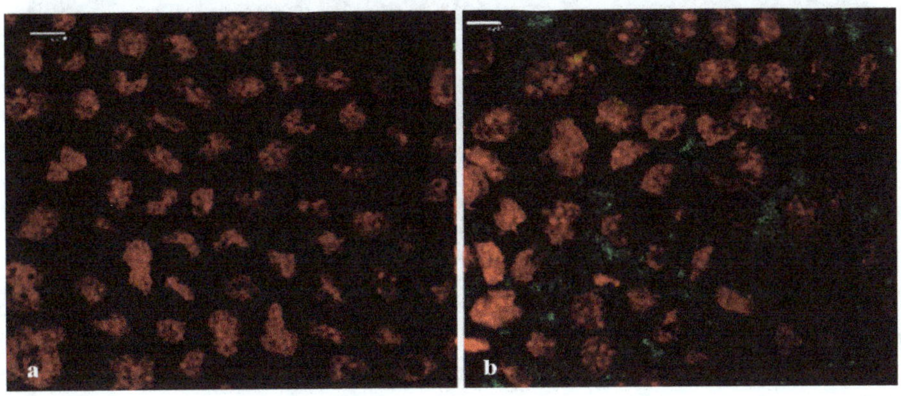

Figure 8. *Cont.*

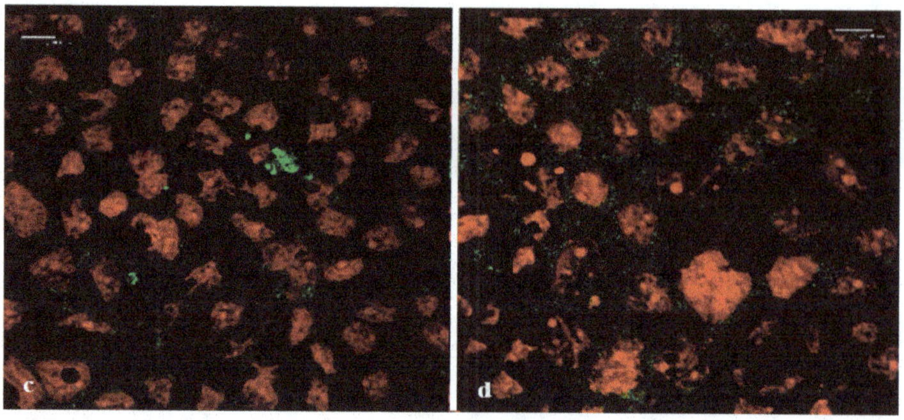

Figure 8. Top-view confocal micrograph images of the Caco-2 cell monolayers on which the FITC-dextran with MW of 4 kDa (FD-4) was applied (**green**: FD-4 and **red**: cell nuclei stained with propidium iodide). (**a**) Negative control (FD-4 alone), (**b**) positive control (0.5% *w*/*v* TMC), (**c**) *A. vera* gel (1.0% *w*/*v*), and (**d**) *A. vera* whole-leaf extract (1.0% *w*/*v*) (Scale bars represents 10 μm).

3.6.2. Visualization of the F-Actin Filaments in the Cytoskeleton

According to Ward et al. [11], disruption of the actin cytoskeleton through modulation of the F-actin structure can cause opening of the tight junctions and an increase in paracellular permeability. The re-arrangement of filamentous actin (F-actin) in the cytoskeleton of the Caco-2 cells was visualized, in order to determine the possible mechanism of action by which the *A. vera* gel and the whole-leaf extract increase the paracellular absorption. The CLSM images in Figure 9 show the F-actin expression in a Caco-2 cell monolayer, after incubation with the TMC (positive control), *A. vera* gel, and whole-leaf extract, and without an absorption enhancer (negative control).

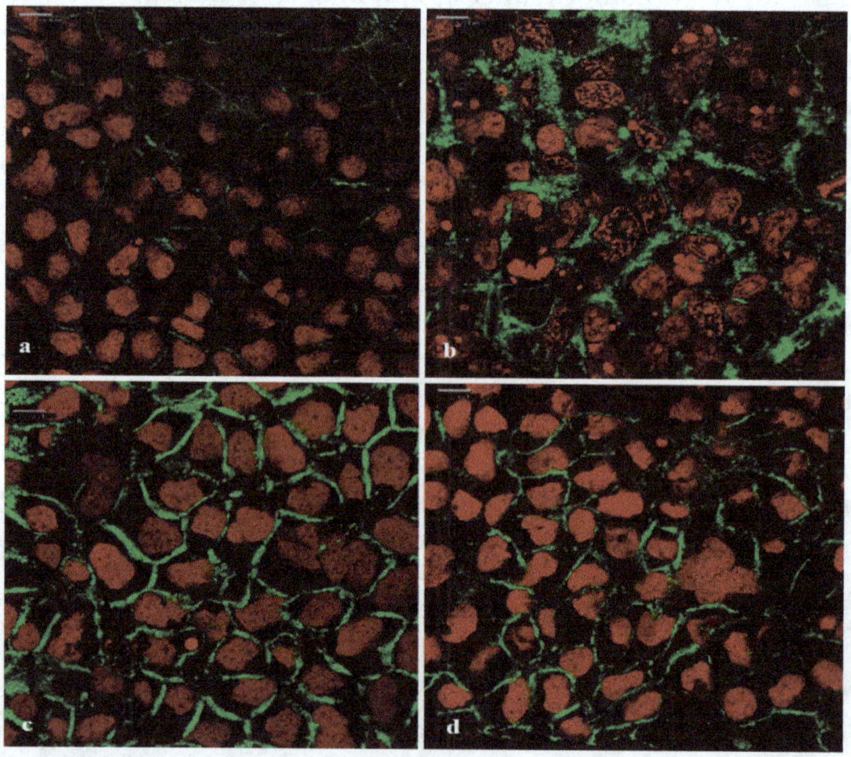

Figure 9. Confocal micrograph images of the filamentous actin (F-actin) distribution in the Caco-2 cell monolayers (**green**: F-actin stained with CytoPainter® Phalloidin iFluor 488 and **red**: cell nuclei stained with propidium iodide). (**a**) Negative control (untreated Caco-2 cell monolayer), (**b**) positive control (0.5% *w*/*v* TMC), (**c**) 1.0% *w*/*v A. vera* gel, and (**d**) 1.0% *w*/*v A. vera* whole-leaf extract (Scale bars represent 10 μm).

In the confocal micrograph images shown in Figure 9, the differences can be seen in the appearance of the F-actin when the Caco-2 cells were treated with *A. vera* gel, *A. vera* whole-leaf extract, and TMC (positive control), as compared to the negative control (untreated cells). The untreated Caco-2 cell monolayer (negative control) showed very little and irregular fluorescence (green) distribution of the F-actin, along the cell borders. In contrast to this, the F-actin fluorescence localization (green) in all the other images was visibly different (Figure 9b–d), which indicates that the F-actin distribution was re-arranged. The rearranged F-actin fluorescence pattern, seen in Figure 9b, is in congruence with previously published research on the effect of TMC (a known tight junction modulator) on the actin cytoskeleton of the Caco-2 cells [56]. The changed fluorescence patterns of the F-actin seen in the Caco-2 cells that were treated with *A. vera* gel (Figure 9c) and the *A. vera* whole-leaf extract (Figure 9d), were similar to that of the TMC. The changed F-actin distribution, therefore, indicates that tight junction modulation occurred in the presence of *A. vera* gel and *A. vera* whole-leaf extract.

4. Conclusions

Tight junction modulation by the *A. vera* gel and *A. vera* whole-leaf extract has previously been suggested, by Chen et al. [32], as a possible mechanism of its action for drug-absorption enhancement. The results obtained from this study confirmed tight junction modulation by the *A. vera* gel and *A. vera* whole-leaf extract, by means of different tests, including TEER reduction, transport enhancement of the FD-4, accumulation of FD-4 between the epithelial cells (i.e., in the intercellular spaces), and F-actin disruption, as determined with confocal laser scanning microscopy.

Author Contributions: Conceptualization, J.H. and L.d.P.; Methodology, A.H., C.W., J.H., and M.G.; Validation, A.H. and C.W.; Investigation, A.H., C.W., and M.G.; Supervision, J.H. and L.d.P.; Writing-Original Draft Preparation, A.H.; Writing-Review & Editing, C.W., M.G., L.d.P., and J.H.; Visualization, A.H. and M.G.; Funding Acquisition, J.H.

Acknowledgments: Thank you to Improve USA Inc. (De Soto, TX, USA) for the kind donation of the *Aloe vera* gel and the whole-leaf extract (Daltonmax700®). Financial support by the North West University (NWU) is, hereby, acknowledged. We want to acknowledge Suria Ellis at the Statistical Service Department of NWU, for the statistical analysis of the permeation data.

References

1. Park, K.; Kwon, I.C.; Park, K. Oral protein delivery: Current status and future prospect. *React. Funct. Polym.* **2011**, *71*, 280–287. [CrossRef]
2. Griffin, B.T.; Guo, J.; Presas, E.; Donovan, M.D.; Alonso, M.J.; O'Driscoll, C.M. Pharmacokinetic, pharmacodynamic and biodistribution following oral administration of nanocarriers containing peptide and protein drugs. *Adv. Drug Deliv. Rev.* **2016**, *106*, 367–380. [CrossRef] [PubMed]
3. Muheem, A.; Shakeel, F.; Jahangir, M.A.; Anwar, M.; Mallick, N.; Jain, G.K.; Warsi, M.H.; Ahmad, F.J. A review on the strategies for the oral delivery of proteins and peptides and their clinical perspectives. *Saudi Pharm. J.* **2016**, *24*, 413–428. [CrossRef] [PubMed]
4. Sánchez-Navarro, M.; Garcia, J.; Giralt, E.; Teixidó, M. Using peptides to increase transport across the intestinal barrier. *Adv. Drug Deliv. Rev.* **2016**, *106*, 355–366. [CrossRef] [PubMed]
5. Zhu, H.; Li, B.V.; Uppoor, R.S.; Mehta, M.; Yu, L.X. Bioavailability and bioequivalence. In *Developing Solid Oral Dosage Forms: Pharmaceutical Theory & Practice*, 2nd ed.; Qiu, Y., Chen, Y., Zhang, G.G.Z., Yu, L., Mantri, R.V., Eds.; Elsevier: Amsterdam, The Netherlands, 2017; pp. 381–397, ISBN 978-01-2802-447-8.
6. Cabrera-Pérez, M.A.; Sanz, M.B.; Sanjuan, V.M.; González-Álvarez, M.; González-Álvarez, I. Importance and applications of cell- and tissue-based in vitro models for drug permeability screening in early stages of drug development. In *Concepts and Models for Drug Permeability Studies*, 1st ed.; Sarmento, B., Ed.; Woodhead Publishing: Cambridge, UK, 2016; pp. 3–29, ISBN 978-00-8100-094-6.
7. Rosenthal, R.; Günzel, D.; Finger, C.; Krug, S.M.; Richter, J.F.; Schulzke, J.; Fromm, M.; Amasheh, S. The effect of chitosan on transcellular and paracellular mechanisms in the intestinal epithelial barrier. *Biomaterials* **2012**, *33*, 2791–2800. [CrossRef] [PubMed]

8. Artursson, P.; Palm, K.; Luthman, K. Caco-2 monolayers in experimental and theoretical predictions of drug transport. *Adv. Drug Deliv. Rev.* **2001**, *46*, 27–43. [CrossRef]
9. Lin, Y.; Chen, C.; Liang, H.; Kulkarni, A.R.; Lee, P.; Chen, C.; Sung, H. Novel nanoparticles for oral insulin delivery via the paracellular pathway. *Nanotechnology* **2007**, *18*, 1–11. [CrossRef]
10. Tscheik, C.; Blasig, I.E.; Winkler, L. Trends in drug delivery through tissue barriers containing tight junctions. *Tissue Barriers* **2013**, *1*, e24565. [CrossRef]
11. Ward, P.D.; Tippin, T.K.; Thakker, D.R. Enhancing paracellular permeability by modulating epithelial tight junctions. *Pharm. Sci. Technol. Today* **2000**, *3*, 346–358. [CrossRef]
12. Lemmer, H.J.R.; Hamman, J.H. Paracellular drug absorption enhancement through tight junction modulation. *Expert Opin. Drug Deliv.* **2013**, *10*, 103–114. [CrossRef]
13. Matter, K.; Balda, M.S. Functional analysis of tight junctions. *Methods* **2003**, *30*, 228–234. [CrossRef]
14. Sun, H.; Chow, E.C.Y.; Liu, S.; Du, Y.; Pang, K.S. The Caco-2 cell monolayer: Usefulness and limitations. *Expert Opin. Drug Metab. Toxicol.* **2008**, *4*, 395–411. [CrossRef] [PubMed]
15. Maher, S.; Mrsny, R.J.; Brayden, D.J. Intestinal permeation enhancers for oral peptide delivery. *Adv. Drug Deliv. Rev.* **2016**, *106*, 277–319. [CrossRef] [PubMed]
16. Lakkireddy, H.R.; Urmannb, M.; Besenius, M.; Werner, U.; Haack, T.; Brun, P.; Alié, J.; Illel, B.; Hortala, L.; Vogel, R.; et al. Oral delivery of diabetes peptides—Comparing standard formulations incorporating functional excipients and nanotechnologies in the translational context. *Adv. Drug Deliv. Rev.* **2016**, *106*, 196–222. [CrossRef] [PubMed]
17. Renukuntla, J.; Vadlapudi, A.D.; Patel, A.; Boddu, S.H.S.; Mitra, A.K. Approaches for enhancing oral bioavailability of peptides and proteins. *Int. J. Pharm.* **2013**, *447*, 75–93. [CrossRef] [PubMed]
18. Mahato, R.I.; Narang, A.S.; Thoma, L.; Miller, D.D. Emerging trends in oral delivery of peptide and protein drugs. *Crit. Rev. Ther. Drug Carrier Syst.* **2003**, *20*, 153–214. [CrossRef]
19. Isoda, H.; Han, J.; Tominaga, M.; Maekawa, T. Effects of capsaicin on human intestinal cell line Caco-2. *Cytotechnology* **2001**, *36*, 155–161. [CrossRef]
20. Kesarwani, K.; Gupta, R. Bioavailability enhancers of herbal origin: An overview. *Asian Pac. J. Trop. Biomed.* **2013**, *3*, 253–266. [CrossRef]
21. Salama, N.N.; Eddington, N.D.; Fasano, A. Tight junction modulation and its relationship to drug delivery. *Adv. Drug Deliv. Rev.* **2006**, *58*, 15–28. [CrossRef]
22. Tatiraju, D.V.; Bagade, V.B.; Karambelkar, P.J.; Jadhav, V.M.; Kadam, V. Natural bioenhancers: An overview. *J. Pharmacogn. Phytochem.* **2013**, *2*, 55–60.
23. Werle, M.; Bernkop-Schnürch, A. Thiolated chitosans: Useful excipients for oral drug delivery. *J. Pharm. Pharmacol.* **2008**, *60*, 273–281. [CrossRef] [PubMed]
24. Vllasaliu, D.; Casettari, L.; Fowler, R.; Exposito-Harris, R.; Garnett, M.; Illum, L.; Stolnik, S. Absorption-promoting effects of chitosan in airway and intestinal cell lines: A comparative study. *Int. J. Pharm.* **2012**, *430*, 151–160. [CrossRef] [PubMed]
25. Boudreau, M.D.; Beland, F.A. An evaluation of the biological and toxicological properties of *Aloe barbadensis* (Miller), *Aloe vera*. *J. Environ. Sci. Health C* **2006**, *24*, 103–154. [CrossRef] [PubMed]
26. Sahu, P.K.; Giri, D.D.; Singh, R.; Pandey, P.; Gupta, S.; Shrivastava, A.K.; Kumar, A.; Pandey, K.D. Therapeutic and medicinal uses of *Aloe vera*: A review. *Pharmacol. Pharm.* **2013**, *4*, 599–610. [CrossRef]
27. Eshun, K.; He, Q. *Aloe vera*: A valuable ingredient for the food, pharmaceutical and cosmetic industries—A review. *Crit. Rev. Food Sci. Nutr.* **2004**, *44*, 91–96. [CrossRef]
28. Hamman, J.H. Composition and applications of *Aloe vera* leaf gel. *Molecules* **2008**, *13*, 1599–1616. [CrossRef]
29. Sánchez-Machado, D.I.; López-Cervantes, J.; Sendón, R.; Sanches-Silva, A. *Aloe vera*: Ancient knowledge with new frontiers. *Trends Food Sci. Technol.* **2017**, *61*, 94–102. [CrossRef]
30. Mascolo, N.; Izzo, A.A.; Borrelli, F.; Capasso, R.; Di Carlo, G.; Sautebin, L.; Capasso, F. Healing powers of aloes. In *Aloes: The genus Aloe*, 1st ed.; Reynolds, T., Ed.; CRC Press: Washington, DC, USA, 2004; pp. 209–238, ISBN 978-04-1530-672-0.
31. Vinson, J.A.; Al Kharrat, H.; Andreoli, L. Effect of *Aloe vera* preparations on the human bioavailability of vitamins C and E. *Phytomedicine* **2005**, *12*, 760–765. [CrossRef]
32. Chen, W.; Lu, Z.; Viljoen, A.; Hamman, J. Intestinal drug transport enhancement by *Aloe vera*. *Planta Med.* **2009**, *75*, 587–595. [CrossRef]

33. Beneke, C.; Viljoen, A.; Hamman, J.H. In vitro drug absorption enhancement effects of *Aloe vera* and *Aloe ferox*. *Sci. Pharm.* **2012**, *80*, 475–486. [CrossRef]
34. Beneke, C.; Viljoen, A.; Hamman, J.H. Modulation of drug efflux by aloe materials: An in vitro investigation across rat intestinal tissue. *Pharmacogn. Mag.* **2013**, *9*, 44–48. [CrossRef]
35. Lebitsa, T.; Viljoen, A.; Lu, Z.; Hamman, J. In vitro drug permeation enhancement potential of Aloe gel materials. *Curr. Drug Deliv.* **2012**, *9*, 297–304. [CrossRef] [PubMed]
36. Cole, L.; Heard, C. Skin permeation enhancement potential of *Aloe vera* and a proposed mechanism of action based upon size exclusion and pull effect. *Int. J. Pharm.* **2007**, *333*, 10–16. [CrossRef] [PubMed]
37. Fox, L.; Gerber, M.; Du Preez, J.L.; Du Plessis, J.; Hamman, J.H. Skin permeation enhancement effects of the gel and whole leaf materials of *Aloe vera*, *Aloe marlothii* and *Aloe ferox*. *J. Pharm. Pharmacol.* **2014**, *67*, 96–106. [CrossRef] [PubMed]
38. Ojewole, E.; Mackraj, I.; Akhundov, K.; Hamman, J.; Viljoen, A.; Olivier, E.; Wesley-Smith, J.; Govender, T. Investigating the effect of *Aloe vera* gel on the buccal permeability of didanosine. *Planta Med.* **2012**, *78*, 354–361. [CrossRef]
39. Djuv, A.; Nilsen, O.G. Caco-2 cell methodology and inhibition of the P-glycoprotein transport of digoxin by *Aloe vera* juice. *Phytother. Res.* **2008**, *22*, 1623–1628. [CrossRef]
40. Jiao, P.; Jia, Q.; Randel, G.; Diehl, B.; Weaver, S.; Milligan, G. Quantitative ^{1}H-NMR Spectrometry Method for Quality Control of *Aloe vera* Products. *J. AOAC Int.* **2010**, *93*, 842–848.
41. Sieval, A.B.; Thanou, M.; Kotzé, A.F.; Verhoef, J.C.; Brussee, J.; Junginger, H.E. Preparation and NMR characterization of highly substituted *N*-trimethyl chitosan chloride. *Carbohydr. Polym.* **1998**, *36*, 157–165. [CrossRef]
42. Hamman, J.H.; Stander, M.; Kotzé, A.F. Effect of the degree of quaternisation of *N*-trimethyl chitosan chloride of absorption enhancement: In vivo evaluation in rat nasal epithelia. *Int. J. Pharm.* **2002**, *232*, 235–242. [CrossRef]
43. Calatayud, M.; Devesa, V.; Montoro, R.; Vélez, D. In vitro study of intestinal transport of arsenite, monomethylarsonous acid, and dimethylarsinous acid by Caco-2 cell line. *Toxicol. Lett.* **2011**, *204*, 127–133. [CrossRef]
44. Bhushani, J.A.; Karthik, P.; Anandharamakrishnan, C. Nanoemulsion based delivery system for improved bioaccessibility and Caco-2 cell monolayer permeability of green tea extract. *Food Hydrocoll.* **2016**, *56*, 372–382. [CrossRef]
45. Alqahtani, S.; Mohamed, L.A.; Kaddoumi, A. Experimental models for predicting drug absorption and metabolism. *Expert Opin. Drug Metab. Toxicol.* **2013**, *9*, 1–14. [CrossRef] [PubMed]
46. Du Toit, T.; Malan, M.M.; Lemmer, H.J.R.; Gouws, C.; Aucamp, M.E.; Breytenbach, W.J.; Hamman, J.H. Combining chemical permeation enhancers for synergistic effects. *Eur. J. Drug Metab. Pharmacokinet.* **2016**, *41*, 575–586. [CrossRef] [PubMed]
47. Pick, D.; Degen, C.; Leiterer, M.; Jahreis, G.; Einax, J.W. Transport of selenium species in Caco-2 cells: Analytical approach employing the Ussing chamber technique and HPLC-ICP-MS. *Microchem. J.* **2013**, *110*, 8–14. [CrossRef]
48. Wahlang, B.; Pawar, Y.B.; Bansal, A.K. Identification of permeability-related hurdles in oral delivery of curcumin using the Caco-2 cell model. *Eur. J. Pharm. Biopharm.* **2011**, *77*, 275–282. [CrossRef] [PubMed]
49. Palumbo, P.; Picchini, U.; Beck, B.; van Gelder, J.; Delbar, N.; DaGaetano, A. A general approach to the apparent permeability index. *J. Pharmacokinet. Pharmacodyn.* **2008**, *35*, 235–248. [CrossRef] [PubMed]
50. Johnson, P.H.; Frank, D.; Costantino, H.R. Discovery of tight junction modulators: Significance for drug development and delivery. *Drug Discov. Today* **2008**, *13*, 261–267. [CrossRef] [PubMed]
51. Kotzé, A.F.; Leußen, H.L.; De Leeuw, B.J.; De Boer, B.G.; Verhoef, J.C.; Junginger, H.E. Comparison of the effect of different chitosan salts and *N*-trimethyl chitosan chloride on the permeability of intestinal epithelial cells (Caco-2). *J. Control Release* **1998**, *51*, 35–46. [CrossRef]
52. Abcam. Immunocytochemistry and Immunofluorescence Protocol: Procedure for Staining of Cell Cultures Using Immunofluorescence. Available online: http://www.abcam.com/protocols/immunocytochemistry-immunofluorescence-protocol (accessed on 9 November 2017).
53. Wu, S.; Don, T.; Lin, C.; Mi, F. Delivery of berberine using chitosan/fucoidan-taurine conjugate nanoparticles for treatment of defective intestinal epithelial tight junction barrier. *Mar. Drugs* **2014**, *12*, 5677–5697. [CrossRef]

54. Abcam. Protocol Booklet: CytoPainter Phalloidin-iFlour 488 Reagent: Instructions for Use for Staining F-Actin in Adherent or Suspension Cells. Available online: http://www.abcam.com/ps/products/176/ab176753/documents/ab176753%20CytoPainter%20Phalloidin-iFluor%20488%20Reagent%20protocol%20v3%20(website).pdf (accessed on 9 November 2017).
55. Dorkoosh, F.A.; Broekhuizen, C.A.N.; Borchard, G.; Rafiee-Tehrani, M.; Verhoef, J.C.; Junginger, H.E. Transport of octreotide and evaluation of mechanism of action of opening the paracellular tight junction using superporous hydrogel polymers in Caco-2 cell monolayers. *J. Pharm. Sci.* **2004**, *93*, 743–752. [CrossRef]
56. Hsu, L.; Ho, Y.; Chuang, E.; Chen, C.; Juang, J.; Su, F.; Hwang, S.; Sung, H. Effects of pH on molecular mechanisms of chitosan-integrin interactions and resulting tight-junction disruptions. *Biomaterials* **2013**, *34*, 784–793. [CrossRef] [PubMed]
57. Abcam. Product Datasheet: Fluoroshield Mounting Medium with Propidium Iodide ab104129. Available online: http://www.abcam.com/fluoroshield-mounting-medium-with-propidium-iodide-20ml-ab104129.html (accessed on 9 November 2017).
58. Kotzé, A.F.; Leußen, H.L.; De Leeuw, B.J.; De Boer, B.G.; Verhoef, J.C.; Junginger, H.E. *N*-trimethyl chitosan chloride as a potential absorption enhancer across mucosal surfaces: In vitro evaluation in intestinal epithelial cells (Caco-2). *Pharm. Res.* **1997**, *14*, 1197–1202. [CrossRef] [PubMed]
59. Thanou, M.; Verhoef, J.C.; Junginger, H.E. Oral drug absorption enhancement by chitosan and its derivatives. *Adv. Drug Deliv. Rev.* **2001**, *52*, 117–126. [CrossRef]

5

Development of Functionalized Carbon Nano-Onions Reinforced Zein Protein Hydrogel Interfaces for Controlled Drug Release

Narsimha Mamidi [1,*], Aldo González-Ortiz [1], Irasema Lopez Romo [2] and Enrique V. Barrera [3,4]

1 Tecnologico de Monterrey, Department of Chemistry and Nanotechnology, School of Engineering and Science, Monterrey 64849, Nuevo Leon, Mexico
2 Tecnologico de Monterrey, Department of Biotechnology, School of Engineering and Science, Monterrey 64849, Nuevo Leon, Mexico
3 Department of Materials Science and NanoEngineering, Rice University, Houston, TX 77005, USA
4 Department of Chemistry, Rice University, Houston, TX 77005, USA
* Correspondence: nmamidi@tec.mx;

Abstract: In the current study, poly 4-mercaptophenyl methacrylate-carbon nano-onions (PMPMA-CNOs = f-CNOs) reinforced natural protein (zein) composites (zein/f-CNOs) are fabricated using the acoustic cavitation technique. The influence of f-CNOs inclusion on the microstructural properties, morphology, mechanical, cytocompatibility, in-vitro degradation, and swelling behavior of the hydrogels are studied. The tensile results showed that zein/f-CNOs hydrogels fabricated by the acoustic cavitation system exhibited good tensile strength (90.18 MPa), compared with the hydrogels fabricated by the traditional method and only microwave radiation method. It reveals the magnitude of physisorption and degree of colloidal stability of f-CNOs within the zein matrix under acoustic cavitation conditions. The swelling behaviors of hydrogels were also tested and improved results were noticed. The cytotoxicity of hydrogels was tested with osteoblast cells. The results showed good cell viability and cell growth. To explore the efficacy of hydrogels as drug transporters, 5-fluorouracil (5-FU) release was measured under gastric and intestinal pH environment. The results showed pH-responsive sustained drug release over 15 days of study, and pH 7.4 showed a more rapid drug release than pH 2.0 and 4.5. Nonetheless, all the results suggest that zein/f-CNOs hydrogel could be a potential pH-responsive drug transporter for a colon-selective delivery system.

Keywords: zein/poly 4-mercaptophenyl methacrylate-carbon nano-onions hydrogels; acoustic cavitation method; pH-responsive drug release; cytocompatibility

---

1. Introduction

Hydrogels are incipient three-dimensional (3D) networking structures that are able to swell in aqueous or non-aqueous fluids without dissolving. The hydrogels have been used in tissue engineering, drug release, material separation, and artificial organs, due to their excellent flexibility, high moisture content, and outstanding viscoelasticity [1]. Various hydrogels have been fabricated from synthetic and/or natural polymers with an emphasis on regenerative medicine, drug delivery, and tissue adhesives [2]. Such developed hydrogels are able to mimic the native extracellular matrix (ECM) and support cellular growth and tissue regeneration [3]. Besides, hydrogels are used in cell-matrix, 3D culturing cell-cell interactions, cellular proliferation, differentiation, and migration [4,5]. In this regard, naturally occurring biopolymers comprising hydrogels have potential advantages over synthetic polymers, including low cost, good cytocompatibility, less immunogenicity, degradability in physiological conditions, and wide availability [6]. Thus, several hydrogels developed from alginate, chitosan, hyaluronic acid, fibrinogen, collagen, and zein have been reported [7–12]. Consequently, it is vital to fabricate plant protein-derived hydrogels for biomedical applications. Zein is a natural plant protein and extracted from corn. Zein is hydrophobic and water-insoluble due to lack of prolamin [13–16]. Zein protein has been used in drug delivery, food packaging, and coatings [15,17]. However, there are some issues, such as shrinkage in water, low mechanical strength, and rapid degradation that impede the biomedical applications of pure zein. Therefore, several chemical modification and physical treatments have been developed to improve the mechanical strength, water-resistance, and plasticity of zein protein [18–22]. Moreover, zein was covalently functionalized with gold nanoparticles, polycaprolactone (PCL), and 3-glycidoxypropyltrimethoxysilane to improve mechanical and degradability, respectively [23–25]. In order to improve the above properties of zein, poly 4-mercaptophenyl methacrylate-carbon nano-onions were incorporated within zein protein to fabricate zein/f-CNOs composite hydrogels.

Carbon-nano-onions (CNOs) are a class of carbon nanomaterials that contain concentric graphitic shells and are described by Ugarte in 1992 [26]. CNOs have been widely used in catalysis, supercapacitors, lithium-ion batteries, cell imaging, and diagnostic, therapeutic, and other biomedical applications because of their good physicochemical properties [27–32]. Among different carbon nanomaterials, CNOs are the most promising carbon material for biomedical applications because of their tolerance to transport in the circulatory systems with negligible toxicity and good cytocompatibility [31]. Moreover, several studies demonstrated that CNOs are highly biocompatible compared to MWCNTs, and CNOs showed less inflammation than CNTs [32]. Pristine CNOs, oxidized CNOs, and PEGylated CNOs are nontoxic and presented more than 85% of cell viability with fibroblasts [33]. Recently, ultra-high molecular weight polyethylene/4-mercaptophenyl methacrylate functionalized carbon nano-onions (UHMWPE/f-CNOs) nanocomposites were developed [34]. The mechanical, cytocompatibile, and thermal properties of the UHMWPE were significantly enhanced in the presence of 0.1 wt% of functionalized CNOs [34]. These outstanding results of f-CNOs motivated us to design and fabricate f-CNOs incorporated zein/f-CNOs hydrogels. Thus, it is of great interest to explore the application of CNOs as a second phase reinforcement in the fabrication of novel hydrogels.

The proper synthetic route of nanomaterials is essential in biomedical application, where the sonochemical method offers an easy path of synthesis. Sonochemistry is an emerging synthetic method to fabricate nanomaterials. Sonochemistry is a simple, facile, and short-time physicochemical method liable to the high-intensity ultrasound and acoustic cavitation phenomenon [35,36]. A sonochemical method has been used to develop several nanomaterials with an emphasis on controlled drug delivery [37,38]. Nonetheless, to the best of our knowledge, the fabrication of plant protein (zein)/f-CNOs composite hydrogels have not yet been established, until now, for controlled drug release. Thus, it is hypothesized that f-CNOs can uniformly disperse and reinforce within the zein matrix by sonochemical method. The homogeneous dispersion of CNOs not only improves the mechanical properties of zein/f-CNOs composite hydrogels but also enhances biodegradability, swelling, drug release, and cytocompatibility.

The aim of the current study is to fabricate poly 4-mercaptophenyl methacrylated CNOs loaded zein protein hydrogels using acoustic cavitation technique. Besides, we will investigate the physicochemical properties, mechanical properties, drug release under physiological conditions, and cytocompatibility of hydrogels.

2. Experimental Section

2.1. Materials and Methods

All the reagents and organic solvents were purchased from commercial suppliers and used without further purification. Zein protein, methacryloyl chloride (MA), *N*-hydroxysuccinimide (NHS), 1-ethyl-3-(3-dimethylaminopropyl) carbodiimide (EDC), 5-Fluorouracil (5-FU), glutaraldehyde (GA), and 2,2′-Azobis(2-methylpropionitrile) (AIBN) were procured from Sigma Aldrich (St. Louis, MO,

USA.). Osteoblast cells were obtained from the American Type Culture Collection (ATCC, Manassas, VA, USA.). Dulbecco's modified Eagle's medium/F12 without phenol red (DMEM/F12), phosphate buffered saline (PBS) pH 7.4, fetal bovine serum (FBS), penicillin/streptomycin, and trypsin were acquired from Gibco Invitrogen (Camarillo, CA, USA.). CellTiter96®AQueous One Solution Cell Proliferation Assay was bought from Promega, (Fitchburg, WI, USA.). LIVE/DEAD Cell Imaging Kit was purchased from Molecular Probes, Life Technologies Corp. (Carlsbad, CA, U.S.A.).

2.2. *Synthesis*

2.2.1. Preparation of Composite Hydrogels

The synthesis of poly 4-mercaptophenyl methacrylated-CNOs was accomplished according to the previous report [34].

Synthesis of CNOs-MP

Briefly, 100 mg of pristine carbon nano-onions were dispersed in 50 mL of anhydrous DMF for 30 min using an ultrasonic bath. Then, 350 mg of *N*-hydroxysuccinimide (NHS) and 350 mg 4-dimethylaminopyridine (DMAP) were added to the dispersion solution and further sonicated for 30 min. After that, 1-ethyl-3-(3-dimethylaminopropyl) carbodiimide (EDC, 570 mg) was added and sonicated for 30 min. Next, 100 mg of 4-mercaptophenol (MP) was added and stirring was continued for 48 h at 60 °C under N_2. After the completion of the reaction (monitored thin layer chromatography), the stirring was stopped and the reaction mixture was cooled to ambient temperature. Next, the supernatant was discarded using centrifugation. The resulting black solid was thoroughly washed with DMF, methanol, DMF/triethylamine (9.9: 01), and ethyl acetate to obtain 4-mercaptophenylated CNOs (CNOs-MP).

Synthesis of CNOs-PMPMA

The mixture of 50 mg of CNOs-MP and 1.0 mL of diisopropylethylamine was dispersed in 50 mL of anhydrous tetrahydrofuran (THF) for 30 min using an ultrasonic bath. Then, 1.0 mL of methacryloyl chloride (MA) was added to the above mixture and stirred at room temperature for 24 h. Subsequently, the supernatant was discarded using centrifugation to attain a black solid. The resulted black solid was washed thoroughly with THF, dichloromethane, and HCl (0.01 M aqueous) to provide monomer CNOs-MPMA as a black solid. Then, 50 mg of CNOs-MPMA and azobisisobutyronitrile (AIBN, 1 wt%) were dissolved in 20 mL of anhydrous THF and sonicated for 30 min. Next, the reaction mixture was stirred at 70 °C for 48 h. Subsequently, the reaction mixture was cooled to ambient temperature and the supernatant was removed by centrifugation to attain CNOs-PMPMA as a black solid. The solid was washed with dichloromethane and diethyl ether and vacuum dried and stored in a desiccator until further use. The functionalized CNOs-PMPMA (f-CNOs) were characterized using ^{1}H-NMR, Raman, TGA, and GPC analysis.

In order to prepare zein/f-CNOs hydrogels, initially, 2 mg/mL of f-CNOs was ultrasonicated for 30 min in water/1,4-dioxane (1:1) to obtain the homogenous dispersion. Then, 1.0 g of zein protein (in 10 mL of water/1,4-dioxane; 1:1) was added into the f-CNOs solution. The resulting reaction mixture was treated with GA (1%, *w*/*w*) as a crosslinking agent under three different reaction conditions as showed in the Table 1.

To prepare the drug-loaded hydrogels, 10 mg/mL of 5-FU was added to the above solutions before the addition of crosslinker to incorporate the drug within the polymer matrix. This could prevent the surface drug loading, burst release, and aid the sustained release.

Table 1. Reaction conditions and fabrication methods of hydrogels.

Entry	Method	Zein/f-CNOs	Cross-Linker (GA)	Time (min.)	Hydrogel [d]
1.	Conventional	(1.0 g/2.0 mg)	(1%, *w/w*)	180 [a]	CZCNOs
2.	Microwave	(1.0 g/2.0 mg)	(1%, *w/w*)	40 [b]	MZCNOs
3.	Acoustic cavitation (ultra-sonic)	(1.0 g/2.0 mg)	(1%, *w/w*)	30 [c]	UZCNOs

[a] The reaction mixture was stirred at 65 °C for 180 min; [b] 500 W of power was applied for 40 min; [c] The reaction mixture was ultra-sonicated for 30 min; [d] The homogeneous reaction mixture was poured into a glass petri dish and left to stand overnight for gel formation.

2.3. Characterizations of Composite Hydrogels

Scanning electron microscopy (SEM, ZEISS EVO®MA 25, Ostalbkreis, Baden-Württemberg, Germany) was used to study the surface morphological properties of composite hydrogels. For this, all the hydrogel samples were flash-frozen in liquid nitrogen and then fractured. Prior to the SEM analysis, the cross-sections of the freeze-dried hydrogel specimens were gold coated. Tensile strength and elongation at break testing were measured to evaluate the mechanical properties of composite hydrogels samples. A tensile testing machine (Instron 3365, Instron, and Norwood, MA, USA.) was used to measure the tensile properties of specimens. The size of the hydrogel sample was 33.0 mm × 6.0 mm × 2.0 mm, and the crosshead speed was 50 mm/min.

To get the information about the functional groups presented in the hydrogel structure, the Fourier transform infrared (FTIR) spectroscopy (Perkin Elmer Universal ATR Sampling Accessory Frontier, Waltham, MA, USA) was used to scrutinize the zein/f-CNOs composite hydrogel specimens in the wavenumber range of 400–4000 cm^{-1} at room temperature.

2.3.1. Dynamic Light Scattering (DLS) and Zeta-Potential Experiments

DLS measurements were recorded using the Malvern Nano-ZS instrument and the data analyzed by Zetasizer software (version 7.12), Malvern Instruments Ltd., Worcestershire, WR14 1XZ, United Kingdom. 500 μg/mL of f-CNOs were probe sonicated in water and DMEM cell medium for 60 min. Then, the final concentration (500 μg/mL) of f-CNOs was diluted into 50, 25, 5, and 1 μg/mL in water and DMEM cell medium to measure the size of the particles. The dispensable zeta potential cuvettes were used to record the Zeta potential measurements. All the zeta measurements were run in triplicate per each sample and averaged to attain the final results.

2.3.2. Swelling of Hydrogels

Swelling ratio measurements of hydrogels were recorded by gravimetrically on a definite amount of dried hydrogel samples. Initially, the freeze-dried and pre-weighed hydrogel samples were immersed in DMEM (pH 7.4) at predetermined time intervals.

The swollen hydrogels were drawn from DMEM and the non-adsorbed medium was soaked mildly with filter paper and weighed with a microbalance. The swelling ratio (SR) was measured using the following equation:

$$SR = \frac{(Ws - Wd)}{Wd} \times 100 \quad (1)$$

where W_s is the weight of hydrogels at equilibrium state and W_d is the weight of the hydrogels at the dry state. The swelling rate of the composite hydrogels was calculated according to the following equation

$$v = \frac{(Wt2 - Wt1)}{Wd(t2 - t1)} \quad (2)$$

where $t1$ and $t2$ were the mean of the swelling time, and W_{t1} and W_{t2} were the weight of the sample at $t1$ and $t2$, and W_d was the weight of dried hydrogels.

2.3.3. In Vitro Degradation of Hydrogels

In vitro degradation of hydrogels was measured with respect to weight loss. For this, initially weighed hydrogel specimens (W_0) were immersed in DMEM (pH 7.4) medium and incubated at 37 °C for 25 days. Then, the samples were taken out from the medium at predetermined time intervals, washed and dried in the desiccator for 12 h and weighed (W_t). The weight loss ratio calculated as $100 \times \frac{W0-Wt}{W0}$. The weight remaining ratio was calculated as $1 - \left[100 \times \frac{W0-Wt}{W0}\right]$.

2.3.4. In Vitro Drug Release from Hydrogels

UV-spectrophotometer (Agilent Technologies, 89090A) was used to measure the 5-FU release from the hydrogel specimens. For this, 30 mg of 5-FU-loaded hydrogel samples were immersed in 10 mL of DMEM (pH 2.0, 4.5, 7.4, and 9.0) and gently incubated at 37 °C. At predetermined time intervals, 2 mL of 5-FU released medium was collected and replaced with 2 mL of fresh DMEM medium to maintain the solution volume constant. The drug release was determined at $\lambda_{max} = 265$ nm to attain 5-FU concentration. The 5-FU release from hydrogel samples against time intervals was established. The pH-values (pH 2.0, 4.5, 7.4, and 9.0) of DMEM medium was adjusted with 1 M HCl or 1 M NaOH. Triplicate measurements were carried out. The drug release (%) was calculated from the following formula:

$$\text{drug release } (\%) = \frac{Mass\ of\ drug\ loaded\ Gel - Mass\ of\ drug\ released}{Mass\ of\ drug\ released}$$

2.3.5. Cytotoxicity Evaluation of Composite Hydrogels

The human osteoblasts (bone-forming cells) were used to evaluate in vitro cytocompatibility of hydrogels. For this, osteoblast cells were cultured on the surface of the hydrogel samples. Cell viability and morphology were also studied.

Cell Viability of Hydrogels

Cell viability was measured using CellTiter96®AQueous One Solution Cell Proliferation Assay. Initially, disk-shaped (~6.3 mm in diameter) hydrogels were prepared and then cut into thin sections and these hydrogel specimens were sterilized by ethanol (70% *v*/*v*) followed by UV irradiation. After that, the sterilized hydrogel specimens were decorated on a 96-well plate and then, human fetal osteoblastic cells (hFOB 1.19) at a density of 1×10^4 cells per well (~3.12×10^4 cells/cm^{-2}) were seeded over the hydrogels. The non-adherent cells were removed on the next day. The cell number was calculated after 1, 2, and 3 days post-seeding, using CellTiter96®. Furthermore, the LIVE/DEAD Cell Staining Kit was used to measure the cell viability of hydrogels and the images were recorded using fluorescence microscopy. The tissue culture plate was used as a control in 96-well plates. The experiments were run in triplicate.

Morphological Evaluations of Osteoblasts on Hydrogels

Prior to cell seeding on 24-well plates, hydrogels were cut into a disk shape. After that, human fetal osteoblastic cells (hFOB 1.19) at a density of 1×10^4 cells/mL were seeded on the surface of hydrogels in DMEM/F12 medium supplemented with 0.3 mg/mL of G418 disulfate salt, 2.5 mM of L-glutamine, 1% of penicillin/streptomycin and 10% of fetal bovine serum. The cells were incubated for 24 h in a humidified atmosphere at 5% CO_2. Then, the medium was transferred from the well plates and washed several times with phosphate buffer solution. After 3 days of incubation, cell images were recorded by an optical microscope (Model IN200A-5M, Amscope, Chino, CA, USA).

2.4. Statistical Analysis

All the experiments were carried out in triplicate and quantitative data were presented as mean ± standard deviation (SD) with $n = 3$. Statistical analysis was determined by one-way analysis of variance (ANOVA) and Tukey's post hoc tests using Minitab17 (Minitab, State College, PA, USA). $p < 0.05$ was considered statistically significant.

3. Results

3.1. Synthesis

Recently, we synthesized poly 4-mercaptophenyl methacrylated CNOs (f-CNOs) starting from the thioester coupling of 4-mercaptophenol with COOH-CNOs followed by methacrylatation and polymerization [34]. Then, UHMWPE/f-CNOs nanocomposites were developed through reinforcing f-CNOs with long-chain UHMWPE. A small quantity of f-CNOs improved the mechanical and cytocompatibility of UHMWPE. The uniform dispersion of f-CNOs particles throughout the hydrogel matrix is necessary to achieve good physicochemical properties of zein/f-CNOs hydrogels. Therefore, f-CNOs were synthesized and zein/f-CNOs (UZCNOs) hydrogels were fabricated by reinforcing f-CNOs within the zein matrix through acoustic cavitation method (Figure 1a). The acoustic cavitation promoted 5-FU loaded UZCNOs hydrogels were crosslinked with GA. The UZCNOs hydrogels were pH sensitive, pH-responsive, and pH 7.4 and pH 9.0 exhibited quicker drug release than pH 2.0 and pH 4.5 medium (Figure 1b). Moreover, the synthesized f-CNOs were dispersed in physiological buffer (DMEM) or aqueous environment and stabilized uniform colloidal dispersion was observed over 12 months (Figure 1c). The digital photo of zein/f-CNOs hydrogel composite is presented in Figure 1d and the inverted image unveils the evidence of the gelation.

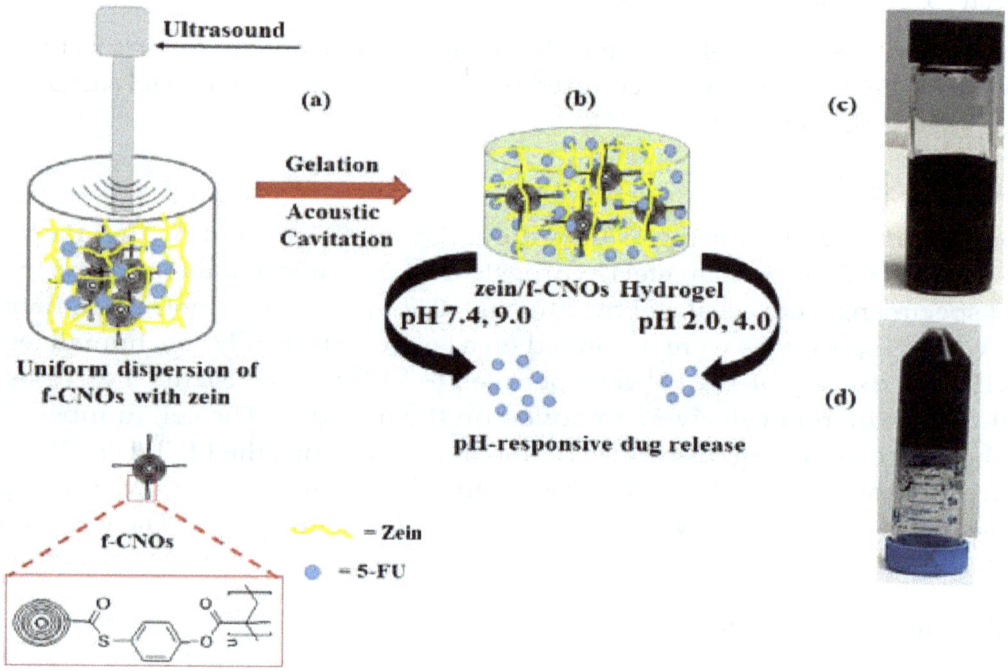

Figure 1. Synthetic illustration of (**a**) hydrogel preparation via acoustic cavitation, (**b**) cartoon diagram of hydrogel, (**c**) digital photograph of uniformly dispersed f-CNOs in DMEM after 1 year, and (**d**) digital photographs of fabricated UZCNOs hydrogel composite. f-CNOs indicates functionalized CNOs.

3.2. Dynamic Light Scattering (DLS) and Zeta-Potential Measurements

The dispersion and stability of pure COOH-CNOs and f-CNOs were scrutinized under physiological environment by DLS measurements. The dispersion of pristine COOH-CNOs particles showed approximately 110 nm, whereas f-CNOs particles exhibited around 147 nm in DMEM (Figure 2a). The particle size of pristine CNOs and f-CNOs was not changed with the concentration and time, indicating a stabilized colloidal dispersion even at relatively high concentrations. Besides, zeta potential measurements of pristine CNOs and f-CNOs were measured in DMEM and water.

The pristine CNOs exhibited ξ-potential values around −35 and −27 mV in DMEM and water, respectively, suggesting that they form uniform dispersions and that the COOH group has a substantial effect on the charge capacity of pristine CNOs (Figure 2b). Accordingly, positive (+ 30 and + 23 mV) ξ-potential values were observed in DMEM, and water, respectively (Figure 2b), indicating the chemical conjugation of the MPMA group on the surface of COOH-CNOs.

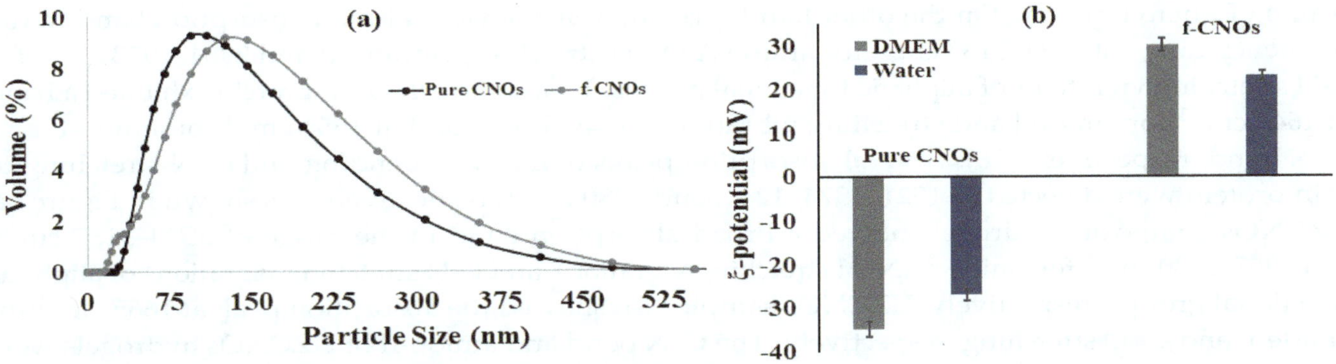

Figure 2. (**a**) Illustration of DLS particle size distribution, and (**b**) ξ-potential measurement of pristine CNOs and f-CNOs dispersions in DMEM.

3.3. SEM Analysis

The SEM analysis was performed to obtain microstructure morphologies of composite hydrogels and the resulting SEM images are illustrated in Figure 3. As shown in the SEM images, CZCNOs, MZCNOs, and UZCNOs hydrogel composites exhibited a porous and continuous structure. However, the porosity and internal morphology of hydrogels were reliant on the fabrication method. Particularly, the conventional thermal method provided CZCNOs showed constrained structure with low porosity (Figure 3a,d). On the other hand, MZCNOs hydrogel provided by microwave radiation showed a somewhat improved porosity (Figure 3b), and the porosity can be observed in the high magnification image of MZCNOs hydrogel (Figure 3e). Whereas UZCNOs hydrogel fabricated by acoustic cavitation exhibited sponge-like structure with good porosity, this porous morphology can restore the water uptake properties of the UZCNOs hydrogel (Figure 3c,f).

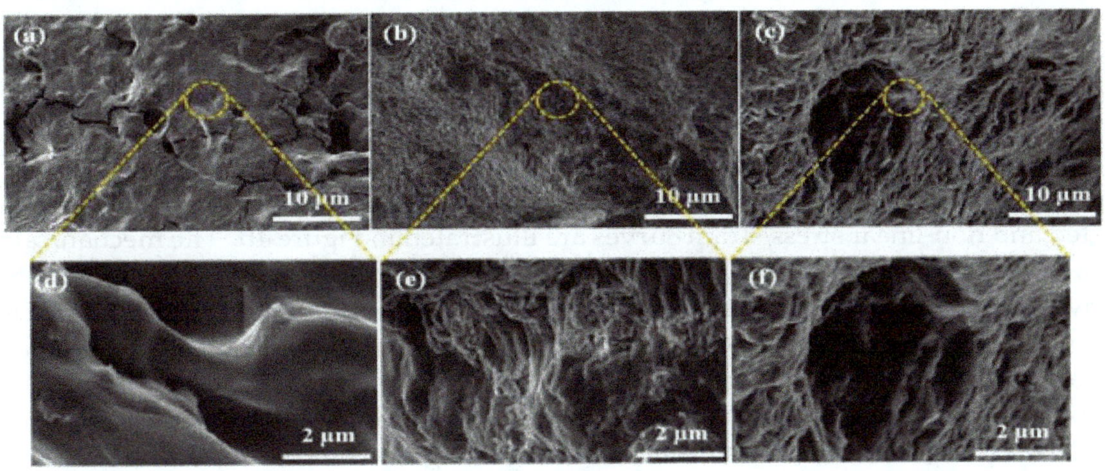

Figure 3. SEM image of composite hydrogel after freeze-drying (**a**,**d**) CZCNOs, (**b**,**e**) MZCNOs, and (**c**,**f**) UZCNOs, respectively. (**d**–**f**) Indicates the high magnification SEM images of CZCNOs, MZCNOs, and UZCNOs hydrogels, respectively.

3.4. FTIR and Tensile Measurements

FTIR analysis was utilized to understand the possible interactions between zein and f-CNOs (Figure 4a). PMPMA chemically conjugated CNOs exhibited a major absorption band at 1745 cm^{-1} for C=O stretching and 1560–1418 cm^{-1} for vibrational starching of the phenyl ring. Besides, 1263–1003 cm^{-1} bands were absorbed for C–O–C stretching and 2960 cm^{-1} for aliphatic C–H stretching of PMPMA moiety. The f-CNOs also showed a sharp peak at 685 cm^{-1} for the C–H bending vibration (out of plane) of phenyl moiety. On the other hand, pristine zein showed a broad absorption band in the frequency range of 3524–3133 cm^{-1} for amide A (N–H stretching vibration) and 2964–2923 cm^{-1} for C-H stretching vibrations of aliphatic functional groups. In addition, the zein protein exhibited a band at 1648 cm^{-1} for amide-I and stretching vibration of C=O bond, and at 1551 cm^{-1} for amide-II and C–N bond, respectively [26]. Several absorption peaks of the N–H bending and C–N stretching of zein protein were detected at 1521–1374, 1241, and 1080 cm^{-1}, respectively. As shown in Figure 4a, UZCNOs composite hydrogel showed a broad absorption band in the range of 3530–3137 cm^{-1}, and 2967–2930 cm^{-1} for amide A (N–H stretching vibration), and C-H stretching vibrations of aliphatic functional groups, respectively. UZCNOs sample also showed the absorption peak at 1665 cm^{-1} for amide-I, and C=O stretching, respectively. The C–N bond and amide-II of UZCNOs hydrogels were detected in the frequency range of 1525–1380 cm^{-1}. Furthermore, UZCNOs hydrogel showed the absorption bands at higher a frequency range for C–N stretching, and N–H bending, respectively. Notably, C–H bending (out of plane) of phenyl moiety (f-CNOs) was absorbed at 690 cm^{-1}.

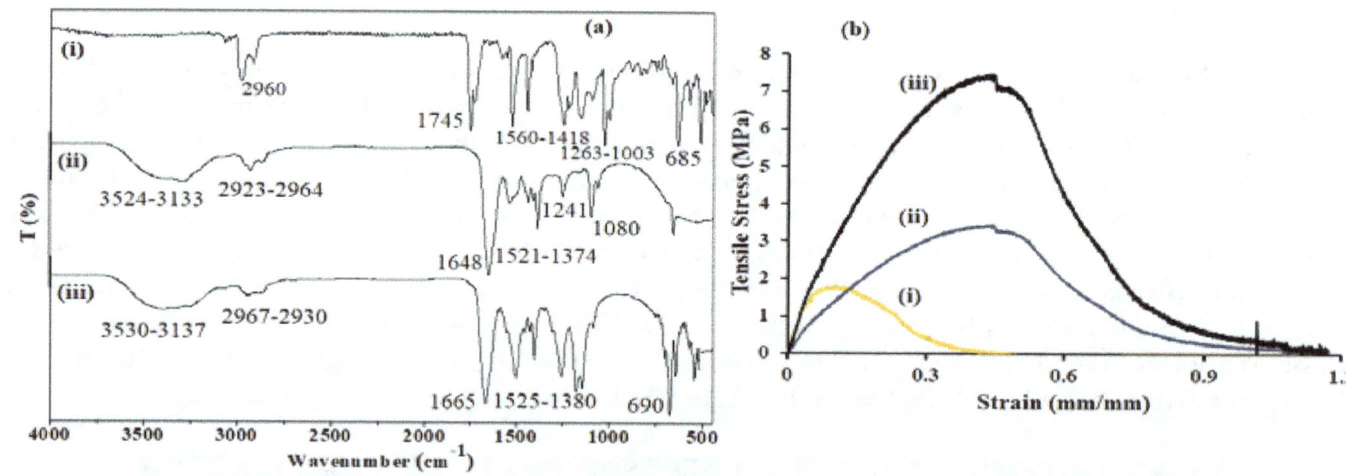

Figure 4. (**a**) FTIR spectra of (i) pure f-CNOs, (ii) pristine zein, and (iii) UZCNOs. (**b**) Tensile graph of (i) CZCNOs, (ii) MZCNOs, and (iii) UZCNOs hydrogels, respectively.

The tolerance of high loads and sustained deformation of the hydrogel are important characteristics in drug delivery applications. Consequently, the mechanical properties of UZCNOs hydrogel composite were recorded and non-linear stress/strain curves are illustrated in Figure 4b. The mechanical properties of UZCNOs hydrogels were significantly ($p < 0.05$) enhanced with the addition of f-CNOs. Specifically, UZCNOs hydrogel composite showed 7.7 ± 0.25 MPa of tensile strength, whereas MZCNOs hydrogel composite exhibited 4.2 ± 1.12 MPa of tensile strength (Figure 4b). These results revealed that UZCNOs hydrogel composite displayed higher tensile strength and lower strain than MZCNOs hydrogel. This could be due to the crosslinking density, electrostatic interactions or hydrogen bonding between f-CNOs and zein protein under acoustic cavitation environment. In addition, the tensile strength of CZCNOs hydrogel was measured (0.98 ± 1.25 MPa) and compared with UZCNOs hydrogel.

3.5. Swelling and Degradation Measurements

Usually, the water absorption of the hydrogel can be influenced by the aggregate structure and chemical structure. Thus, the swelling ratio and swelling rate of the fabricated hydrogels with different methods were measured using the gravimetric method and the results were presented in Figure 5a,b, respectively. From Figure 5a, it can be seen that the percentage swelling of the composite hydrogels was more than 150%. Particularly, UZCNOs hydrogel synthesized by acoustic cavitation and MZCNOs synthesized by microwave radiation showed the higher mass swelling ratio (>255%), this indicates that f-CNOs have a detrimental effect on the swelling ratio. Besides, the swelling rate of hydrogels was measured and is illustrated in Figure 5b. According to Figure 5, the swelling rates of the all the composite hydrogels were gradually decreased and reached equilibrium values, which indicates that the swelling behavior of hydrogels could be controlled with a short period for zein/f-CNOs hydrogels. Subsequently, this can be a rapid absorbent.

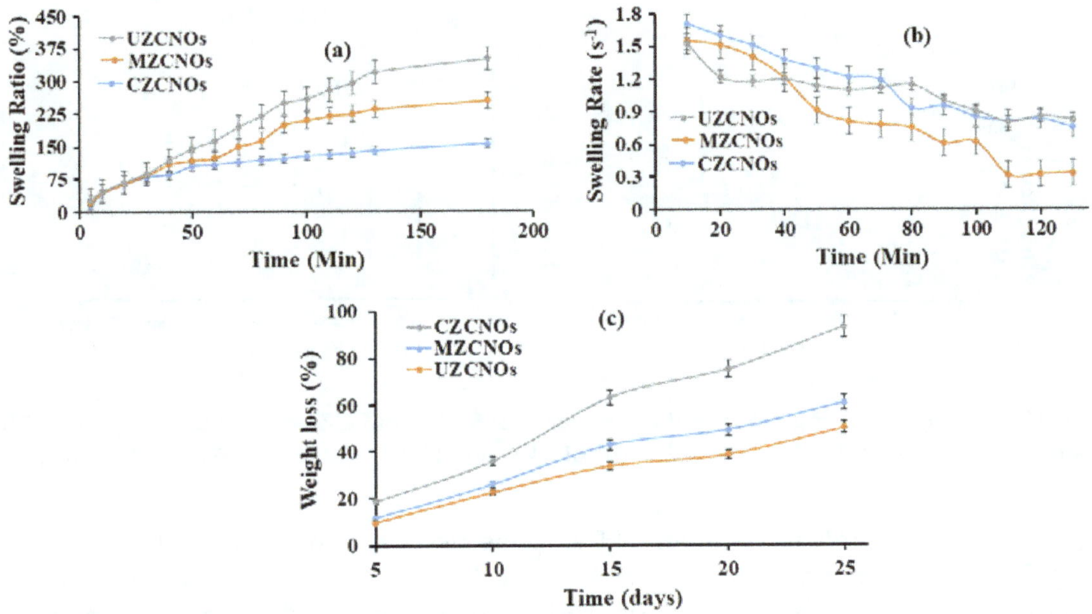

Figure 5. (**a**) Swelling ratio, (**b**) swelling rate, and (**c**) degradation curves of (i) CZCNO, MZCNOs, and UZCNOs hydrogels, respectively, in DMEM (pH 7.4) at room temperature.

The biodegradation characteristics of composite hydrogels display an important role in drug delivery and tissue engineering. Consequently, the degradation of hydrogels was measured in DMEM (pH 7.4) at 37 °C and the results are illustrated in Figure 5c. The CZCNOs hydrogel showed approximately 93% of degradation in 25 days of incubation. This could be due to the existence of weak electrostatic interactions and a difference in crosslinking density under the conventional method. On the other hand, MZCNOs and UZCNOs hydrogels showed sustained weight loss up to 25 days of incubation (Figure 5c). The UZCNOs hydrogel exhibited a lower degradation rate than MZCNOs hydrogels. Specifically, UZCNOs hydrogel showed around 50% of degradation in 25 days of study. This could be due to the strong electrostatic interactions and higher crosslinking density under acoustic cavitation. Whereas MZCNOs hydrogel exhibited approximately 61% of degradation in 25 days of study.

3.6. PH-Responsive Drug Release

In vitro release of 5-FU from composite hydrogels was performed by immersing the 5-FU loaded hydrogels in DMEM at pH 2.0, 4.5, 7.4, and 9.0. The drug release curves are presented in Figure 6. Initially, the 5-FU release from CZCNOs, MZCNOs, and UZCNOs hydrogels was measured at pH 2.0 over 15 days (Figure 6a). Under these conditions, composite hydrogels showed prolonged drug release. Particularly, the CZCNOs sample exhibited approximately 52% and the MZCNOs sample showed 69%

of drug release over 15 days of study (Figure 6a). On the other hand, the UZCNOs sample showed 85% of drug release over 15 days at pH 2.0.

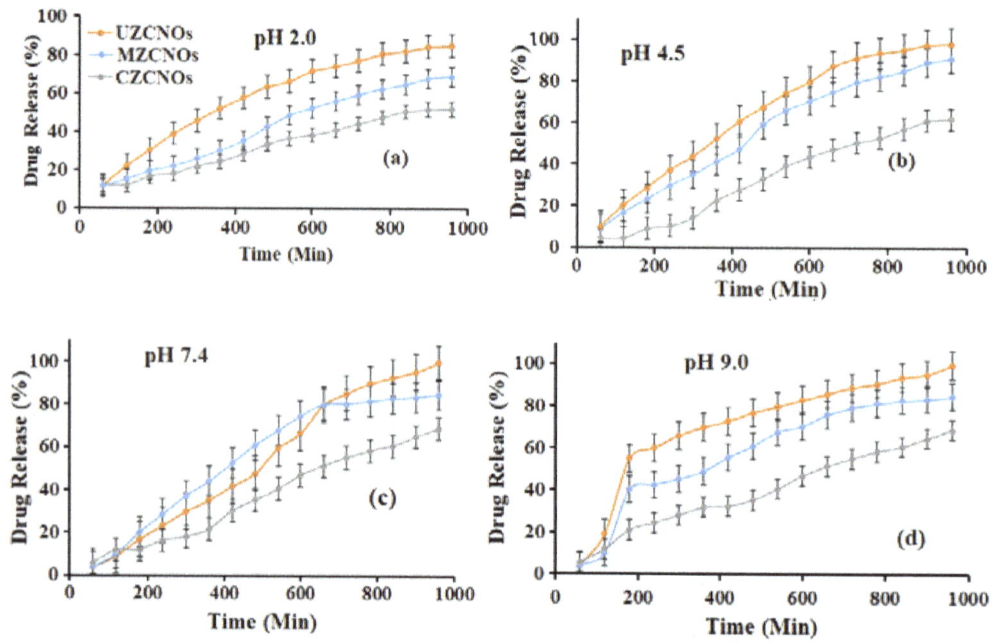

Figure 6. The graph illustrating the cumulative release of 5-FU from CZCNOs, MZCNOs, and UZCNOs composite hydrogels in DMEM at (**a**) pH 2.0, (**b**) pH 4.5, (**c**) pH 7.4, and (**d**) pH 9.0 at 37 °C, respectively.

To improve the drug release profile, pH 4.5 was used and measured the 5-FU release from composite hydrogel specimens (Figure 6b). As expected, CZCNOs hydrogel specimen exhibited around 62% of drug release over 15 days of study, which improved 8% of drug release at pH 4.5 (Figure 6b). The MZCNOs hydrogels sample showed around 91% of 5-FU release after 15 days of study and 20% of drug release was improved by changing pH 2.0 to pH 4.5., whereas the UZCNOs hydrogel sample synthesized by acoustic cavitation method exhibited approximately 94% of drug release at pH 4.5 over 15 days of incubation and reached plateau (Figure 6b).

In addition, 5-FU release was carried out in DMEM at pH 7.4 at room temperature (Figure 6c). This pH environment is defensible to the normal cells and reduces drug loss during drug transportation. Besides, pH 7.4 can control drug release behavior of hydrogel specimens while they present at the cytoplasm of normal cells or intracellular environment. The CZCNOs hydrogel showed around 67% of sustained drug release over 15 days of study. The MZCNOs hydrogel exhibited 85% of sustained drug release, whereas UZCNOs hydrogel samples displayed approximately 97% of sustained drug release over 15 days of study and reached a plateau.

Furthermore, 5-FU release was measured at pH 9.0 and the results are illustrated in Figure 6d. The UZCNOs hydrogel specimen showed approximately 52% of burst release on the third day of study. After that, around 99.9% of the drug was released in 15 days of study and reached a plateau (Figure 6d). On the other hand, MZCNOs hydrogels showed around 40% of burst release on the third day, followed by 85% of sustained drug release over 15 days of study, which is very similar to the pH 7.4 study (Figure 6d). Finally, CZCNOs hydrogels showed approximately 70% of sustained drug release over 15 days of incubation (Figure 6d).

3.7. *In Vitro Cytocompatibility Measurements*

The CellTiter96®AQueous One Solution was used to measure the cell viability of composite hydrogels and the results are depicted in Figure 7. The osteoblast cells were cultured on the pre-sterilized hydrogels specimens. On the first day of incubation, very similar cell viability was observed in CZCNOs, MZCNOs, and UZCNOs composite hydrogels. On the second day of study, MZCNOs, and UZCNOs hydrogel samples showed slightly improved cell viability, whereas CZCNOs hydrogel sample exhibited comparable viability on the same day of study (Figure 7). However, on the third day of incubation, the UZCNOs hydrogel specimen exhibited a better cell viability than the MZCNOs and CZCNOs hydrogel specimens.

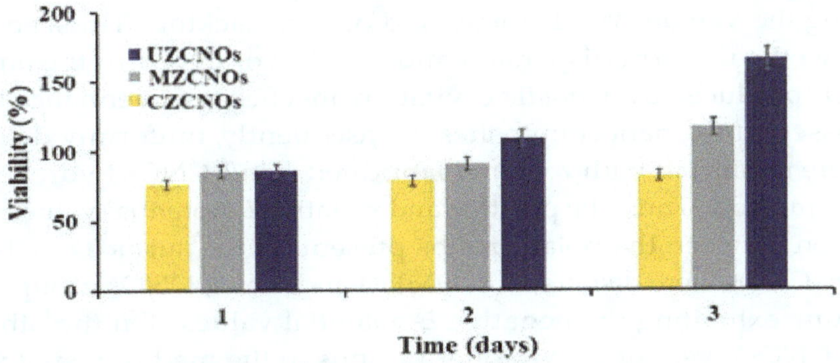

Figure 7. Cell viability of CZCNOs, MZCNOs, and UZCNOs composite hydrogels. Data represent mean ± SD ($n = 3$). Statistically significant difference ($p < 0.05$) was observed between the cell viability parameters of CZCNOs, MZCNOs, and UZCNOs samples.

The LIVE/DEAD kit was also utilized to evaluate the cytotoxicity of f-CNOs in zein/f-CNOs composite hydrogels and the resulting optical images are depicted in Figure 8. The cell culture plate was used as a controller and it exhibited some DEAD cells after three days of study (Figure 8a). The CZCNOs hydrogel sample showed a decent percentage (77 ± 1.30%) of LIVE cells along with some of the DEAD cells (Figure 8b). The MZCNOs hydrogel sample displayed approximately 93 ± 0.81% of LIVE cells along with a small number of DEAD cells (Figure 8c). Interestingly, UZCNOs sample exhibited more than 97 ± 0.41% of LIVE cells (Figure 8d).

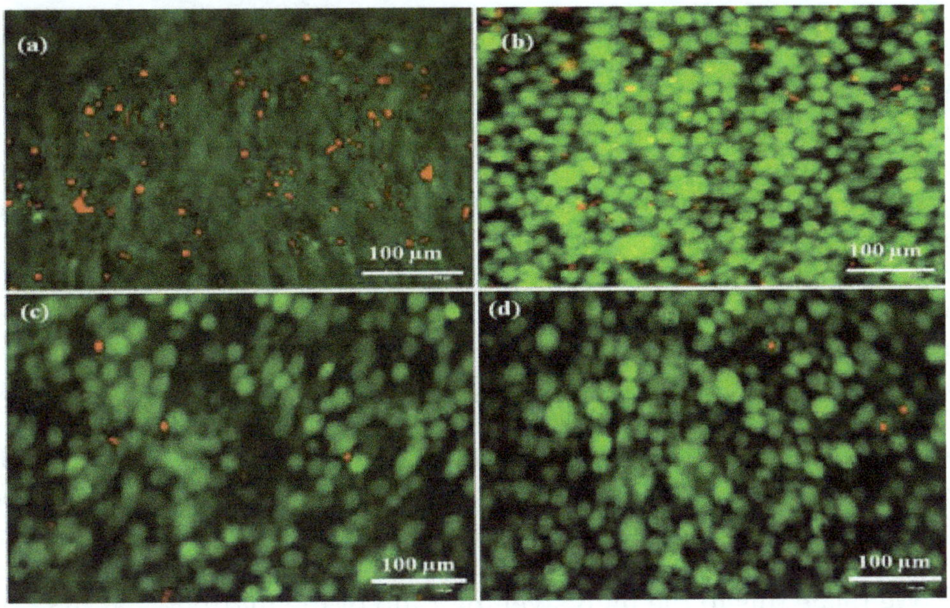

Figure 8. Optical images of osteoblast cells on the surface of zein/f-CNOs composite hydrogels after 3 days of study: (**a**) The control (tissue culture plate), (**b**) CZCNOs, (**c**) MZCNOs, and (**d**) UZCNOs; green indicates LIVE cells, and red indicates DEAD, respectively. Scale bar = 100 μm.

4. Discussion

The homogeneous colloidal dispersion measurements suggested that the functionalized CNOs could stabilize in the aqueous environment. The acoustic cavitation wave or acoustic cavitation is the superlative stringent source of exfoliation of 2D nanomaterials. The fluctuation of pressure in the liquid environment generates the acoustic cavitation that creates bubble growth followed by bubble collapse and finally internal turbulence. This ultrasound energy renovates into high temperature and pressure. Ultrasound waves transfer through carbon nanoparticles (CNOs) which are held by weak interactions, including the Van der Waals forces and/or π–π stacking. Thus, acoustic cavitation is a good choice to achieve the uniform dispersion and stability of CNOs in the aqueous environment. Colloidal stable CNOs produced by acoustic cavitation are effective to enhance the electrical, tensile, and biocompatible assets of the nanocomposites. Consequently, uniformly dispersed and colloidal stabilized f-CNOs were reinforced with zein and fabricated zein/f-CNOs hydrogel composite through the acoustic cavitation method. Thus, the positive and negative ξ-potential values described the proton exchange phenomenon between the polar groups present on the surface of CNOs and the solvent system. When COOH-CNOs were dispersed in DMEM and water, CNOs groups were able to donate protons to the medium, exhibiting the negative ξ-potential values. On the other hand, chemically conjugated CNOs (f-CNOs) were unable to offer protons to the medium, switching the ξ-potential to positive values. The SEM analysis of UZCNOs hydrogel exhibited a sponge-like structure with porous morphology.

All these absorption bands of pristine zein were altered in the FTIR spectrum of UZCNOs hydrogel composite, suggesting that there were hydrophobic interactions or π-π stacking between the zein protein and f-CNOs. Thus, UZCNOs hydrogel composite showed a peak at 1665 cm^{-1} for C=O stretching vibration and amide-I, whereas, 1525 cm^{-1} for amide II and the C–N bond, respectively. Likewise, the N–H bending and C–N stretching peaks of UZCNOs hydrogel were shifted to a higher frequency range, which reveals that f-CNOs were completely blended within the hydrogel matrix. Thus, FTIR spectra show physicochemical interactions between zein protein and f-CNOs. The tensile results suggest that the UZCNOs hydrogel produced by acoustic cavitation has exhibited approximately seven times higher tensile strength than CZCNOs hydrogel produced by a conventional stirring method. Accordingly, the mechanical measurements reveal that the hydrogel fabrication method could be critical to obtaining enhanced tensile properties.

The percentage of the swelling ratio of the CZCNOs hydrogel synthesized by the traditional stirring method was significantly lower than UZCNOs and MZCNOs (Figure 5a). This could be due to the difference in crosslinking density. By comparing the swelling results from Figure 5a, it can be revealed that the swelling ratio of CZCNOs hydrogel was remarkably lower than MZCNOs and UZCNOs hydrogels, which indicates that the crosslinking density was higher for hydrogels fabricated by radiation and acoustic cavitation. The UZCNOs hydrogels showed the lowest degradation in 25 days of incubation. This could be due to the existence of moderate electrostatic interactions and the difference in crosslinking density under the microwave method. Overall, the fabrication method had a considerable impact on the degradation measurements.

The UZCNOs hydrogels exhibited higher drug release than MZCNOs and CZCNOs hydrogels at pH 2.0 and 4.5. This could be due to the π-π stacking and Van der Waal forces between hydrogels and 5-FU. These characteristics might have slowed the diffusion rate of 5-FU from the composite hydrogels. Besides, it is hypothesized that the solubility and diffusion of 5-FU dawdled in the presence of f-CNOs. Moreover, the fabrication method, lower swelling ratio, and mobility of f-CNOs played a key role in the drug release measurements. In addition, UZCNOs hydrogel showed improved drug release (97%) at pH 7.4. We relate this to the high swelling ratio of the hydrogels at pH 7.4. Furthermore, the 5-FU release rate is significantly proportional to the swelling behavior of the hydrogel network. Whereas at pH 9.0 we did not see a significant improvement in the drug release of MZCNOs and CZCNOs specimens by increasing from pH 7.4 to pH 9.0, however, the UZCNOs hydrogel sample exhibited burst release followed by sustained drug release up to 15 days of study. It could be due to the hydrophilic nature of 5-FU within the gel matrix, which led to faster diffusion from the hydrogel into the medium.

The drug release results at pH 7.4 and 9.0 are attributed to π–π stacking of 5-FU molecules on the surface of composite hydrogels. 5-FU is a chemotherapeutic agent and is used clinically for colorectal carcinoma and there is a great need for colon-specific controlled delivery systems to treat directly at a disease site in the colon [39]. The results of in vitro 5-FU release from zein/f-CNOs suggest that the UZCNOs could be a prospective pH-sensitive transporter for colon-specific drug delivery. It is well known that the natural pH environment of the gastrointestinal tract differs from acidic (stomach) to slightly basic (intestinal). Particularly, the gastrointestinal tract increases its pH environment from the stomach (pH 1.4–3.0) to the terminal ileum (pH 7.5 ± 0.5). Such pH environment decreases to 6.4 ± 0.6 at the beginning of the colon, which slightly rises to pH 6.6 ± 0.8 in the middle of the colon and reaches 7.0 ± 0.7 in the left colon [40]. Therefore, it is important to consider the pH environment of the gastrointestinal tract while designing peroral dosage forms. The pH-responsive release of 5-FU from the UZCNOs hydrogels could indicate that zein/f-CNOs composite has an admirable protective effect for the oral delivery system of peptides and other drugs, which are easily ruined by gastric acid. Thus, the loaded drug can be released in a lesser amount from the hydrogel as it travels through the stomach. After reaching the colon, a significant amount of drug retained in the gel matrix could be released from the hydrogel.

Besides, UZCNOs hydrogels displayed higher cell viability ($p < 0.05$) than MZCNOs and CZCNOs hydrogels. This could be due to the enhanced tensile strength, lower degradation, higher hydrophobicity, and crosslinking density of UZCNOs hydrogel synthesized by acoustic cavitation method. The cell viability results revealed that the percentage of cell viability was dependent on the fabrication method of hydrogels. Moreover, cell viability suggests that UZCNOs composite hydrogels would useful as potential drug transporters with good cytocompatibility.

The LIVE/DEAD results suggest that the cell growth was considerably enhanced with f-CNOs inclusion and cells were extensively attached on the surface of the composite hydrogels. This could be due to the excellent cytocompatibility behavior and less degradability of f-CNOs. Overall, UZCNOs hydrogels exhibited better cell growth than a controller, MZCNOs, and CZCNOs samples. The LIVE/DEAD measurements also suggest a positive effect of f-CNOs on the osteoblast cells. Moreover, spherical cellular morphology was also observed on the surface of the hydrogels due to a contact angle with the cell medium, surface morphology, and surface chemical interactions of cells with hydrogels. In addition, it is also posited that the homogeneous colloidal dispersion of f-CNOs within the hydrogel matrix and wrapping with zein produced strengthened zein/f-CNOs hydrogels with amenable cytocompatibility. Nonetheless, improved mechanical strength, admiral cytocompatibility, the pH-responsive sustained drug release, and good pH-sensitivity of UZCNOs hydrogels can be useful as potential drug transporters for oral colon delivery systems and cartilage tissue engineering.

Author Contributions: Conceptualization, N.M.; methodology, A.G.-O.; formal analysis, I.L.R.; investigation, N.M., A.G.-O., I.L.R., and E.V.B.; resources, data curation, writing—original draft preparation, project administration, and funding acquisition, N.M.; writing—review and editing, E.V.B.

Acknowledgments: We gratefully acknowledge Consejo Nacional de Ciencia y Tecnología de México (CONACYT) for the materials and Tecnologico de Monterrey for the infrastructure facilities.

References

1. Sangeetha, K.; Thamizhavel, A.; Girija, E.K. Effect of gelatin on the in situ formation of Alginate/Hydroxyapatite nanocomposite. *Mater. Lett.* **2013**, *91*, 27–30. [CrossRef]
2. Annabi, N.; Tamayol, A.; Uquillas, J.A.; Akbari, M.; Bertassoni, L.E.; Cha, C.; Camci-Unal, G.; Dokmeci, M.R.; Peppas, N.A.; Khademhosseini, A. 25th anniversary article: Rational design and applications of hydrogels in regenerative medicine. *Adv. Mater.* **2014**, *26*, 85–124. [CrossRef] [PubMed]

3. Alge, D.L.; Anseth, K.S. Bioactive hydrogels: Lighting the way. *Nat. Mater.* **2013**, *12*, 950–952. [CrossRef]
4. Yue, K.; Trujillo-de Santiago, G.; Alvarez, M.M.; Tamayol, A.; Annabi, N.; Khademhosseini, A. Synthesis, properties, and biomedical applications of gelatin methacryloyl (GelMA) hydrogels. *Biomaterials* **2015**, *73*, 254–271. [CrossRef] [PubMed]
5. West, J.L. Protein-patterned hydrogels: Customized cell microenvironments. *Nat. Mater.* **2011**, *10*, 727–729. [CrossRef] [PubMed]
6. Silva, R.; Fabry, B. Boccaccini, A.R. Fibrous protein-based hydrogels for cell encapsulation. *Biomaterials* **2014**, *35*, 6727–6738. [CrossRef] [PubMed]
7. Zhang, Z.; Zhang, R.; Zou, L.; McClements, D.J. Protein encapsulation in alginate hydrogel beads: Effect of pH on microgel stability, protein retention and protein release. *Food Hydrocoll.* **2016**, *58*, 308–315. [CrossRef]
8. Hamid, H.; Sara, M.; Samuel, M.H.; Alan, E.T. Chitosan based hydrogels and their applications for drug delivery in wound dressings: A review. *Carbohydr. Polym.* **2018**, *199*, 445–460. [CrossRef] [PubMed]
9. Dorsey, S.M.; McGarvey, J.R.; Wang, H.; Nikou, A.; Arama, L.; Koomalsingh, K.J.; Kondo, N.; Gorman, J.H.; Pilla, J.J.; Gorman, R.C.; et al. MRI evaluation of injectable hyaluronic acid-based hydrogel therapy to limit ventricular remodeling after myocardial infarction. *Biomaterials* **2015**, *69*, 65–75. [CrossRef] [PubMed]
10. Thanavel, R.; Seong, S.A.A. Fibrinogen and fibrin based micro and nano scaffolds incorporated with drugs, proteins, cells and genes for therapeutic biomedical applications. *Int. J. Nanomed.* **2013**, *8*, 3641–3662.
11. Ravichandran, R.; Islam, M.M.; Alarcon, E.I.; Samanta, A.; Wang, S.; Lundstrom, P.; Hilborn, J.; Griffith, M.; Phopase, J. Functionalised type-I collagen as a hydrogel building block for bio-orthogonal tissue engineering applications. *J. Mater. Chem. B.* **2016**, *4*, 318–326. [CrossRef]
12. Labib, G. Overview on zein protein: A promising pharmaceutical excipient in drug delivery systems and tissue engineering. *Expert Opin. Drug Deliv.* **2018**, *15*, 65–75. [CrossRef] [PubMed]
13. Apoorva, G.; Mandeep, S.B. Ag Nanometallic Surfaces for Self-Assembled Ordered Morphologies of Zein. *ACS Omega.* **2018**, *3*, 10851–10857. [CrossRef]
14. De Folter, J.W.J.; Van Ruijven, M.W.M.; Velikov, K.P. Oil-in-water Pickering emulsions stabilized by colloidal particles from the water-insoluble protein zein. *Soft Matter.* **2012**, *8*, 6807–6815. [CrossRef]
15. Paliwal, R.; Palakurthi, S. Zein in controlled drug delivery and tissue engineering. *J. Control. Release* **2014**, *189*, 108–122. [CrossRef] [PubMed]
16. Zhang, Y.; Cui, L.; Che, X.; Zhang, H.; Shi, N.; Li, C.; Chen, Y.; Kong, W. Zein-based films and their usage for controlled delivery: Origin, classes and current landscape. *J. Control. Release* **2015**, *206*, 206–219. [CrossRef]
17. Lin, J.; Li, C.; Zhao, Y.; Hu, J.; Zhang, L.M. Co-electrospun nanofibrous membranes of collagen and zein for wound healing. *ACS Appl. Mater. Interfaces* **2012**, *4*, 1050–1057. [CrossRef]
18. Wang, Y.; Padua, G.W. Nanoscale characterization of zein self-assembly. *Langmuir* **2012**, *28*, 2429–2435. [CrossRef]
19. Chen, Y.; Ye, R.; Xu, H. Physicochemical Properties of Zein-Based Films by Electrophoretic Deposition Using Indium Tin Oxide Electrodes: Vertical and Horizontal Electric Fields. *Int. J. Food Prop.* **2016**, *19*, 945–957. [CrossRef]
20. Dong, F.; Zhang, M.; Tang, W.W.; Wang, Y. Formation and mechanism of superhydrophobic/hydrophobic surfaces made from amphiphiles through droplet-mediated evaporation-induced self-assembly. *J. Phys. Chem. B* **2015**, *119*, 5321–5327. [CrossRef]
21. Hao, L.; Lin, G.; Chen, C.; Zhou, H.; Chen, H.; Zhou, X. Phosphorylated Zein as Biodegradable and Aqueous Nanocarriers for Pesticides with Sustained-Release and anti-UV Properties. *J. Agric. Food Chem.* **2019**, *67*, 9989–9999. [CrossRef] [PubMed]
22. Mamidi, N.; Romo, I.L.; Leija Gutiérrez, H.M.; Barrera, E.V.; Elías-Zúñiga, A. Development of forcespun fiber-aligned scaffolds from gelatin-zein composites for potential use in tissue engineering and drug release. *MRS Commun.* **2018**, *8*, 885–892. [CrossRef]
23. Verdolotti, L.; Lavorgna, M.; Oliviero, M.; Sorrentino, A.; Iozzino, V.; Buonocore, G.; Iannace, S. Functional zein-siloxane biohybrids. *ACS Sustain. Chem. Eng.* **2014**, *2*, 254–263. [CrossRef]
24. Yoosaf, M.A.P.; Jayaprakash, A.; Ghosh, S.; Jaswal, V.S.; Singh, K.; Mandal, S.; Shahid, M.; Yadav, M.; Das, S.; Kumar., P. Zein film functionalized with gold nanoparticles and the factors affecting its mechanical properties. *RSC Adv.* **2019**, *9*, 25184–25188. [CrossRef]
25. Wu, Q.; Yoshino, T.; Sakabe, H.; Zhang, H.; Isobe, S. Chemical modification of zein by bifunctional polycaprolactone (PCL). *Polymer* **2003**, *44*, 3909–3919. [CrossRef]

26. Ugarte, D. Curling and closure of graphitic networks under electron-beam irradiation. *Nature* **1992**, *359*, 710–713. [CrossRef]
27. Han, F.D.; Yao, B.; Bai, Y.J. Preparation of carbon nano-onions and their application as anode materials for rechargeable lithium-ion batteries. *J. Phys. Chem. C.* **2011**, *115*, 8923–8927. [CrossRef]
28. Pech, D.; Brunet, M.; Durou, H.; Huang, P.H.; Mochalin, V.; Gogotsi, Y.; Taberna, P.L.; Simon, P. Ultrahigh-power micrometre-sized supercapacitors based on onion-like carbon. *Nat. Nanotechnol.* **2010**, *5*, 651–654. [CrossRef]
29. Mykhailiv, O.; Zubyk, H.; Plonska-Brzezinska, M.E. Carbon nano-onions: Unique carbon nanostructures with fascinating properties and their potential applications. *Inorg. Chim. Acta* **2017**, *468*, 49–66. [CrossRef]
30. Frasconi, M.; Marotta, R.; Markey, L.; Flavin, K.; Spampinato, V.; Ceccone, G.; Echegoyen, L.; Scanlan, E.M.; Giordani, S. Multi-Functionalized Carbon Nano-onions as Imaging Probes for Cancer Cells. *Chem A Eur. J.* **2015**, *21*, 19071–19080. [CrossRef]
31. Camisasca, A.; Giordani, S. Carbon nano-onions in biomedical applications: Promising theranostic agents. *Inorg. Chim. Acta* **2017**, *468*, 67–76. [CrossRef]
32. Yang, M.; Flavin, K.; Kopf, I.; Radics, G.; Hearnden, C.H.A.; McManus, G.J.; Moran, B.; Villalta-Cerdas, A.; Echegoyen, L.A.; Giordani, S.; et al. Functionalization of carbon nanoparticles modulates inflammatory cell recruitment and NLRP3 inflammasome activation. *Small* **2013**, *9*, 4194–4206. [CrossRef] [PubMed]
33. Luszczyn, J.; Plonska-Brzezinska, M.E.; Palkar, A.; Dubis, A.T.; Simionescu, A.; Simionescu, D.T.; KalskaSzostko, B.; Winkler, K.; Echegoyen, L. Small noncytotoxic carbon nano-onions: First covalent functionalization with biomolecules. *Chem - A Eur. J.* **2010**, *16*, 4870–4880. [CrossRef] [PubMed]
34. Mamidi, N.; Gamero, M.R.M.; Castrejón, J.V.; Zúníga, A.E. Development of ultra-high molecular weight polyethylene-functionalized carbon nano-onions composites for biomedical applications. *Diam. Relat. Mater.* **2019**, *97*, 107435. [CrossRef]
35. Rooze, J.; Rebrov, E.V.; Schouten, J.C.; Keurentjes, J.T.F. Dissolved gas and ultrasonic cavitation—A review. *Ultrason. Sonochem.* **2013**, *20*, 1–11. [CrossRef]
36. Wu, J.; Zhu, Y.J.; Cao, S.W.; Chen, F. Hierachically nanostructured mesoporous spheres of calcium silicate hydrate: Surfactant-free sonochemical synthesis and drug-delivery system with ultrahigh drug-loading capacity. *Adv. Mater.* **2010**, *22*, 749–753. [CrossRef]
37. Li, Z.F.; Yang, T.; Lin, C.M.; Li, Q.S.; Liu, S.F.; Xu, F.Z.; Wang, H.Y.; Cui, X.J. Sonochemical Synthesis of Hydrophilic Drug Loaded Multifunctional Bovine Serum Albumin Nanocapsules. *ACS Appl. Mater. Interfaces* **2015**, *7*, 19390–19397. [CrossRef]
38. Li, Z.; Du, X.; Cui, X.; Wang, Z. Ultrasonic-assisted fabrication and release kinetics of two model redox-responsive magnetic microcapsules for hydrophobic drug delivery. *Ultrason Sonochem.* **2019**, *57*, 223–232. [CrossRef]
39. Krishnaiah, Y.S.R.; Khan, M.A. Strategies of targeting oral drug delivery systems to the colon and their potential use for the treatment of colorectal cancer. *Pharm. Dev. Technol.* **2012**, *17*, 521–540. [CrossRef]
40. Amidon, S.; Brown, J.E.; Dave, V.S. Colon-Targeted Oral Drug Delivery Systems: Design Trends and Approaches. *AAPS PharmSciTech* **2015**, *16*, 731–741. [CrossRef]

6

Electrospinning of Cyclodextrin Functional Nanofibers for Drug Delivery Applications

Fuat Topuz * and Tamer Uyar *

Institute of Materials Science & Nanotechnology, UNAM-National Nanotechnology Research Center, Bilkent University, 06800 Ankara, Turkey

* Correspondence: fuat.topuz@rwth-aachen.de (F.T.); tamer@unam.bilkent.edu.tr (T.U.)

Abstract: Electrospun nanofibers have sparked tremendous attention in drug delivery since they can offer high specific surface area, tailored release of drugs, controlled surface chemistry for preferred protein adsorption, and tunable porosity. Several functional motifs were incorporated into electrospun nanofibers to greatly expand their drug loading capacity or to provide the sustained release of the embedded drug molecules. In this regard, cyclodextrins (CyD) are considered as ideal drug carrier molecules as they are natural, edible, and biocompatible compounds with a truncated cone-shape with a relatively hydrophobic cavity interior for complexation with hydrophobic drugs and a hydrophilic exterior to increase the water-solubility of drugs. Further, the formation of CyD-drug inclusion complexes can protect drug molecules from physiological degradation, or elimination and thus increases the stability and bioavailability of drugs, of which the release takes place with time, accompanied by fiber degradation. In this review, we summarize studies related to CyD-functional electrospun nanofibers for drug delivery applications. The review begins with an introductory description of electrospinning; the structure, properties, and toxicology of CyD; and CyD-drug complexation. Thereafter, the release of various drug molecules from CyD-functional electrospun nanofibers is provided in subsequent sections. The review concludes with a summary and outlook on material strategies.

Keywords: cyclodextrin; electrospinning; drug delivery; nanofibers; cyclodextrin-inclusion complexes; essential oils; electrospun nanofibers; poly-cyclodextrin; antibacterial; antibiotics

---

1. Introduction

Electrospun nanofibers of synthetic, natural, and hybrid systems have been widely exploited as drug delivery materials due to their high specific surface area, which allows enhanced drug loading and ability to modulate release profiles by structural tuning [1–11]. They can be engineered in various shapes, textures, and sizes with diameters down to a few nanometers. Further, the fiber surface can be modified with specific functional ligands or molecules to hinder them from the nonspecific adsorption of proteins or make them cell adhesive via decoration with cell binding ligands [3,12,13]. Drugs can be loaded into electrospun nanofibers by blending prior to electrospinning or using specific chemistry for the controlled release of drugs from the fiber matrix [14,15]. Although there are many pros of electrospun nanofibers for drug delivery applications, they cannot serve as injectable drug reservoirs. On the other hand, the drug-loaded nanowebs or fiber-deposited meshes are quite promising as wound dressing materials [11,12]. Apart from their physical protection to the injured tissue, they can provide the sustained release of the entrapped drugs to achieve wound debridement and wound healing simultaneously [16]. In this regard, comprehensive reviews on the use of electrospun nanofibers for wound healing are available [16,17]. Likewise, the use of CyD-based hydrogel materials for wound dressing has been reviewed in detail [18]. As most drugs are hydrophobic compounds and thus not intrinsically water soluble, the incorporation of a considerable amount of drug molecules into electrospun nanofibers while maintaining their activity can be problematic. In this context, the use of CyD enhances the solubility of the embedded drugs while keeping them stable and bioavailable for enhanced therapy results. The drug release can take place as CyD/drug ICs, if CyD are not chemically attached to the material, or by altering the surrounding conditions that lead to entropically unfavorable inclusion complexation.

The use of drug-loaded electrospun mats as implant materials has taken considerable interest in wound healing. The release of the embedded drugs can take place with the degradation of nanofibers. With that, the entrapped drug molecules can be released from the fiber matrix. Particularly, the use of some specific drugs can accelerate wound healing process and reduce pain. Furthermore, the drug release can be tuned by the structure of the fiber components: sustained drug release can be obtained for the electrospun fibers made by hydrophobic polymers or structurally tuned fiber systems. In one example, core-sheath structured nanofibers with core-loading of hydroxycamptothecin (HCPT) were used on mice via intratumoral implantation [19]. The use of hydroxypropyl β-CyD (HP-β-CyD) molecules as an additive significantly fastened the HCPT release and allowed the higher degradation of emulsion electrospun fibers. The higher release of the loaded HCPT was ascribed to the distribution pattern of HP-β-CyD and HCPT within the fibers. In another example, CyD inclusion complexes (CyD:ICs) with perfluoroperhydrophenanthrene (PFP) as oxygen carriers to cells seeded on the electrospun scaffolds of poly(carbonate urethane) (PCU) and polycaprolactone (PCL) [20]. The ICs of PFP and CyD significantly increased the amount of the dissolved oxygen. Such a concept can be exploited in in vivo applications to fasten the healing of wounded tissues.

In the electrospinning, the texture, size, and structure of nanofibers can be tailored over electrospinning parameters and polymer formulation [21]. Such control on the fiber structure endows them with enhanced performance in drug loading and allows the sustained release of the embedded drug molecules. In this regard, several polymer-based fiber systems were implemented in drug delivery applications [1,22]. Particularly, biocompatible polymers are preferably chosen since they do not release any toxic products during their use. In this regard, polycaprolactone (PCL), poly-L-lactic acid (PLLA), and polycaprolactone/poly(ethylene oxide) (PCL/PEO) are the most widely used polymeric materials [23–26]. The degradation of such nanofibers takes place over hydrolysis, starting from the surface to the core through surface erosion without leaving any toxic byproducts [27]. Along with the fiber degradation, the entrapped drug molecules are released from the fiber matrix. The sustained drug release from such polymers is greatly influenced by the structural features of polymers (e.g., hydrophobicity and glass-transition temperature (T_g)) and the type of the used spinneret system. In this context, a comprehensive review on the sustained release of drugs from electrospun nanofibers was reported by Chou et al., in which the release from uniaxial and coaxial nanofibers from various polymers was deliberately discussed [28]. When hydrophilic electrospun nanofibers are used, the degradation mostly follows bulk erosion with the breakage of hydrolytically labile bonds. In other words, the bulk erosion takes place once the water diffusion is much faster than the scaffold degradation, followed by mass loss throughout the bulk of the material [29].

The crucial problems in drug delivery applications are (i) uncontrolled release of drug molecules (i.e., burst release), (ii) unsustainable drug delivery, (iii) low drug loading, and (iv) low stability and bioavailability of drugs. In this regard, the electrospinning can minimize these problems to some extent because of its unique features, including easy to use with tailored-made fiber properties and applicability to a wide range of materials, such as polymers, composites, and ceramics with fiber sizes ranging from nanometer to micrometer. Further, the functionalization of electrospun nanofibers with pharmaceutical excipients, such as CyD, improves their performance in drug delivery applications. CyD comprise unique features that are often desired in drug delivery carriers. For instance, drug molecules can be entrapped into the hydrophobic molecular-environment of CyD by inclusion-complexation, which dramatically increases the stability of drug molecules under harsh conditions, e.g., high temperature, sunlight, and pH [30]. Further, such complexation remarkably increases their water solubility since many drugs are hydrophobic molecules. Most importantly, for a drug molecule to be pharmacologically active, it should have significant water solubility and lipophilicity to be able to permeate biological membranes through passive diffusion so that no accumulation occurs that can give rise to toxicity. In this regard, lipophilic CyD may assist them in crossing the biological membranes through component extraction or fluidization and can minimize the immunogenic response of body [31]. Further, the surface of the electrospun nanofibers becomes crucial for their in vivo applications since the biocompatibility of the nanofibers and their interactions with the immune system are greatly defined by their surface chemistry. Undesired protein adsorption may occur rapidly when the material is implanted. The adsorbed proteins can denature on hydrophobic surfaces and thus affect the immune system and wound healing. Hence, the surface chemistry becomes a highly critical factor when the fiber mats are intended to be used in in vivo drug delivery.

CyD-functional electrospun nanofibers have been engineered using different approaches. Although most research has been focused on CyD/drug inclusion-complexes (ICs)-embedded polymeric electrospun nanofibers, the recent decade has witnessed significant advances in the polymer-free electrospinning of CyD and their use in drug delivery applications. Functional electrospun nanofibers were also produced using poly-cyclodextrin (polyCyD) molecules in the fiber matrix. In this regard, various active agents either with anticancer, antibacterial, antioxidant or anthelmintic properties have been incorporated into such nanofibers and exploited in drug delivery systems. In the first part of this review, some of the intriguing features of CyD and the mechanism of inclusion-complexation and drug solubility/stability are given. Afterward, several approaches based on CyD-functional nanofibers for drug delivery applications are discussed. The review ends with a future outlook and concluding remarks.

2. Electrospinning

Electrospinning is a versatile process that relies on the jetting of a viscous solution or polymer melt under an electrical field [32]. With the evaporation of solvent molecules, the solidified jet is directed to a collector by electrical forces. During the electrospinning, the fiber is subjected to many different forces, including aerodynamic, inertial, gravitational, rheological, and tensile forces [33,34]. Once an electrical voltage is applied, free charges in the solution lead to the movement and rapidly transfer a force to the electrospinning solution to flow. In this regard, the surface tension, viscoelasticity, and charge density of electrospinning solutions are the key factors for the formation of electrospun nanofibers. The texture, morphology, and size of the nanofibers depend on the processing parameters and solution properties. Mostly, polymeric solutions were used to produce continuous electrospun fibers due to their high viscosity and the presence of intra- and intermolecular interactions. Sometimes, because of the instability of the jet of polymer solutions, the formation of beaded fibers can be observed [35–37]. However, with increasing viscosity or tailoring other solution parameters, bead-free electrospun nanofibers can be obtained [37]. Further, various additives can be incorporated in the electrospinning solution to produce functional nanofibers.

The fiber stability can be provided using either hydrophobic molecules or cross-linking approaches to attain water-insoluble fiber meshes. The main advantages of the electrospinning process are as follows: (i) easy to operate, (ii) adaptability to various polymeric systems, and (iii) suitability to prepare the nanofibers with various diameters, textures, and structures. Figure 1 shows a general representation of an electrospinning setup together with some important processing parameters and nanofibers in various forms. The presence of additives can lead to nanofibers with different morphologies. Various nanoparticles can be loaded in the electrospinning solutions by blending to yield hybrid fibers, or the thermal treatment of nanofibers impregnated with inorganic or metallic precursors. Using different spinneret systems, hollow, core-shell, and triaxial fiber structures can be obtained. Particularly, the co-axial fibers show better sustained release profiles than uniaxial fiber systems as the outer shell acts as a molecular gate in the transport of drug molecules. The fiber size can simply be adapted by the electrospinning parameters or solution conductivity while the solution properties allow the fabrication of ultrafine fibers having diameters in the nanoscale with different morphologies and textures (Figure 1). In general, increasing the polymer concentration, and flow rate causes the formation of larger nanofibers [38]. On the other hand, the fiber diameter decreases with increasing distance between the needle and collector and solution conductivity [38]. In this regard, the addition of salts is a common approach to produce thinner nanofibers for various polymeric systems [39].

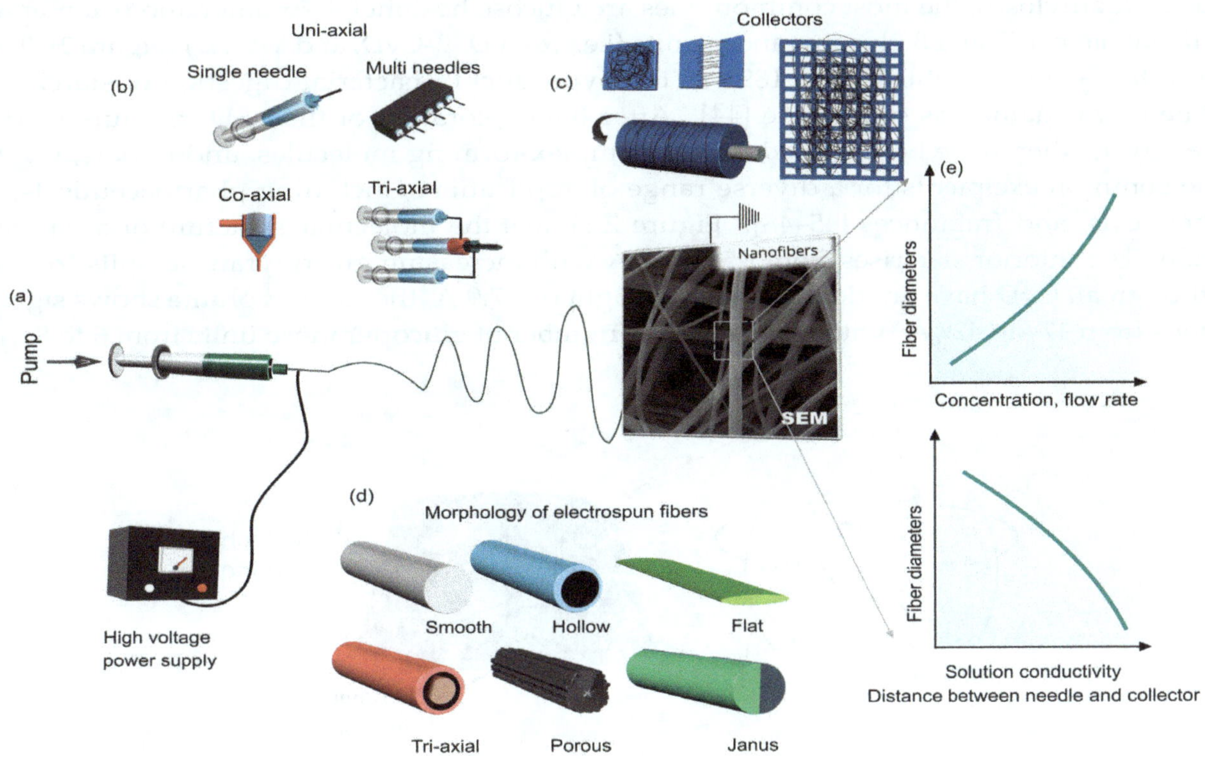

Figure 1. An electrospinning setup with important parameters is shown. (**a**) A cartoon scheme of an electrospinning system with the scanning electron micrograph of electrospun fibers, (**b**) common spinneret systems used in electrospinning, (**c**) collector types, (**d**) the morphology of electrospun fibers, and (**e**) diagrams showing the influence of electrospinning process parameters and solution properties on the electrospun fibers.

3. Cyclodextrins

Cyclodextrins (CyD) are cyclic oligosaccharides of glucopyranose formed during enzyme-catalyzed degradation of starch by glucosyltransferase over chain splitting and intramolecular rearrangement [40]. The molecular structure of CyD resembles a torus-like molecular ring, of which the interior is partially hydrophobic, while the exterior is hydrophilic because of many hydroxyl groups [41]. The inner cavity of CyD accommodates small hydrophobic molecules or portions of large compounds that can fit into their cavities [42]. Owing to their complexation with a wide spectrum of lipophilic molecules, CyD have been implemented in diverse applications, including solubilization enhancers, drug delivery, textile and food industry, tissue engineering, and allied applications [41].

CyD molecules do not elicit an immune response, have low toxicity, and hence are extensively used in bio-related fields, particularly to improve the bioavailability of drugs. In the following section, brief information is provided on the structure, properties, and toxicology of CyD and their inclusion-complexation with guest molecules.

3.1. Structure and Properties of Cyclodextrins

Due to the $^4C_1$ chair conformation (all equatorial groups in $^4C_1$ become axial and vice versa) of each glucopyranose unit, CyD have a shape of a hollow truncated cone, of which the cavity interior has a partial hydrophobic character because of hydrogen atoms of C-3, C-5, and the oxygen atoms of the glycosidic link [43]. Whereas the exterior of CyD is hydrophilic owing to the presence of several hydroxyl groups. Although the existence of numerous CyD with various ring sizes in the class of cycloamyloses, the most common ones are glucose hexamer, heptamer and octamer, which respectively have 6, 7, and 8 glucopyranose units (i.e., α-CyD, β-CyD, and γ-CyD) (Figure 2). The first reference to CyD was published in 1891 as the byproduct of bacterial digestion of starch, and at that time it was named as cellulosine [44]. After the exploration of their 3D structure in 1942 by X-ray analysis, they have been considered as complex-forming molecules, and to date, CyD have become common excipients for a diverse range of applications, including pharmaceuticals, foods, agrochemicals, and fragrances [45–48]. Figure 2 shows the molecular structure of a native CyD molecule. The interior size rises from ~5 to ~8 Å with increasing glucopyranose units from 6 to 8. Even though all CyD have an identical cavity height of ~7.9 Å, the cavity volume shows significant variations from 174 to 427 $Å^3$ with increasing the number of glucopyranose units from 6 to 8.

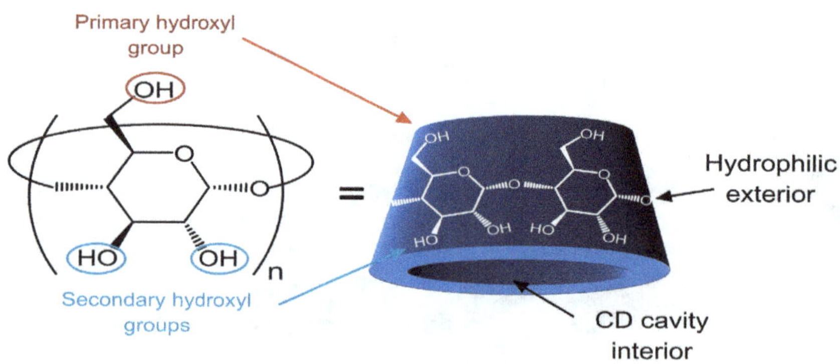

	α-CyD	β-CyD	γ-CyD
Number of glucose	6	7	8
Molecular weight (g/mol)	973	1135	1297
Water solubility (g/L)	145	18.5	232
Internal diameter (Å)	4.7-5.3	6.0-6.5	7.5-8.3
External diameter (Å)	14.6	15.4	17.5
Cavity volume ($Å^3$)	174	262	427
Height (Å)	7.9	7.9	7.9

Figure 2. The chemical structure and the representative cartoon illustration of a native cyclodextrin (CyD) molecule in the 3D form. The general characteristics of CyD are given in the inset table [49].

Due to intermolecular hydrogen bonds, native CyD are not very water-soluble compounds. Particularly, β-CyD molecule has very limited water solubility (~18.5 g/L) while α-CyD and γ-CyD molecules have better water solubility at 145 and 232 g/L, respectively. The poor solubility of β-CyD is originated by the formation of a hydrogen-bond network between the secondary hydroxyl groups [50]. To enhance the water-solubility of the native CyD, they have been chemically modified with different functional groups via amination, esterification, or etherification to break 2-OH-3-OH hydrogen bonds. This also causes the loss of crystallization due to the formation of a statistically substituted material that is made up of many isomeric components with the resultant amorphous, highly soluble end-product. The relatively hydrophobic character of the cavity interior makes CyD ideal molecular carriers of numerous hydrophobic molecules, whose size should be small enough to fit into the cavity. In this context, CyD can form host-guest complexes with a diverse range of organic molecules, inorganic ions, rare gases, and coordination compounds [51–54]. For interested readers, comprehensive reviews on all aspects of CyD and their applications in drug delivery are available [40,55,56].

3.2. Toxicological Issues of Cyclodextrins

For their bio-related applications, CyD must possess some critical conditions, such as biocompatibility and biodegradation. CyD are biocompatible pharmaceutical excipients and have found a wide spectrum of biological use. Even though they have many applications, there are some critical remarks that must be taken into account in their in vivo use. CyD are relatively stable molecules against degradation by human enzymes, and, in this regard, it was reported that after intravenous uptake of CyD by humans, they are excreted intact via the kidney. On the other hand, CyD can be degraded by bacterial and fungal enzymes (i.e., amylases), and hence, in the body, CyD are metabolized in the colon before excretion. The toxicity of CyD arises from their administration route; for instance, for mice exposed to CyD intravenously, the dose that causes 50% death (LD_{50}) is 1.0 g/kg, 0.79 g/kg, and more than 4.0 g/kg for α-CyD, β-CyD, and γ-CyD, respectively [57,58]. Particularly, the uptake of high β-CyD content caused toxicity because of its low water solubility (i.e., 18.5 g/L) [59]. The poor water solubility of β-CyD led to microcrystalline precipitation in the kidney. Further, β-CyD altered the cell membrane permeability by leading hemolysis because of the binding and extraction of cholesterol through inclusion-complexation [60]. Likewise, Zimmer et al. reported that HP-β-CyD interact with cholesterol crystals and dissolve them, which enhance oxysterol production and promote the anti-inflammatory reprogramming of macrophages [61]. Moreover, β-CyD damage renal cells by the extraction of cholesterol from kidney membrane and lead to nephrotoxicity [62]. In vivo studies showed the insignificant amount of CyD adsorbed from the intestinal tract in intact form. The major part of orally administered CyD is metabolized in the colon, and the primary metabolites are further metabolized to CO_2 and H_2O. Because of structural differences between native CyD and CyD derivatives, the adsorption, distribution, and excretion of CyD might have different profiles. Even though the oral administration of CyD did not reveal any significant toxicity, some studies reported their adverse effects on long-term parenteral administration. In this regard, Kantner et al. reported subcutaneous long-term administration of HP-β-CyD with a daily dose of 200 mg/kg resulted in increased bone resorption and bone loss [63]. Even at low dosages (50 mg/kg), minor changes in bone metabolism were also observed. The 2-hydroxypropylation of β-CyD minimizes these toxic effects due to high water solubility of the resultant compound with the condition of less than 1.5% unmodified β-CyD presence. The native β-CyD have been approved in the USA as Generally Recognized as Safe (GRAS) [64]. Likewise, the modified CyD, particularly hydroxypropyl (HP) β-CyD and sulfobutyl ether (SBE) β-CyD, are also included in the FDA (Food and Drug Administration) list as approved chemicals for human use [65]. The metabolism of CyD inclusion complexes (ICs) on oral administration of CyD-ICs, they rapidly dissociate, and the guest molecule leaves the cavity [66]. Thereafter, CyD and guest molecules are involved in the normal biological pathway to be metabolized and excreted from the body. Overall, CyD are generally non-toxic chemicals and can potentially be used for many different biological applications.

3.3. Mechanism of Cyclodextrin Inclusion-Complexation and Drug Solubility

Many drug molecules are poorly soluble molecules in water and, hence, have affinity to complex with CyD. As the inner cavity of CyD molecules has partial hydrophobic character, they can accommodate small lipophilic molecules into their cavities and significantly enhance their water-solubility via inclusion-complexation. The main driving force of the inclusion-complexation relies on hydrophobic interactions between guest molecules and the CyD cavity. Further, other forces, such as van der Waals and dipole-dipole interactions may also be involved in the inclusion-complexation [67,68]. The outer surface of CyD forms hydrogen bonds with water to make them water-soluble. In the inclusion-complexation, intermolecular interactions occur between

CyD and guest molecules as partial or the complete penetration of a guest molecule into the CyD cavity. Figure 3a depicts a guest molecule entrapped in the CyD cavity, driven by inclusion-complexation. The inclusion-complexation may also occur in diverse ways as shown in Figure 3a. Depending on the conditions, one guest molecule can complex with two CyD molecules or vice versa (i.e., two guest molecules with one CyD). The interaction between CyD and guest molecule is in an equilibrium directed by an equilibrium constant (K_c). Figure 3b displays the phase solubility plot for guest molecules, where the increased solubility is associated with the CyD concentration. Each line highlights the type of inclusion-complex (IC) formed, as well as its stoichiometry. Linear line (shown in pink color (i)) represents the formation of soluble IC, while the line in orange color (ii) depicts the formation of IC with limited solubility.

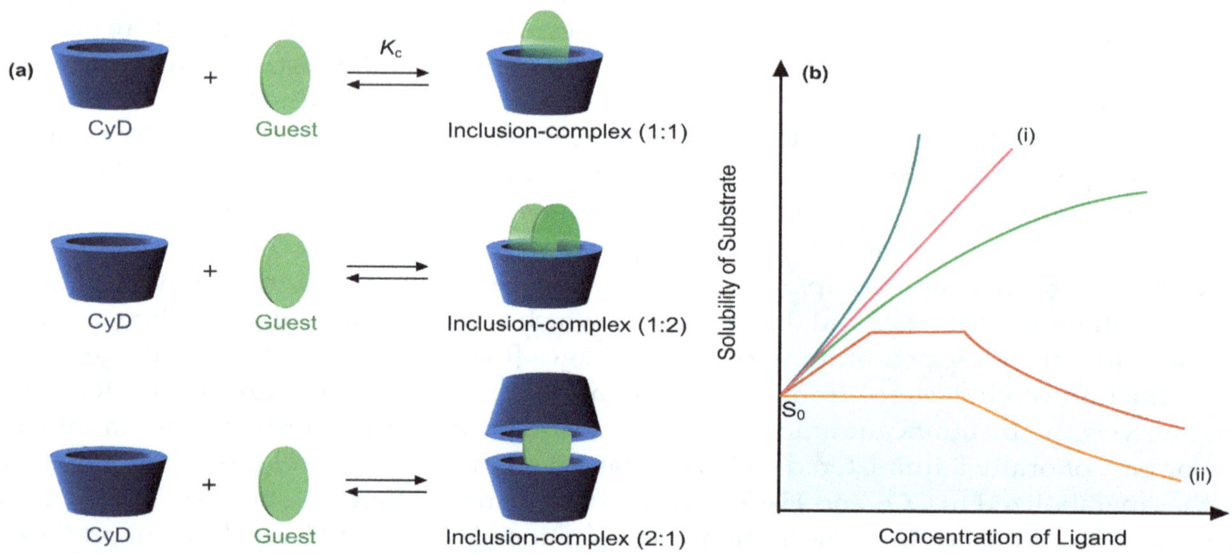

Figure 3. (**a**) The inclusion complex formation between CyD and guest molecules at various stoichiometries. (**b**) The plot shows a phase solubility of guest molecules; (i) represents the formation of soluble inclusion-complex (IC), and (ii) denotes the formation of IC with limited solubility.

Many studies have reported that the inclusion-complexation is governed by van der Waals, electrostatic forces, hydrophobic interactions, hydrogen bonding, and the release of conformational strain [43,69–71]. Some parameters define the strength and relative stability of the complexation. Particularly, the size of cavity and guest molecule, the presence of modified groups in the CyD structure, polarity, and substitution groups on the guest molecule, and environmental conditions, such as medium, ionic strength, and temperature, are prominent factors that can affect the relative strength of inclusion-complexation [72,73]. Normally, a CyD molecule exists in a hydrated form in water—that is, CyD cavity accommodates many water molecules. In the presence of a guest molecule, the replacement between high-energy water molecules and a hydrophobic guest is favored because of an energetically unfavored state of water molecules in the hydrophobic cavity, [41,74]. In general, α-CyD forms complexes with aliphatic chains and molecules (e.g., PCL and poly(ethylene glycol) (PEG)) [75–77], whereas larger cavity of the β-CyD allows host-guest complexes with aromatic rings, such as polycyclic aromatic hydrocarbons (PAHs) [78,79] and essential oils [80,81].

3.4. Drug Stability and Release from Cyclodextrin Inclusion Complexes

One of the currently important issues in drug delivery is the stability of drug molecules on exposure to some harsh conditions. Particularly, biological drugs are sensitive because of their limited stability upon oral administration and during subsequent circulation. They have low bioavailability and short therapeutic half-lives [82]. In this regard, the CyD cavity is enrolled as a shield to protect them from degradation and increase their bioavailability. CyD are stable molecules and can maintain their torus-like molecular structure even at basic pH values [83]. Further, the pyrolysis of CyD molecules starts over 300 °C, implying their thermal stability at high temperature conditions [84]. The inner cavity of CyD molecules accommodates various hydrophobic small molecules and increases their thermal stability. In this regard, various volatile substances (e.g., essential oils) were treated with CyD molecules to form inclusion-complexes for extending their shelf-lives [85,86]. Major benefits of CyD in their drug delivery are (i) increasing the water solubility, stability and bioavailability, (ii) reducing the evaporation of volatile active agents, (iii) low degree of hemolysis, and (iv) avoiding admixture incompatibilities [50].

Hydrophobic and van der Waals interactions are the main dominant driving forces for inclusion-complexation [87]. Therefore, the stability of CyD-ICs is highly dependent on the surrounding conditions that influence these interactions: if pH, ionic strength and temperature of the medium change, guest molecules may leave the CyD cavity because of an energetically unfavored state [72]. This can also be achieved by altering other conditions, making CyD-IC thermodynamically unfavorable.

4. Cyclodextrin Functional Electrospun Nanofibers for Drug Delivery Systems

Various CyD-functional electrospun nanofiber-based materials have been reported as drug delivery systems. These include the blending of polymers with CyD/drug ICs and using CyD-based polymers with drugs. Further, the electrospun nanofibers of only CyD/drug ICs were also performed without the requirement of a polymeric carrier. Due to the absence of a polymeric component, such nanostructured materials present high loading of active agents complexed with CyD for their use in drug delivery. In the following sections, we subcategorize CyD-functional electrospun nanofibers by means of their route of preparation.

4.1. Cyclodextrin-Drug Encapsulated Electrospun Polymeric Nanofibers for Drug Delivery Applications

This is the simplest method to engineer drug-encapsulated electrospun nanofibers through the blending of components (i.e., CyD, drug and polymeric matrix). Generally, CyD and drug are mixed to form inclusion complexes (ICs), and then, blended with the polymer solution, of which the electrospinning produces drug-encapsulated nanofibers. The inclusion-complexation with CyD motifs significantly enhances the water solubility of drug molecules so that high loading capacities can be achieved. In this regard, the Uyar research group reported naproxen (NAP)-CyD ICs loaded PCL nanofibers [88]. Naproxen (NAP), a non-steroidal anti-inflammatory drug, is used in the treatment of pain, inflammation, and fever [89,90]. Due to its lipophilic nature, it is practically insoluble in water at low pH, while it becomes soluble at high pH. To make them water-soluble under mild conditions, their ICs were prepared by slowly adding β-CyD into the aqueous solution of NAP, and the solution was stirred overnight in water until it became cloudy. Thereafter, the solution was freeze-dried, and IC powder was obtained. The complexation between CyD and NAP significantly enhanced the water solubility of NAP. The ICs were mixed with PCL solution and electrospun to form nanofibers. The mean diameter of PCL nanofibers slightly increased from ~335 to ~390 nm with the incorporation of NAP-β-CyD ICs. The release studies showed enhanced release of NAP from NAP-β-CyD ICs encapsulated PCL nanofibers when compared to the pristine NAP-loaded PCL nanofibers prepared in the absence of CyD. Likewise, Akduman et al. reported naproxen-CyD embedded polyurethane nanofibers and observed that the complete release of NAP from the only polyurethane fiber matrix took 120 h while the use of β-CyD or HP-β-CyD reduced the delivery time for NAP to ~36 and 5 h, respectively [91]. The difference in the release profiles from both CyD was due to the solubility difference of β-CyD and HP-β-CyD; HP-β-CyD has much higher water solubility than the unsubstituted β-CyD.

The Uyar research group also reported hydroxypropyl cellulose (HPC) nanofibers impregnated with sulfisoxazole/CyD ICs [92]. Sulfisoxazole (SFS) is a sulfonamide drug with antibiotic properties [93]. Because of its low water solubility (i.e., <0.1 g per 100 mL), it was mixed with HP-β-CyD to form inclusion-complexation, which significantly increased the water solubility of SFS for enhanced therapy results. Thereafter, ICs were mixed with HPC, and the resultant mixture was electrospun to obtain ultrafine nanofibers. The IC-loaded nanofibers had a mean fiber diameter of 60 ± 25 nm, while sole SFS-loaded nanofibers (i.e., produced in the absence of CyD) sized 90 ± 40 nm, suggesting the use of ICs as an additive reduced the fiber diameter. However, the incorporation of IC did not make any significant impact on the fiber morphology. Although the initial release of SFS from the fiber matrix was fast, the complete release process took 12 h. The inclusion-complexation increased the release rate of SFS than those released from the HPC fiber matrix in the absence of CyD. Further, a sandwich-like fiber system was engineered by placing HPC/SFS/HP-β-CyD-IC nanofibers between PCL nanowebs. This nanofiber system slowed the release rate of SFS than the fiber prepared without PCL nanofibers. Tonglairoum et al. reported clotrimazole (CZ) loaded nanofibers through electrospinning [94]. A multicomponent fiber system containing CZ-loaded polyvinylpyrrolidone (PVP)/hydroxypropyl-β-cyclodextrin (HP-β-CyD) was prepared, and the fiber surface was coated with chitosan-cysteine (CS-SH)/poly(vinyl alcohol) (PVA) to increase the mucoadhesive properties and achieve the sustained release of CZ from the nanofibers. CZ-loaded nanofibers were successful in killing *Candida* significantly faster than the commercially used CZ lozenges at 5, 15, and 30 min and were safe for 2 h incubation. The release profiles of the embedded CZ did not show significant variations, and 80–90% release was observed after 480 min. Overall, the nanofibers showed promising results in the treatment of oral candidiasis.

Voriconazole (VRC) is a triazole antifungal agent loaded as ICs with HP-β-CyD into poly(vinyl alcohol) (PVA) nanofibers and used for ophthalmic delivery [95]. The VRC-loading capacity could be enhanced with increasing CyD content. The total release of VRC took about 8 h from the nanofibers. Ocular irritation tests were performed on rabbit samples, and the Draize eye test results revealed that there was no ocular discomfort after the administration of the VRC nanofibers and VRC solution, suggesting that VRC-loaded PVA/HP-β-CyD composite nanofibers are promising non-irritant materials. Siafaka et al. reported voriconazole-loaded PCL nanofibers in the presence of β-CyD [96]. The ICs of VRC and β-CyD were mixed with PCL solution and electrospun to form nanofibers. VRC with various concentrations (5–20 wt.%) were loaded into nanofibers. All nanofibers showed an initial burst release of the VRC over 80%. The burst release was decreased with increasing VRC content. The nanofibers showed antifungal properties with the inhibition of *Candida albicans*. Opanasopit and co-workers reported fast releasing polyvinylpyrrolidone (PVP)/CyD composite nanofibers for the taste-masked meloxicam [97]. Meloxicam (MX) is a nonsteroidal anti-inflammatory drug molecule that is intended to be used in treating rheumatoid arthritis [98]. CyD molecules were blended to improve the fiber stability. MX was mixed with the CyD, and then PVP solution, of which the electrospinning led to nanofibers. In another CyD-based drug delivery system, electrospun mats were developed using PVP and HP-β-CyD/MX ICs [99]. MX was mixed with CyD molecules and electrospun in the presence of PVP in different solvent systems (dimethylformamide (DMF) and ethyl alcohol (EtOH)). HP-β-CyD molecules significantly improved the solubility of MX. A fast disintegration time and the burst release of MX were observed in an EtOH-based system. Furthermore, EtOH-based fiber system rapidly dissolved in the mouth. Cytotoxicity tests showed that the EtOH-system was much safer than the DMF-based system. Overall, the study showed a composite fiber of PVP and HP-β-CyD is ideal for fast-dissolving drug delivery to increase palatability of dosage forms.

Recently, Monteiro et al. reported tetracycline/β-CyD IC loaded PCL nanofibers [100]. Tetracycline (TCN) is a common drug used for periodontal disease treatment [101]. After the preparation of TCN/β-CyD ICs, they were incorporated in PCL solution and electrospun to form nanofibers. The half of the embedded-TCN released as a burst from the matrix and then a slow release profile was observed. Total release of the entrapped TCN took 350 min. The nanofibers showed antimicrobial activity against *Aggregatibacter actinomycetemcomitans* and *Porphyromonas gingivalis*. TCN was also released in a sustained manner from CyD-free electrospun fibers of PCL/Zein [102,103] and PCL/poly(ethylene-*co*-vinyl acetate) (PEVA) [104,105]. The incorporation of PCL into the zein fibers slowed the release rate of TCN. TCN release could also be tuned by multi-layered electrospun fibrous mats. In this regard, Alhusein et al. showed that the sustained release of TCN from triple-layered fibers of PCL and PEVA when TCN loaded PEVA fibers were used in the middle covered by TCN-free PCL fibers from both sides [105]. This dramatically reduced the burst release of TCN, demonstrating the importance of drug localization on the release profile. In this context, a detailed review on the controlled release of drugs, including TCN, from PCL-based fibers was reported by Blagbrough and colleagues [106]. Chen and coworkers used silk-fibroin based electrospun nanofibers impregnated with HP-β-CyD as the carrier of Tamoxifen [107]. Tamoxifen (TAM) is a selective estrogen receptor modulator and acts as antiestrogen by binding to the estrogen receptors to inhibit the growth of the malignant mammary tumors in some tissues [108]. It is also effective in patients with ER-positive metastatic breast cancer [109]. TAM was mixed with HP-β-CyD molecules to form ICs to make it water-soluble. Thereafter, the solution was mixed with silk-fibroin and electrospun to form composite fibers. The inclusion-complexation significantly decreased the fiber diameter. The effective loading of TAM was confirmed by the Raman analysis of the fibers. The release results showed that the TAM first dissociated from the ICs, and then, was subsequently released from the fiber matrix. The release occurs slowly, and 50% release was observed after two weeks of incubation, suggesting that the presented concept can be intended as a promising local drug delivery system for breast cancer therapy. Souza et al. recently reported PCL nanofibers impregnated with β-CyD-silver sulfadiazine ICs [110]. Silver sulfadiazine (SAg) pertains to a sulfanilamide class of chemicals and is known for its topical antimicrobial properties, and is commonly used for the treatment of infected burns [111]. After inclusion-complexation with β-CyD, the solution was electrospun in acetic acid to form fibers, whose diameters showed great variations depending on the components; the solution of 15 wt.% PCL led to nanofibers with a mean diameter 358 nm, while IC-loaded PCL nanofibers possessed a mean diameter of 892 nm, suggesting the IC incorporation led to a dramatic increase in the fiber diameter. The release studies showed that, after one day, ca. 80% of SAg was released from CyD-free PCL fibers, while the respective value was 66% from the IC-loaded PCL fibers. The nanofibers demonstrated antibacterial properties against *S. aureus* and *E. coli*.

Core-shell electrospun nanofibers impregnated with CyD functionalities have also been investigated in drug delivery applications. Generally, co-axial nanofibers promoted the sustained release of the entrapped drugs than the uniaxial fibers. In this regard, the Uyar research group reported the preparation of the core-shell nanofibers of curcumin/CyD IC and polylactic acid (PLA) [112]. The core of the nanofibers was IC of CyD and curcumin (CUR), while the shell layer was PLA. The formation of core-shell fiber structure was confirmed by TEM analysis with a contrast difference on the fibers. The slow release of CUR was achieved by core-shell nanofiber structure and the inclusion-complexation of CUR with HP-β-CyD provided high solubility. The embedded CUR showed antioxidant activity on the scavenging of 2,2-diphenyl-1-picrylhydrazyl (DPPH) radicals. CUR was also loaded into poly(vinyl alcohol) (PVA) nanofibers in a form of their complexes with CyD molecules [113]. The in vitro studies showed rapid diffusion of curcumin in the first hour followed by slower release. The nanofibers with low CUR loads showed faster release profiles. Another curcumin-loaded nanofiber system with multifunctional additives was developed using poly (L-lactic acid-*co*-ε-caprolactone) (PLACL) and Aloe Vera (AV), MgO nanoparticles, curcumin and β-CyD as a candidate material for breast cancer therapy [114]. These multifunctional nanofibers were tested with Michigan Cancer Foundation-7 (MCF-7) breast cancer cells. Depending on the fiber constituents, the proliferation of MCF-7 cells showed a clear decrease by 66% in PLACL/AV/MgO/CUR with respect to PLACL/AV/MgO nanofibrous scaffolds on day 9. The results demonstrated that 1% CUR interacting with MgO nanoparticles exhibited higher inhibition of MCF-7 cells among all other nanofibrous scaffolds, demonstrating their effectiveness for breast cancer therapy. Another PLLA-based nanofibers with CyD functionalities were prepared for the release of hydroxycamptothecin (HCPT) [115]. HCPT is an antitumor drug with poor water solubility, which restricts its use in clinical applications. The solution of PLLA and PEG was mixed with HP-β-CyD and HCPT and electrospun into nanofibers whose diameters slightly decreased from 780 to 700 nm in contrast to those nanofibers prepared in the absence of CyD and HCPT. The homogenous distribution of HCPT in the fiber matrix was confirmed by confocal analysis. The release studies revealed the initial burst release of ca. 15%, followed by a gradual release over 20 days. Increasing the HCPT content boosted the release percentage while the addition of higher CyD content minimized the burst release of HCPT. Recently, Masoumi et al. reported ciprofloxacin/CyD-encapsulated PCL nanofibers [116]. Ciprofloxacin (CIP) is an antibiotic drug molecule with poor water solubility and low dissolution rate, which limit its bioavailability [117]. CIP was mixed with α-CyD or β-CyD to form ICs and thereafter added to PCL solution. The electrospinning of these composite mixtures led to bead-free electrospun nanofibers loaded with CIP. The release tests were performed at pH = 7.2, and the released CIP content showed variations depending on the CyD-type and the preparation route of ICs; sonication-driven IC-loaded PCL fiber showed better release rate than those prepared without sonication. This can be ascribed to a higher amount of CIP entrapped in the CyD cavity under sonic energy.

The ICs of antifungal drug griseofulvin (GSV) [118], antipsychotic drug (aripiprazole) [119] and phytochemical (asiaticoside) [120] with CyD were also mixed with various polymeric matrices and electrospun to form drug-loaded nanofibers. The Uyar research group reported allyl isothiocyanate loaded PVA nanofibers and investigated their antibacterial properties [121]. The ICs of antibacterial agent allyl isocyanate (AITC) and β-CyD were loaded into the electrospun nanofibers of PVA. CyD molecules significantly stabilized AITC during the electrospinning because of inclusion-complexation. The release experiments were performed at three different temperatures (30, 50 and 75 °C) in gas phase, and the release was dramatically increased with higher temperature. The nanofibers showed antibacterial properties with the significant inhibition of *E. coli* and *S. aureus*. AITC/CyD ICs were also embedded in the electrospun nanofibers of soy protein isolate (SPI), PEO or PLLA [122]. Fiber morphologies were affected by the AITC concentration used. The AITC release was negligible under dry conditions but increased dramatically as relative humidity rose. Luo et al. reported CyD functional polymeric nanofibers for sequential release of vascular disrupting and chemotherapeutic agents from electrospun nanofibers [123]. Combretastatin A-4 (CA4) and hydroxycamptothecin (HCPT) were loaded in the nanofibers of poly(ethylene glycol)-polylactide (PELA) in the presence of HP-β-CyD. The sequential release of CA4 and HCPT could achieve a sequential killing of endothelial and tumor cells. Anthelmintic drugs were also released from CyD functional electrospun fibers. In this context, Vigh et al. reported flubendazole/HP-β-CyD IC embedded PVP nanofiber webs with enhanced oral bioavailability [124]. A forty milligram could be released in 15 min, and the administration of the nanofiber system led to an increased plasma concentration profile in rats in contrast to the practically non-absorbable crystalline flubendazole. This can be ascribed to the effect of the embedded CyD, which prevented the crystallization of flubendazole. Doxorubicin (DOX), a chemotherapy medicine, was released from the PLLA nanofibers in the form of their ICs with methylated-β-CyD in parallel to their release from CyD-free PLLA fibers [125]. The results showed that the use of CyD molecules led to controlled release, and 17% decrease in the burst release was observed, followed by a quantifiable sustained release up to two days. Metoclopramide hydrochloride (MH), a drug molecule that has been used to treat nausea and vomiting, was incorporated into HP-β-CyD functional PVA nanofibers, and the release of MA was performed in a phosphate buffer (pH = 6.8) at 37 °C [126]. 90% Release of MA took place in 1 min due to burst release of MA. CyD-functional electrospun nanofibers were also used for the delivery of proteins. In one example, β-lactamase BlaP protein was mixed with the solution of chitosan/PEO containing CyD molecules, and the resultant mixture was electrospun into fibers [127]. CyD were used to increase the protein stability. In the absence of protein, spindle-shaped fibers were formed. However, the protein addition gave rise to smooth, bead-free nanofibers. The activity of the β-lactamase tested over the hydrolysis of nitrocefin, and enhanced hydrolysis was observed for the CyD functional nanofibers, demonstrating that the embedded CyD stabilized the protein in the fiber matrix.

A blending method was also applied for the preparation of essential oil loaded CyD functional electrospun fibers. Essential oils are plant-derived phytochemicals with antibacterial and antimicrobial properties [128,129]. They have also shown antimutagenic and antifungal activities [130]. Opanasopit and colleagues reported plai oil/HP-β-CyD IC [131] and herbal oil/ HP-β-CyD IC [132] loaded PVP nanofibers and monitored release profiles of the oil from the fiber matrix. The release of plai oil from the fiber matrix demonstrated burst release and subsequent sustained release over 24 h. The release rate changed between 10 and 30% in 24 h depending upon the oil load in the fiber. The release of herbal oil took less than one minute. Lin et al. reported cinnamon essential oil (CEO)/CyD loaded PEO nanofibers [133]. In this regard, first CEO/β-CyD proteoliposomes were prepared by using a thin-lipid film evaporation-ultrasonic hydration-freeze and thaw technique. Afterwards, they mixed with PEO and electrospun to form bead-free nanofibers (Figure 4A). The CEO release studies were performed in ethanol, and the amount of CEO released from the fiber matrix was measured by GC-MS. In the presence of *Bacillus cereus*, the release of CEO was significantly enhanced. The CEO release from the nanofibers was about 30% in 96 h, whereas this increased to 80% in the presence of *B. cereus*. A similar effect was observed at higher temperature, which enhanced the release rate of CEO (Figure 4C). The resultant nanofibers showed significant inhibition against the growth of *B. cereus* due to the antibacterial property of CEO.

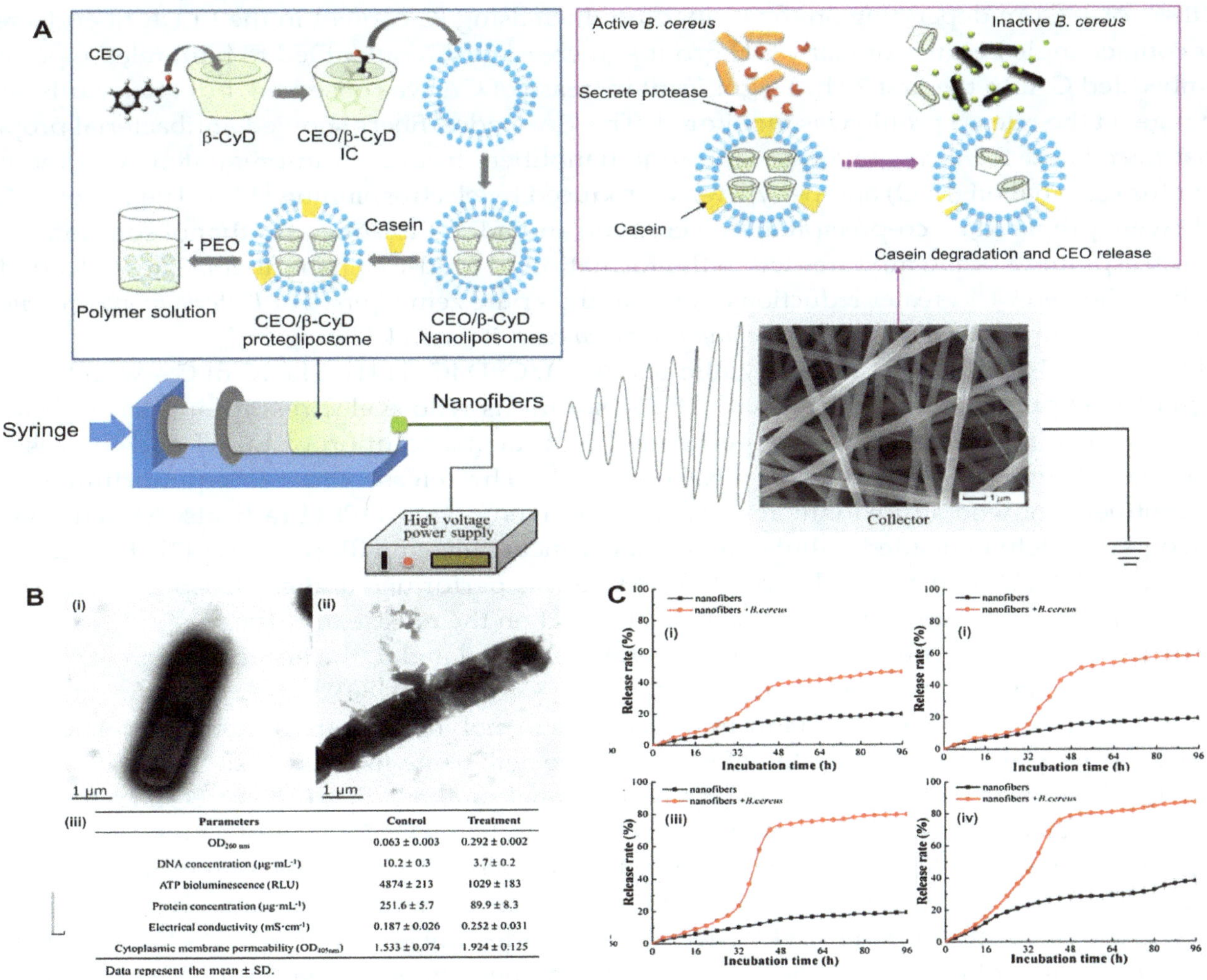

Parameters	Control	Treatment
$OD_{260\ nm}$	0.063 ± 0.003	0.292 ± 0.002
DNA concentration (μg·mL^{-1})	10.2 ± 0.3	3.7 ± 0.2
ATP bioluminescence (RLU)	4874 ± 213	1029 ± 183
Protein concentration (μg·mL^{-1})	251.6 ± 5.7	89.9 ± 8.3
Electrical conductivity (mS·cm^{-1})	0.187 ± 0.026	0.252 ± 0.031
Cytoplasmic membrane permeability (OD_{405nm})	1.533 ± 0.074	1.924 ± 0.125

Data represent the mean ± SD.

Figure 4. **(A)** Cartoon schemes of the production of CEO/β-CyD proteoliposomes incorporated poly(ethylene oxide) (PEO) fibers and *B. cereus* proteinase triggered cinnamon essential oil (CEO) delivery from CEO/β-CyD proteoliposomes. **(B)** TEM images of *B. cereus* before **(i)** and after the treatment **(ii)** of CEO/β-CyD proteoliposomes. **(iii)** The respective analysis results on the release of *B. cereus* cell constituents and the cell membrane permeability before and after proteoliposomes treatment. **(C)** The release rate of CEO/β-CyD proteoliposomes nanofibers stored at different temperatures 4 °C **(i)**, 12 °C **(ii)**, 25 °C **(iii)**, and 37 °C **(iv)** for 4 days. The figure was reproduced from [133] with the permission of Elsevier, 2017.

The cinnamon essential oil (CEO) was also encapsulated in PVA/β-CyD nanofibers, and in this context, the ICs of cinnamon and β-CyD were mixed with PVA solutions and electrospun to form nanofibers with a mean diameter of 240 ± 40 nm [134]. CyD molecules notably increased the thermal stability of CEO after complexation. Due to the intrinsic antimicrobial property of CEO, the nanofibers exhibited strong antimicrobial activity against *E. coli* and *S. aureus*. Furthermore, the entrapment in fiber systems prolonged the shelf-life of CEO. Cinnamon/β-CyD ICs were also loaded into PLLA fibers, and the nanofibers showed antimicrobial properties [135]. The same research group also reported an identical fiber system using lysozyme as an additive and observed the enhancement of the antimicrobial activity of cinnamon essential oil-loaded electrospun nanofilm by the incorporation of lysozyme [136]. Recently, Munhuweyi et al. reported that cinnamon and oregano essential oils–loaded PVA-CyD nanofibers [137]. The ICs of essential oils with β-CyD molecules were prepared and mixed PVA solutions, of which the electrospinning led to nanofibers varying between 120 and 180 nm in diameter depending on essential oil loading. Liu et al. reported cinnamaldehyde/CyD loaded PLLA fibers via electrospinning [138]. Cinnamaldehyde (CA) pertains to the class of essential oils and is known for its antibacterial and antioxidant properties [139]. The ICs of the β-CyD and CA were mixed with PLA and electrospun into fibers of 4–6 μm depending on the IC loading. Increasing IC content in the PLLA fiber decreased water contact angle because of many OH groups. Increasing IC content led to high release percent of the embedded CA. In the first 20 h, a significant increase of CA was observed, but afterwards, almost no change on the release profile was monitored. The CA-loaded fibers showed antibacterial properties against *E. coli* and *S. aureus*. Likewise, ultrafine nanofibers from zein impregnated with the ICs of eucalyptus essential oil (EEO) and β-CyD were produced by electrospinning [140]. The ICs of EEO and β-CyD were prepared by co-precipitation technique and added to aqueous ethanol solutions of zein. The electrospinning of the mixtures led to the formation of bead-free nanofibers. The IC-loaded zein nanofibers showed 24% greater reduction of growth than pure zein fibers. For *Listeria monocytogenes*, the growth reduction was 28.5%, and for *Staphylococcus aureus*, it was 24.3%.

PLLA was also used as a carrier of gallic acid (GA)/CyD ICs [141]. The IC of GA with HP-β-CyD molecules was prepared and mixed with PLLA solutions whose electrospinning led to bead-free nanofibers. The release studies were performed in aqueous solution of EtOH and increased GA release was observed with increasing EtOH content. The release came to equilibrium after 4 h. The nanofibers showed antioxidant activity in the scavenging of DPPH radicals. Mascheroni et al. reported perillaldehyde-loaded pullulan nanofibers functionalized with β-CyD [142]. The blending of pullulan and β-CyD with embedded perillaldehyde was performed and electrospun. The release of volatile perillaldehyde showed a profound effect of RH on the release profile.

The Uyar research group has reported several studies related to the encapsulation of CyD ICs of volatile active agents such as essential oils (e.g., eugenol [85], geraniol [86]) or fragrance/flavor molecules (e.g., menthol [143–145], vanillin [146]) into electrospun polymeric nanofibers in order to enhance the temperature stability and shelf-life of such volatile active agents. Likewise, hexanal, a naturally occurring volatile compound, released from CyD-functional xanthan fibers. The CyD-functional xanthan fibers showed faster release of hexanal than pure xanthan fibers [147]. Moreover, a type of vitamin E (α-tocopherol), an antioxidant, was incorporated into PLLA nanofibers after its complexation with γ-CyD molecules [148]. The PLLA/α-tocopherol/γ-CyD nanofibers showed antioxidant properties. The Uyar research group has also reported β-CyD/quercetin ICs loaded poly(acrylic acid) (PAA) nanofibers [149]. The electrospinning of the mixture of PAA, β-CyD and quercetin led to well-tuned nanofibers with a mean diameter of 270 nm. The nanofibers showed a burst release of almost all quercetin molecules. The nanofibers showed antioxidant activity due to the embedded quercetin. Kingshott and colleagues reported retinyl acetate (RA) release from β-CyD functional PVA nanofibers [150]. The ICs of β-CyD and RA were incorporated into PVA nanofibers to enhance the shelf-life and thermal stability of RA. The release of RA was very slow, reaching 90% after 3 months. The general overview of the CyD/drug ICs loaded polymeric electrospun nanofibers was summarized in Table 1, where the composition of the fiber matrix and drug molecules were given, along with release data.

Table 1. General overview of CyD/drug ICs embedded polymeric electrospun nanofibers used in drug delivery.

CyD Type	Polymer Additive	Active Molecule	Release Data	Ref
β-CyD	PCL	Naproxen (NAP)	Higher NAP release with CyD	[88]
β-CyD, HP-β-CyD	Pellethane (TPU)	Naproxen (NAP)	10 h (NAP-TPU), 32 h (NAP/β-CyD/TPU), 120 h (NAP, HP-β-CyD/TPU)	[91]
HP-β-CyD	Hydroxypropyl cellulose (HPC)	Sulfisoxazole (SFS)	720 min (PCL-PCL-HPC/SFS/HP-β-CyD-IC-NF), >720 min (HPC/SFS/HP-β-CyD-IC-NF)	[92]
HP-β-CyD	PVP, PVA, Thiolated chitosan (CS-SH)	Clotrimazole (CZ)	For all nanofibers 80% in 480 min	[94]
HP-β-CyD	PVA	Voriconazole (VRC)	8 h for 100% release	[95]
β-CyD, HP-β-CyD	PVP	Meloxicam (MX)	For all nanofibers, 20 min for 100% release	[97]
HP-β-CyD	PVP	Meloxicam (MX)	Rapid release (<10 min)	[99]
β-CyD	PCL	Tetracycline (TCN)	Drug release occurred up to 2 weeks	[100]
HP-β-CyD	Silk fibroin (SF)	Tamoxifen (TAM)	10% in 22 days in PBS, 50–60% in PBS-EtOH (30%) in 22 days)	[107]
β-CyD	PCL	Silver sulfadiazine (SAg)	80% release from PCL/SAg, 66% release from PCL/SAg/β-CyD	[110]
HP-β-CyD	PLLA	Curcumin (CUR)	Higher release at pH of 1. CyD increased drug release.	[112]
β-CyD	PVA	Curcumin (CUR)	Higher drug content increased the release rate.	[113]
β-CyD	Poly (L-lactic acid-co-ε-caprolactone) (PLACL)	Curcumin (CUR)	1% CUR interacting with MgO nanoparticles showed higher inhibition of breast cancer cells.	[114]
HP-β-CyD	Poly(DL-lactic acid)–poly(ethylene glycol) (PELA)	Hydroxycamptothecin (HCPT)	Higher CyD content increased release rate. The release was slow and took many weeks.	[115]
α-CyD and β-CyD	PCL	Ciprofloxacin	Higher release with initial higher drug loading	[116]
SBE-β-CyD	PEO	Aripiprazole (ARP)	Rapid release in 2 min	[119]
HP-β-CyD	Cellulose acetate	Asiaticoside (AC)	Higher release with CyD and initial burst release within 300 min	[120]
β-CyD	PVA	Allyl isothiocyanate (AITC)	Higher release at 75 °C and followed by 50 and 30 °C.	[121]
β-CyD	PEO	Allyl isothiocyanate (AITC)	Higher release with increasing relative humidity	[122]
HP-β-CyD	Poly(ethylene glycol)-polylactide (PELA)	Combretastatin A-4 (CA4) and hydroxycamptothecin (HCPT)	Sustained release of CA4 over 30 days, fibers showed significant antitumor efficacy and tumor vasculature destruction	[123]
HP-β-CyD	PVP	Flubendazole	The release of a dose of 40 mg in 15 min	[124]
M-β-CyD	PLLA	Doxorubicin (DOX)	17% Decrease in the burst release was observed and followed by a quantifiable sustained release up to 2 days.	[125]
HP-β-CyD	PVA	Metoclopramide hydrochloride (MH)	Burst release: 90% release in 2 min	[126]

Table 1. *Cont.*

CyD Type	Polymer Additive	Active Molecule	Release Data	Ref
β-CyD derivative	Chitosan	β-Lactamase BlaP protein	CyD increased the stability of the embedded protein	[127]
HP-β-CyD	PVP	Plai oil	The release rate ranged was in the order of 10% > 20%~30% plai oil within 24 h.	[131]
HP-β-CyD	PVP	Herbal oil	Very rapid release: 50% release in 1 min	[132]
β-CyD	PEO	Cinnamon (CEO)	Controlled release in nanofibers via bacterial protease.	[133]
β-CyD	PVA	Cinnamon (CEO)	Nanofibers showed excellent antimicrobial activity against *E. coli* and *S. aureus*.	[134]
β-CyD	PLA	Cinnamon (CEO)	High antimicrobial activity due to released CEO	[135]
β-CyD	PVA	Cinnamon (CEO)	Stronger antimicrobial activity with incorporated lysozyme	[136]
β-CyD	Chitosan and PVA	Oregano and cinnamon EOs	Lower release of Oregano EO than CEO	[137]
β-CyD	PLA	Cinnamaldehyde (CA)	Higher release with increasing CA content	[138]
β-CyD	Zein	Eucalyptus EO	Higher antimicrobial activity with increasing EEO content	[140]
HP-β-CyD	PLA	Gallic acid	Increasing release rate with CyD incorporation	[141]
β-CyD	Pullulan	Perillaldehyde	Higher release with increasing humidity	[142]
α-CyD	Xanthan	Hexanal	CyD increased the release rate	[147]
γ-CyD	PLA	α-Tocopherol (α-TC)	CyD increased higher release of α-TC.	[148]
β-CyD	PAA	Quercetin	Nanofibers showed enhanced release rate than the films	[149]
β-CyD	PVA	Retinyl acetate (RA)	Slower release with CyD incorporation	[150]

4.2. Poly-Cyclodextrin Functional Electrospun Nanofibers for Drug Delivery Systems

CyD can be cross-linked or polymerized in controlled or noncontrolled routes to form cyclodextrin based polymeric materials (poly-cyclodextrin (polyCyD)). Further, CyD can be functionalized with polymerizable groups to produce controlled CyD polymers. The poly-cyclodextrin (polyCyD) was also electrospun to form nanofibers to be used in drug delivery applications. In this regard, Oliveira et al. reported coaxial nanofibers based on polyCyD associated with poly(methacrylic acid) (PMAA) for the release of hydrophilic drug, propranolol hydrochloride (PROP) [151]. The nanofibers were cross-linked with thermal treatment at 170 °C for 48 h to obtain water-insoluble polyCyD nanofibers (Figure 5a–c). The biocompatibility of the nanofibers was explored over fibroblast cells, and high cell viability was observed. The interaction between CyD and drug molecules was explored and found to be spontaneous. The burst release of the encapsulated PROP could be modulated by coaxial electrospinning. Uniaxial nanofibers produced with PMAA/polyCyD (80:20 *w*/*w*) and (60:40 *w*/*w*) released 30% and 35% PROP in 8 h, while sole PMAA nanofibers released 100% dose in 15 min. Further, coaxial nanofibers made by polyCyD/PROP core and a shell of PMAA showed better sustained release. In another study, polyCyD was used for the release of fluconazole from the uniaxial nanofibers of polyCyD mixed with PCL and PVP [152]. The nanofibers were further coated with a hydrophobic poly(hexamethyldisiloxane) (polyHMDSO) for tailoring the fiber dissolution and the respective drug release rate. The coating process was performed under mild condition plasma polymerization. Unlike non-coated fibers, which rapidly released the drug payload, polyHMDSO-coated nanofibers prolonged drug releasing time to 24 h. The coated nanofibers were tested with bacteria, and the results showed that they could inhibit the in vitro growth of *Candida albicans*. Another polyCyD-based electrospun nanofiber system was developed using a polymer of HP-β-CyD/citric acid mixed with chitosan to obtain polyelectrolyte complexes [153]. Triclosan was mixed with polyHP-β-CyD to form ICs, and thereafter, chitosan was added to the solution. The nanofibers were cross-linked with a treatment at 90 °C for 4 h and demonstrated antimicrobial activity against the growth of *S. aureus* and *E. coli* for longer periods of time.

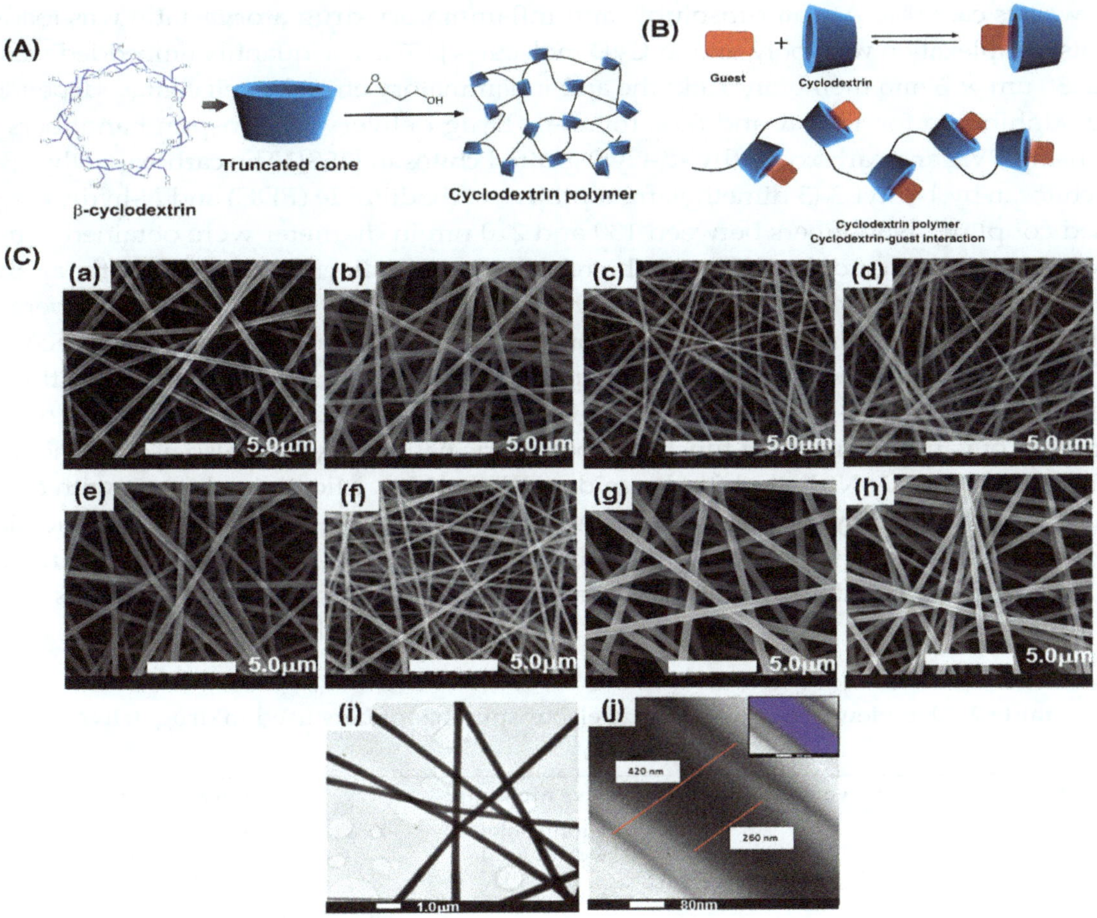

Figure 5. Cartoon schemes of (**A**) the synthesis pathway of CyD polymers and (**B**) their complexation with guest molecules. (**C**) scanning electron microscopy (SEM) and transmission electron microscopy (TEM) images of uni- and co-axial PMAA/polyCyD fibers: (**a**) SEM uniaxial–PMAA; (**b**) SEM uniaxial–PMAA + PROP; (**c**) SEM uniaxial PMAA/polyCyD (80:20); (**d**) SEM uniaxial PMAA/polyCyD (80:20) + PROP; (**e**) SEM uniaxial PMAA/polyCyD (60:40); (**f**) SEM uniaxial PMAA/polyCyD (60:40) + PROP; (**g**) SEM coaxial–shell (PMAA) and core (polyCyD); (**h**) SEM coaxial–shell (PMAA) and core (polyCyD + PROP); (**i**) TEM coaxial–shell (PMAA) and core (polyCyD + PROP); and (**j**) TEM coaxial–shell (PMAA) and core (polyCyD + PROP). The figure was reproduced from [151] with the permission of Elsevier, 2015.

Hydrophobic CyD-based polymers were also used for drug delivery applications. In this regard, Heydari et al. reported the controlled release of vitamin B2 from hydrophobic peracetyl-β-CyD polymer (Acβ-CyDP) based electrospun nanofibers [154]. Acβ-CyDP was synthesized by the acetylation of epichlorohydrin functional β-CyD polymer in the mixture of acetic acid and pyridine at 100 °C for 7 h. The electrospinning of Acβ-CyDP in the mixture of acetone and DMF (3:2, *v/v*) led to thin nanofibers, of which the diameters remained nearly stable even with increasing the polymer concentration from 8 to

25 wt.%, demonstrating no clear influence of CyD content on the diameters of the resultant fibers. The cumulative release of vitamin B2 from the fiber matrix was explored at two different pH values (1.2 and 7.4), and the results revealed enhanced release at pH = 1.2. The release of vitamin B2 gradually occurred, and 60 and 40% of the vitamin diffused out of the nanofibers after 170 h for the solutions having pH of 1.2 and 7.4, respectively. Nada et al. used a CyD cross-linked gelatin fiber matrix for the carrier of chloramphenicol [155]. Chloramphenicol is an antibiotic, which may lead to bone marrow suppression and influences red blood cells [156]. The oxidation of β-CyD led to polyaldehyde β-CyD, and it was used to cross-link gelatin. The nanofibers showed antimicrobial activities against *Staphylococcus aureus* (Gram positive) and *Pseudomonas aeruginosa* (Gram negative bacteria) and *Candida albicans*. After two days, the release was as ca. 90%. A water-insoluble anti-inflammatory drug atorvastatin was loaded in PCL fibers after its complexation with poly-amino-CyD molecules [157]. The quantity embedded was estimated (70–90 μg in 30 μm × 6 mm membrane) and the anti-inflammatory effect by cell contact-dependent release reached 60% inhibition for TNF-α and 80% for IL-6. Drug delivery electrospun nanofibers were also developed using PVA and carboxymethyl-β-CyD grafted chitosan [158]. The carboxymethyl-β-CyD was grafted on chitosan by 1-ethyl-3-(3-dimethylaminopropyl) carbodiimide (EDC) and *N*-hydroxysuccinimide (NHS) based coupling. Nanofibers between 130 and 210 nm in diameter were obtained. The presence of CyD molecules in the nanofibers slowed the release rate of salicylic acid (SA). After an initial burst release of SA, the release percentage reached over 80% after 24 h. CyD-functional fibers were also produced by the electrospinning of a CyD functional polymer and an antibiotic drug vancomycin [159]. The CyD-functional polymer was synthesized by poly(ethylene-vinyl alcohol) (pEVOH)/thiol-modified CyD and a bifunctional cross-linker *N*-(p-maleimidophenyl) isocyanate (PMPI). The fibers showed the sustained release of vancomycin. CyD-functional polymeric nanofibers were also used to the delivery of a common insect repellent, *N,N*-diethyl-3-toluamide (DEET) [160]. Micro-sized fibers with a diameter of 2.8 ± 0.8 μm were obtained by the electrospinning of a water-soluble β-CyD/pyromellitic dianhydride (PMDA) polymer and thereafter loaded with DEET in diethyl ether. The release data were obtained by TGA analysis, which revealed a sustained release of all DEET in two weeks. The details related to the polyCyD/drug nanofibers for drug delivery were summarized in Table 2.

Table 2. Overview of polyCyD/drug electrospun nanofibers used in drug delivery.

CyD Type	Polymer Additive	Active Molecule	Release Data	Ref
PolyCyD	PMAA	Propranolol hydrochloride (PROP)	40% Release (uniaxial PMAA:polyCyD (60:40, 80:20), 20% release from coaxial fibers	[151]
PolyCyD	PCL, PVP	Fluconazole	Burst release ((FLU-poly-α-CyD)-IC/PCL and (FLU-poly-β-CyD)-IC/PCL mats showed a burst of 85% in the first 15 min)	[152]
HP-β-CyD	Chitosan, citric acid (as cross-linker)	Triclosan	Higher release at lower pH (5.5), 80% release in 10 h	[153]
PolyCyD (peracetyl-β-CyD polymer)	-	Vitamin B2	60% (pH = 1.2) and 40% (pH = 7.4) release after 170 h	[154]
Poly aldehyde β-CyD (PA-β-CyD).	Gelatin	Chloramphenicol	Burst release for gelatin/drug (90% in 30 min), 90% release in 48 h for 7.5 and 10 wt.% PA-β-CyD	[155]
Poly-amino-β-CyD	PCL	Atorvastatin calcium trihydrate	TNF-α inhibition reached about 60% at 48 h (no dose effect), and up to 80% for IL-6, depending on the dose	[157]
Chitosan grafted carboxymethyl-β-CyD (CM β-CyD)	Chitosan	Salicylic acid	90% after 24 h at 37 °C, 84% after 24 h at 20 °C	[158]
Thiolated CyD	pEVOH/sH-CyD/PMDI	Vancomycin	Slow release	[159]
β-CyD	β-CyD/PMDA polymer	*N,N*-diethyl-3-toluamide (DEET)	Sustained release of all loaded DEET in 2 weeks.	[160]

4.3. Polymer-Free Cyclodextrin Electrospun Nanofibers for Drug Delivery Systems

Drug-loaded electrospun CyD nanofibers can also be prepared without using a polymeric carrier matrix. The electrospinning of polymer-free CyD/drug IC solutions can produce uniform nanofibers, which are solely based on CyD molecules and their ICs with drug molecules. As these electrospun nanofibers are mostly uncross-linked and hydrophilic, rapid release profiles were observed, along with the fast-dissolving fiber character. The electrospinning of CyD molecules takes place over their aggregates, which are governed by numerous hydrogen bonds. The Uyar research group has pioneered polymer-free electrospinning of nanofibers from CyD and CyD-IC based systems. The first paper was reported in 2010 [161], and it has been shown that highly concentrated (140–160 wt.%) solutions of methylated β-CyD (M-β-CyD) molecules either in water or dimethylformamide (DMF) form large aggregates driven by hydrogen bonds, which is the key factor for uniform fiber formation during electrospinning process [161]. In a later study, polymer-free nanofibers were successfully electrospun from three different CyD derivatives—HP-β-CyD, HP-γ-CyD and M-β-CyD—in three different solvent systems—water, DMF, and dimethylacetamide (DMAc) [162]. The polymer-free nanofibers from native CyD were also produced, in which electrospinning was carried out for α-CyD and β-CyD in alkaline aqueous systems [83], and γ-CyD nanofibers were electrospun from a dimethyl sulfoxide (DMSO)/water solvent system [163]. The Uyar research group has also shown that the electrospinning of uniform nanofibers could be produced from CyD-ICs without using a polymer carrier, in which triclosan/CyD ICs system was successfully electrospun into uniform and bead-free nanofibers [164]. In another study, antibacterial properties of electrospun nanofibers from triclosan/CyD IC using two different CyD derivatives (HP-β-CyD and HP-γ-CyD) were also reported [165]. Triclosan/CyD ICs electrospun nanofibers showed better antibacterial properties in the inhibition of growth of Gram-negative (*E. coli*) and Gram-positive (*S. aureus*) bacteria than pure triclosan.

Essential oils are widely implemented in medical, food, cosmetic, and allied applications due to their antibacterial, antiseptic, antifungal, and antioxidant properties [139]. The Uyar research group has made significant contributions in the fabrication of essential oil loaded CyD functional nanofibers, and several studies related to the polymer-free electrospinning of essential oils/CyD ICs were reported. Since the most of them are slightly water soluble, the use of CyD molecules in the nanofiber form can offer bulk materials loaded essential oils. Very recently, Celebioglu et al. has reported the electrospinning of CyD-camphor IC nanofibers [166]. Camphor-loaded CyD nanofibers rapidly dissolved in water because of their uncross-linked hydrophilic nature. Despite the fact that camphor is a volatile molecule, it can be preserved in the CyD cavity during electrospinning, and the molar ratio after electrospinning was calculated as ~1.00/0.65 and ~1.00/0.90 in HP-β-CyD/camphor-IC and HP-β-CyD/camphor-IC nanofibers, respectively. The camphor release from HP-β-CyD-IC and HP-γ-CyD-IC nanofibers in gas phase was monitored at two different temperatures (37 and 75 °C) using gas chromatography-mass spectrometry (GC-MS) for 4 h, where the higher temperature enhanced the release rate of camphor because of the diffusion coefficient increment of camphor molecules. Another important essential oil, eugenol, was complexed within CyD nanofibers [167]. The ICs of three cyclodextrin derivatives (HP-β-CyD, HP-γ-CyD, and M-β-CyD) with eugenol were prepared in water and electrospun to form nanofibers. Inclusion-complexation significantly enhanced water solubility and increased the thermal stability of volatile eugenol. Due to their hydrophilic and uncross-linked nature, CyD nanofibers rapidly dissolve in water. The eugenol-loaded CyD nanofibers showed a higher antioxidant capacity than eugenol itself, suggesting enhanced antioxidant activity of the fibers than the powder form of eugenol. Essential oils, *p*-cymene and cineole, were also embedded in polymer-free CyD nanofibers in the form of CyD-ICs [168]. Electrospun nanowebs were produced by the ICs of *p*-cymene and cineole with two modified cyclodextrins (HP-β-CyD and HP-γ-CyD). The thermal stability of both *p*-cymene and cineole increased with inclusion-complexation. On contact, the nanofibers rapidly dissolved in water. Linalool, a natural ingredient of many essential oils, was also loaded into CyD nanofibers as ICs through electrospinning [169]. Well-tuned nanofibers were obtained with antibacterial properties. Antibacterial limonene-loaded polymer-free CyD nanofibers were prepared by electrospinning [170]. Modified cyclodextrins (M-β-CyD, HP-β-CyD and HP-γ-CyD) and limonene were mixed to form ICs. The computational and experimental results revealed the molar ratio of the CyD-limonene was 1:1. The released limonene from M-β-CyD/limonene-IC was less than the nanofibers of HP-β-CyD/limonene-IC and HP-γ-CyD/limonene-IC due to the higher amount of the preserved limonene in the nanofiber. 25% limonene was released from M-β-CyD/limonene-IC nanofibers, whereas the nanofibers of HP-β-CyD/limonene-IC and HP-γ-CyD/limonene-IC released 51 and 88 wt.% limonene in 100 days, respectively. Inclusion-complexation significantly enhanced the thermal stability of the entrapped active molecules. The nanofibers significantly inhibited the growth of *S. aureus* and *E. coli* because of the antibacterial property of limonene. In addition, the nanofibers rapidly dissolved in water because of the polymer-free nature of hydrophilic CyD derivatives. Geraniol-CyD ICs-loaded nanofibers were also reported by the Uyar research group without the requirement of any polymer carrier [171]. Bead-free nanofibers were obtained using three different CyD types e.g., HP-β-CyD, M-β-CyD, and HP-γ-CyD. Even though geraniol is a volatile molecule, it could be preserved in the nanofibers in the range of ∼60–90% depending on formulation parameters. The release studies were either performed at room temperature or short term at high temperature (37, 50, and 75 °C), and the results revealed M-β-CyD /geraniol-IC complex loaded nanofibers released less geraniol than the nanofibers of HP-β-CyD/geraniol-IC and HP-γ-CyD/geraniol-IC, suggesting the strongest inclusion-complexation occurred between M-β-CyD and geraniol. The nanofibers showed antibacterial properties in the sense of the inhibition of growth of *E. coli* and *S. aureus* because of the released geraniol from the fiber matrix. Furthermore, the nanofibers showed enhanced antioxidant activity to those of pure geraniol because of its low water solubility. Likewise, thymol-loaded CyD nanofibers were prepared as ICs of CyD (M-β-CyD, HP-β-CyD, and HP-γ-CyD) [172]. Due to the volatile nature of thymol, it was entrapped in the CyD cavity to enhance its thermal stability. Thymol-loaded CyD nanofibers showed more rapid dissolution in water than hydrophobic thymol. Due to the antioxidant properties of thymol, the respective nanofibers were tested by DPPH radical scavenging, and high scavenging capacity was observed. Polymer-free CyD nanofibers were also electrospun from their ICs with volatile flavor agents e.g., menthol [173] and vanillin [174], and vitamins e.g., vitamin E [175] with enhanced solubility and prolonged shelf-life. Recently, Uyar and colleagues reported the polymer-free electrospinning of carvacrol/CyD ICs [176]. Carvacrol is a phenolic component of plant essential oils and has antioxidant and antimicrobial properties [177,178]. The ICs of carvacrol with HP-β-CyD or HP-β-CyD were electrospun into fibers. These fast dissolving fibers showed enhanced antioxidant activity with an increase content of carvacrol.

In order to develop a fast-dissolving drug/CyD IC nanofibrous system, the ICs of sulfisoxazole (SFS) and sulfobutyl ether β-CyD (SBE_7-β-CyD) were prepared in water, and thereafter, electrospun into nanofibers in the form of self-standing flexible nanofibrous webs (Figure 6) [179]. In parallel, the ICs of SBE_7-β-CyD and SFS were prepared as powder. On contact with water, the entrapped SFS was released from the polymer nanofibers, along with the disintegration of the fibers (Figure 7). The polymer-free nanofibers of SBE_7-β-CyD-SFS ICs showed faster dissolution than the powder form of the SBE7-β-CyD-SFS ICs, and pure SFS was not soluble in water in the absence of CyD (Figure 7). These fast dissolving CyD functional fiber nanowebs can be implemented if the rapid release of water-insoluble drugs, as the case here with SFS, is desired.

Another fast-dissolving polymer-free fiber system loaded with poorly soluble diclofenac sodium was reported by Balogh et al. [180]. The fibers rapidly dissolved in water (within 2 min). Spironolactone, a diuretic drug with antiandrogenic properties, was complexed with CyD and electrospun into nanofibers without the requirement of any polymeric carrier [181]. The resultant nanofibers rapidly dissolved in water, and the system allowed high loading of lipophilic spironolactone. An interesting

CyD based polymer-free fiber system for drug delivery applications was developed using modified γ-CyD molecules. Yu et al. modified γ-CyD with phenylacetic acid and performed electrospinning from the mixed solution of dichloromethane (DCM) and dimethylformamide (DMF) (8:2, *v*/*v*) to form fibers (Figure 8) [182]. The bead-free, water insoluble ultrafine fibers with a diameter range of 1–2 μm were obtained. Unlike other polymer-free CyD fibers, these fibers did not show rapid dissolution. In vitro cell tests revealed the fibers are biocompatible. Several drug molecules (doxorubicin, fluorescein isothiocyanate-dextran (FITC-dextran), recombinant human insulin (FITC-labeled insulin), and chlorin) were loaded by simply incubating the fibers in the solutions of the respective drug molecules. ~50% of Release of the entrapped drug molecules was observed from the fiber matrix in one month, demonstrating their slow release (Figure 8E). Chlorin-loaded fibers were also exploited for in vivo drug release in mice, and on day 28, the complete release of chlorin was observed because of the disappearance of its fluorescence signal. The general overview of polymer-free CD/drug ICs fibers for drug delivery was summarized in Table 3.

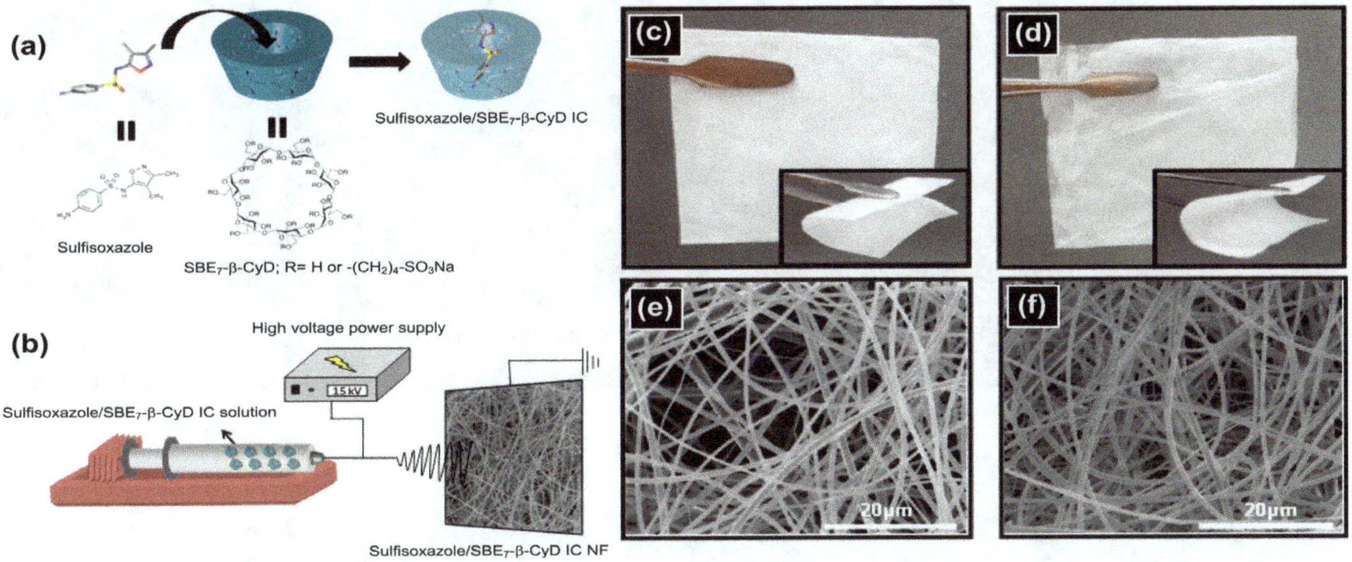

Figure 6. (**a**) Cartoon illustration of inclusion-complexation between CyD and sulfisoxazole (SFS). The chemical structure of sulfisoxazole and SBE$_7$-β-CyD with a schematic representation of sulfisoxazole, SBE$_7$-β-CyD and their IC, (**b**) schematic representation of the electrospinning of SFS/SBE$_7$-β-CyD-IC NF. Photographs of electrospun (**c**) SBE$_7$-β-CyD nanofibers, (**d**) SFS/SBE$_7$-β-CyD-IC nanofibers, and SEM images of (**e**) SBE$_7$-β-CyD NF, (**f**) SFS/SBE$_7$-β-CyD-IC nanofibers. The figure was reproduced from [179] with the permission of Elsevier, 2017.

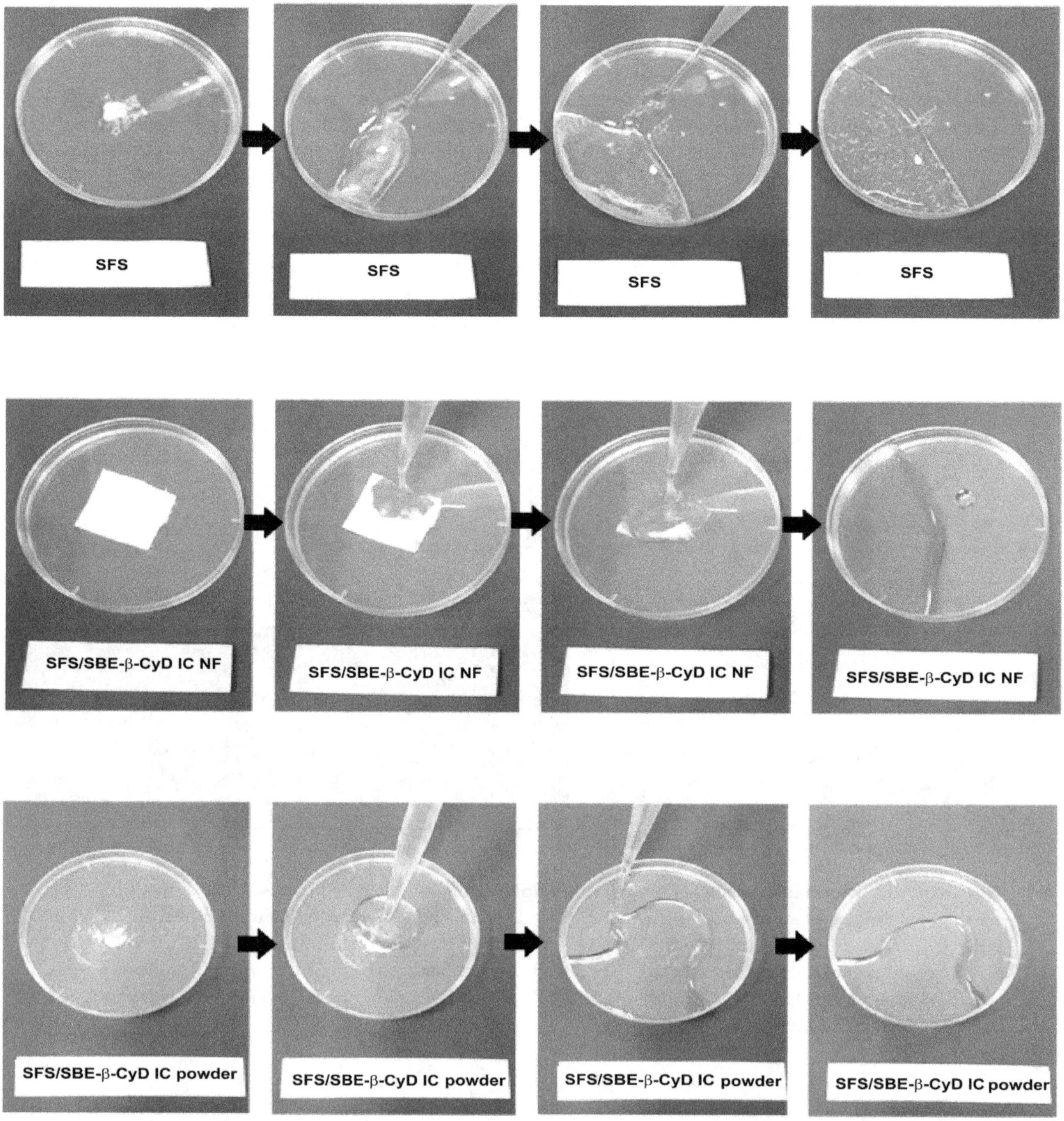

Figure 7. Typical water-solubility of the drug loaded polymer-free CyD fibers. The representative photos of the SFS and SFS/ SBE_7-β-CyD IC powder and SFS/ SBE_7-β-CyD IC nanofibers on exposure to water. The figure was reproduced from [179] with the permission of Elsevier, 2017.

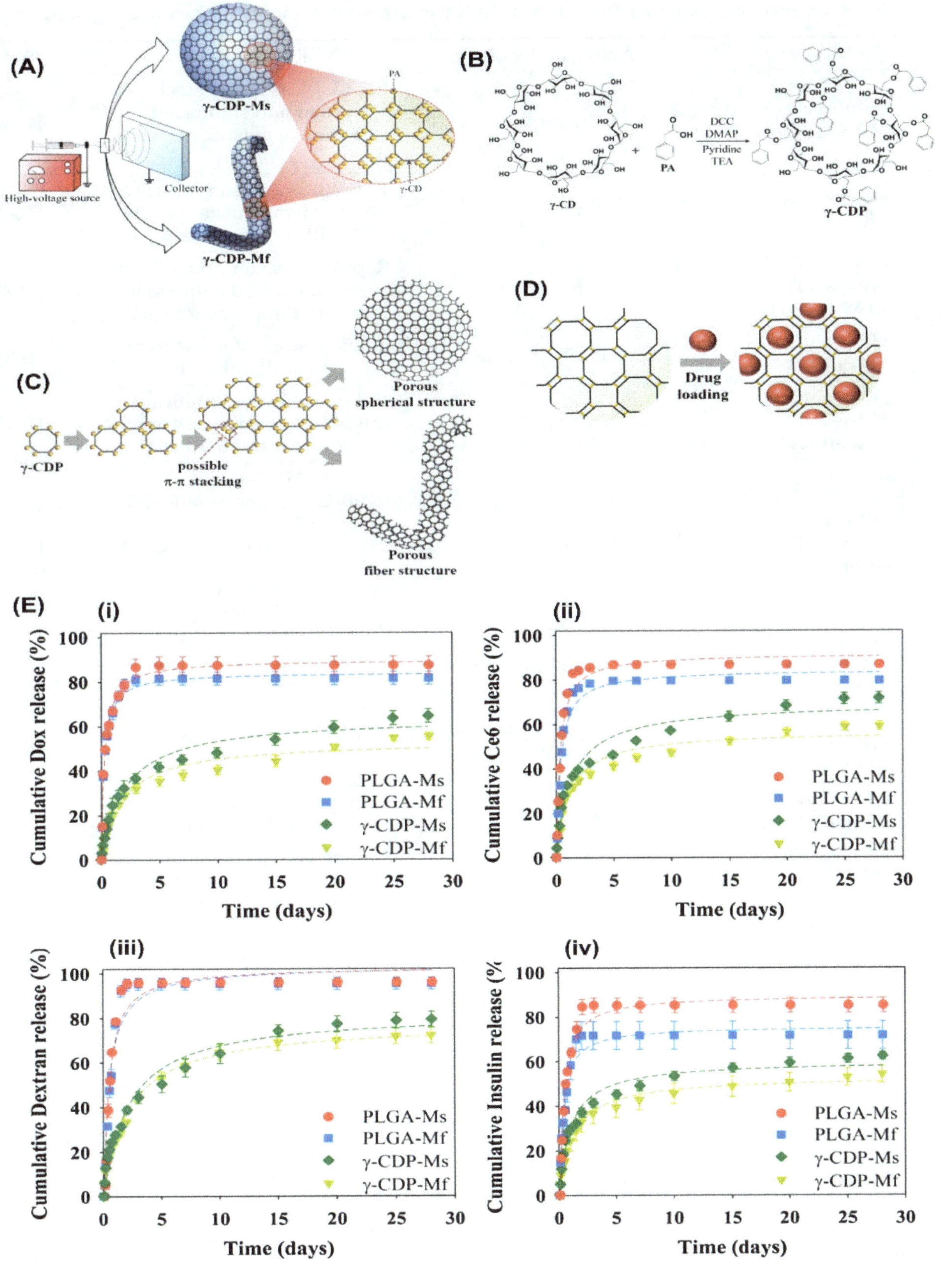

Figure 8. (**A**) A schematic representation of the electrospinning and electrospraying of γ-CyDPs. (**B**) The synthesis pathway of γ-CyDP. (**C**) Cartoon schemes of γ-CyDP-microspheres (Ms) or γ-CyDP microfibers (Mf) with porous structure and (**D**) their drug loading. (**E**) The cumulative molecule (**i**) Dox, (**ii**) Ce6, (**iii**) dextran, and (**iv**) insulin release (wt. %) from PLGA-Ms, PLGA-Mf, γ-CyDP-Ms, and γ-CyDP-Mf (n = 3). The figure was reproduced from [182] with the permission of Elsevier, 2018.

Table 3. Overview of polymer-free CyD/drug ICs electrospun nanofibers used in drug delivery.

CyD type	Active molecule	Release data	Ref
HP-β-CyD, HP-γ-CyD	Triclosan	Rapid release on contact with water and significant inhibition against *E. coli* and *S. aureus*	[165]
HP-β-CyD, HP-γ-CyD	Camphor	In gas phase, faster release at higher temp., faster for the HP-β-CyD system	[166]
HP-β-CyD, HP-γ-CyD, and M-β-CyD	Eugenol	Rapid release on contact with water, enhanced antioxidant activity than eugenol itself	[167]
HP-β-CyD, HP-γ-CyD	Cineole and *p*-cymene	Rapid release along with the fiber dissolution	[168]
HP-β-CyD, HP-γ-CyD, and M-β-CyD	Linalool	Rapid release, significant inhibition against the growth of *E. coli* and *S. aureus*	[169]
HP-β-CyD, HP-γ-CyD and M-β-CyD	Limonene	25% Release M-β-CyD/limonene-IC-NF, 51% release HP-β-CyD/limonene-IC-NF, 88% release HP-γ-CyD/limonene-IC-NF in 100 days	[170]
HP-β-CyD, HP-γ-CyD and M-β-CyD	Geraniol	Long-term stability of geraniol in gas phase	[171]
HP-β-CyD, HP-γ-CyD and M-β-CyD	Thymol	Immediately on contact with water	[172]
HP-β-CyD, HP-γ-CyD	Menthol	Rapid release along with the fiber dissolution	[173]
HP-β-CyD, HP-γ-CyD and M-β-CyD	Vanillin	Immediately on contact with water, enhanced antioxidant activity with nanofibers	[174]
HP-β-CyD	Vitamin E	Rapid and enhanced release, higher antioxidant activity with CyD	[175]
HP-β-CyD, HP-β-CyD	Carvacrol	Rapid release on contact with water	[176]
SBE_7-β-CyD	Sulfisoxazole	Rapid and enhanced release of sulfisoxazole on contact with water	[179]
HP-β-CyD	Diclofenac sodium	Release in few minutes	[180]
HP-β-CyD	Spironolactone	Total release in 1 h	[181]
Phenylacetic-β-CyD	Doxorubicin, fluorescein isothiocyanate-dextran (FITC-dextran), recombinant human insulin (FITC-labeled insulin) and chlorin e6	50% Release of drugs in vitro in 30 days, ~100% release of chlorin in vivo on day 28	[182]

5. Concluding Remarks and Future Outlook

Electrospinning has become a dynamic, rapidly changing field that can affect human lives in diverse ways. It allows for the production of electrospun nanofibers with tailored-made properties to address problems in the environment, biomedicine, textile, and food industries. High specific surface area, ease of operation, adaptability, tunable fiber texture, and a wide size spectrum make the electrospun nanofibers potential drug carriers with many intrinsic benefits, including enhanced drug loading, controlled release of drugs, and a short diffusion pathway. Further, processing parameters and structural modification allow tuning the fiber structure for the sustained release of drug molecules—for example, in the case of co-axial nanofibers with the drugs-embedded in the core. In this regard, various drug molecules with anticancer, antibiotic, antimicrobial, or antioxidant properties were incorporated into electrospun fibers, mostly using their ICs with CyD. The non-specific incorporation of such drug molecules can cause undesired release profiles, low drug loadings, activity loss of environmentally sensitive drugs, or other problems. In this regard, the incorporation of biocompatible nanocarriers into such systems allows the fabrication of high-performance drug delivery nanomaterials. Toward this goal, CyD molecules have found a large application area because of their unique 3D structure, which endows nanofibers with distinct features e.g., enhanced drug solubility, stability, and bioavailability useful in drug delivery applications. Furthermore, they do not provoke the immune system and have low toxicities to mammals. Hence, they have become important excipients in pharmaceutical applications. Native CyD, particularly β-CyD, have ideal cavity size related to complex with a wide range of chemicals but have significant issues related to the poor water solubility of native CyD. These drawbacks of β-CyD can be mitigated by chemical modifications to produce highly soluble derivatives, such as hydroxypropyl functional-CyD. CyD-functional electrospun nanofibers were prepared by either blending of CyD-drug complexes with polymers or using CyD polymers with another polymer carrier or standalone. CyD molecules could also be electrospun without the requirement of a carrier polymer. In the latter case, CyD and guest molecules were mixed to form ICs and their electrospinning produced polymer-free nanofibers with high drug loading. However, these fibers, on contact, rapidly dissolve in water and release the entrapped drug molecules in the form of CyD-drug ICs without any control on drug release. Tables 1–3 give the characteristics of some selected examples on CyD functional electrospun nanofibers used in drug delivery applications. All these fiber systems have their own pros and cons. Still, there is a growing interest to engineer CyD-functional drug delivery systems that deliver therapeutics in a safe, effective, and targeted fashion. The most of researches in this field concentrated on the blending of CyD-drug ICs with various polymers. This route produces CyD-drug IC loaded polymeric nanofibers with longer dissolution time depending on the structural properties of polymeric carrier in the fiber. The CyD-drug ICs can also be electrospun in the absence of a polymer. However, such fibers rapidly dissolve on contact with water, and drug molecules are released in the forms of CyD-drug ICs. In contrast to both methods, the polyCyD fibers can be engineered and used in drug delivery with a better control on release profiles. A schematic overview of the CyD-functional nanofibers was shown in Figure 9, where important parameters of the relevant synthesis routes are pointed out. Each preparation approach comprises different benefits. While polymer-free CyD nanofibers are simpler to produce, they suffer from the instant water solubility. However, in this context, hydrophobically-modified CyD can offer water-insoluble polymer-free fiber meshes. On the other hand, polyCyD functional nanofibers have certain difficulties in the synthesis of functional CyD derivatives and their polymers. Regardless of preparation route, the ability to tune fiber structure should facilitate the sustained release of drugs, such as through co-axial electrospinning.

The use of CyD in electrospun nanofibers for drug delivery systems are likely to find increasing interest in the coming years. Currently, there are significant advances in polyCyD electrospun nanofibers produced without the need of any additional polymeric carrier. These water insoluble nanofibers exhibited the efficient removal of water micropollutants, e.g., methylene blue, because of their high active CyD contents [183]. In the future, such nanofibers may find applications in drug delivery. Further, a stimulus can be applied for the release of drug molecules from the CyD cavity in a controllable fashion. Likewise, CyD-containing polymers, particularly those contain CyD as pendent motifs on the polymer backbone can offer promising results for the sustained release of drugs from the fiber matrix depending on the hydrophobicity of the polymer. In this regard, cross-linked nano-porous β-CyD polymers showed enhanced IC constant as high as 10^9 M^{-1} than those uncross-linked ones (native β-CyD, 10^3 M^{-1}) [184]. Beside their use in in vitro drug release applications, CyD-functional electrospun materials will find more applications as implant materials in tissue engineering. Unlike CyD-free electrospun fibers, the functionalization of electrospun fibers with CyD can improve their properties in terms of high drug loading, increased stability, and bioavailability of the payloads in the body.

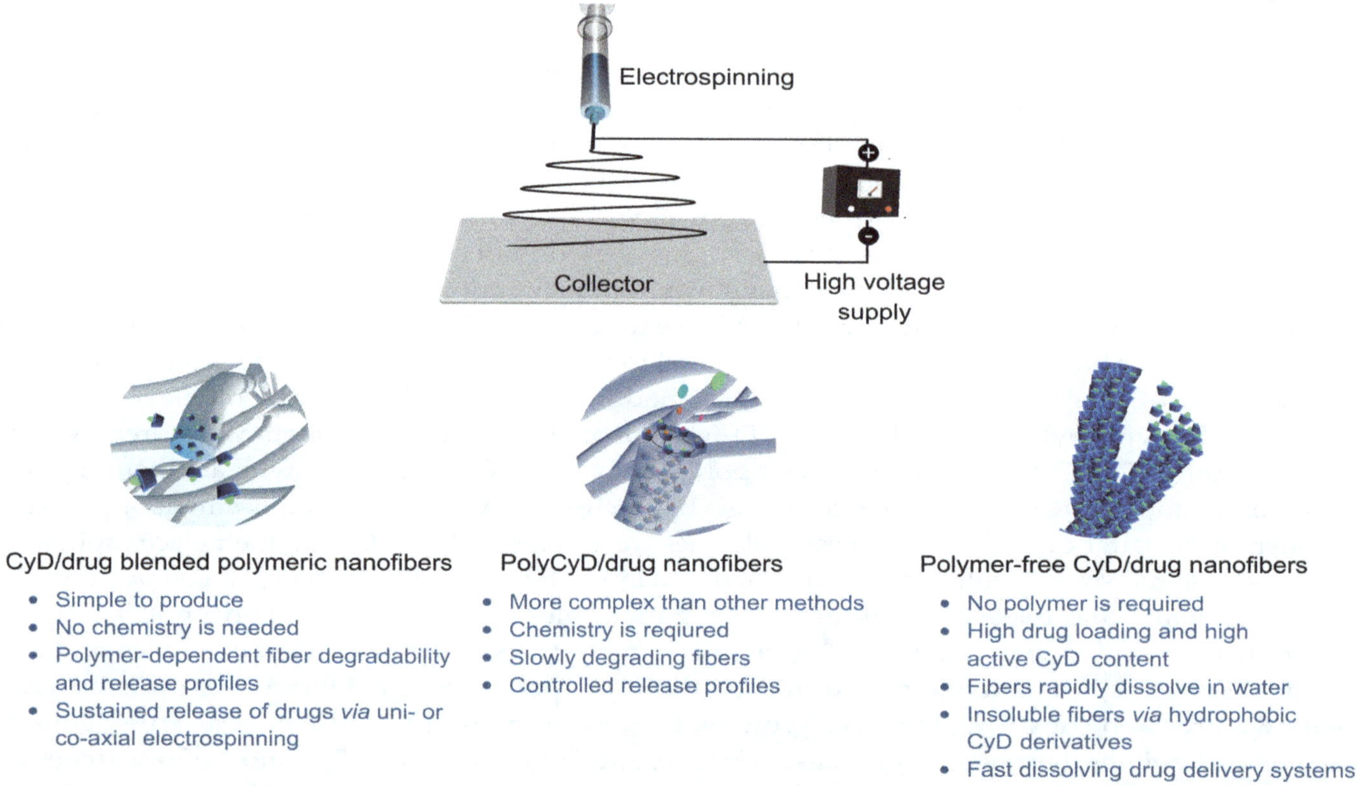

Figure 9. Cartoon illustration of CyD-functional electrospun nanofibers used for drug delivery applications.

To conclude, drug delivery is a dynamic and complex process and can be adapted to meet the needs of the targeted application. Advanced drug delivery therapy requires nontoxic pharmaceutical excipients to provide high drug loading and keeps the drugs stable, active, and accessible for bioavailability. In this regard, CyD-functional nanofibers would be one of the best material systems for drug delivery applications since they offer intrinsic features of both electrospun nanofibers and CyD possessing a hydrophobic molecular-environment for drug entrapment. CyD, thus, significantly increase water solubility of hydrophobic drug molecules (i.e., for high drug loading) and shield drug molecules from physiological degradation or elimination for bioavailability while nanofiber form offers high specific surface area, ease of operation, and further control on the nanofiber form for the sustained release of the entrapped drug molecules. As the electrospinning produces tailored nanostructured materials with further control mechanisms on drug release, the utilization of CyD-functional electrospun materials will increase to meet the demands of advanced drug delivery systems.

Author Contributions: F.T. and T.U. conceived the review. F.T. with the supervision of T.U. analyzed the references and wrote the manuscript. T.U. revised and reviewed the manuscript.

Abbreviations

Ac-β-CyDP	Peracetyl-β-CyD polymer
AITC	Allyl isocyanate
AV	Aloe Vera
CEO	Cinnamon essential oil
CIP	Ciprofloxacin
CUR	Curcumin
CyD	Cyclodextrins
CZ	Clotrimazole
DDS	Drug Delivery System
DPPH	2,2-Diphenyl-1-picrylhydrazyl
E. coli	*Escherichia coli*
EEO	Eucalyptus essential oil
EtOH	Ethanol
FDA	Federal Drug Administration
GC-MS	Gas chromatograph mass spectrometry
HCPT	Hydroxycamptothecin
HPC	Hydroxypropyl cellulose
HP-β-CyD	Hydroxypropyl-β-cyclodextrin
IC	Inclusion-Complex
MX	Meloxicam
M-β-CyD	Methyl-β-Cyclodextrin
NAP	Naproxen
PCL	Polycaprolactone
PEG	Poly(ethylene glycol)
PEO	Poly(ethylene oxide)
PLACL	Poly (L-lactic acid-*co*-ε-caprolactone)
PLLA	Poly (L-lactic acid)
PMAA	Poly(methylacrylic acid)
PolyCyD	Polycyclodextrin
PROP	Propranolol hydrochloride
PS	Polystyrene
PVA	Poly(vinyl alcohol)
RA	Retinyl acetate
RH	Relative humidity
S. aureus	*Staphylococcus aureus*
SA	Salicylic acid
SAg	Silver sulfadiazine
SFS	Sulfisoxazole
TAM	Tamoxifen
TCN	Tetracycline
VRC	Voriconazole

References

1. Zeng, J.; Xu, X.; Chen, X.; Liang, Q.; Bian, X.; Yang, L.; Jing, X. Biodegradable electrospun fibers for drug delivery. *J. Control. Release* **2003**, *92*, 227–231. [CrossRef]
2. Sill, T.J.; von Recum, H.A. Electrospinning: Applications in drug delivery and tissue engineering. *Biomaterials* **2008**, *29*, 1989–2006. [CrossRef] [PubMed]
3. Yoo, H.S.; Kim, T.G.; Park, T.G. Surface-functionalized electrospun nanofibers for tissue engineering and drug delivery. *Adv. Drug Deliv. Rev.* **2009**, *61*, 1033–1042. [CrossRef] [PubMed]

4. Kenawy, E.-R.; Bowlin, G.L.; Mansfield, K.; Layman, J.; Simpson, D.G.; Sanders, E.H.; Wnek, G.E. Release of tetracycline hydrochloride from electrospun poly(ethylene-co-vinylacetate), poly(lactic acid), and a blend. *J. Control. Release* **2002**, *81*, 57–64. [CrossRef]
5. Zeng, J.; Yang, L.; Liang, Q.; Zhang, X.; Guan, H.; Xu, X.; Chen, X.; Jing, X. Influence of the drug compatibility with polymer solution on the release kinetics of electrospun fiber formulation. *J. Control. Release* **2005**, *105*, 43–51. [CrossRef] [PubMed]
6. Katti, D.S.; Robinson, K.W.; Ko, F.K.; Laurencin, C.T. Bioresorbable nanofiber-based systems for wound healing and drug delivery: Optimization of fabrication parameters. *J. Biomed. Mater. Res. Part B Appl. Biomater.* **2004**, *70B*, 286–296. [CrossRef] [PubMed]
7. Wenguo, C.; Yue, Z.; Jiang, C. Electrospun nanofibrous materials for tissue engineering and drug delivery. *Sci. Technol. Adv. Mater.* **2010**, *11*, 014108.
8. Deng-Guang, Y.; Xia-Xia, S.; Chris, B.-W.; Kenneth, W.; Li-Min, Z.; Bligh, S.W.A. Oral fast-dissolving drug delivery membranes prepared from electrospun polyvinylpyrrolidone ultrafine fibers. *Nanotechnology* **2009**, *20*, 055104.
9. Bognitzki, M.; Czado, W.; Frese, T.; Schaper, A.; Hellwig, M.; Steinhart, M.; Greiner, A.; Wendorff, J.H. Nanostructured fibers via electrospinning. *Adv. Mater.* **2001**, *13*, 70–72. [CrossRef]
10. He, C.L.; Huang, Z.M.; Han, X.J.; Liu, L.; Zhang, H.S.; Chen, L.S. Coaxial electrospun poly(L-lactic acid) ultrafine fibers for sustained drug delivery. *J. Macromol. Sci. Part B* **2006**, *45*, 515–524. [CrossRef]
11. Uyar, T.; Kny, E. *Electrospun Materials for Tissue Engineering and Biomedical Applications: Research, Design and Commercialization*; Elsevier: New York, NY, USA; Woodhead Publishing: Sawston/Cambridge, UK, 2017; ISBN 9780081010228.
12. Grafahrend, D.; Heffels, K.-H.; Beer, M.V.; Gasteier, P.; Möller, M.; Boehm, G.; Dalton, P.D.; Groll, J. Degradable polyester scaffolds with controlled surface chemistry combining minimal protein adsorption with specific bioactivation. *Nat. Mater.* **2010**, *10*, 67. [CrossRef] [PubMed]
13. Choi Ji, S.; Messersmith Phillip, B.; Yoo Hyuk, S. Decoration of electrospun nanofibers with monomeric catechols to facilitate cell adhesion. *Macromol. Biosci.* **2013**, *14*, 270–279. [CrossRef] [PubMed]
14. Pires, L.R. 9-electrospun fibers for drug and molecular delivery a2-guarino, vincenzo. In *Electrofluidodynamic Technologies (Efdts) for Biomaterials and Medical Devices*; Ambrosio, L., Ed.; Woodhead Publishing: Sawston/Cambridge, UK, 2018; pp. 157–177.
15. Yu, D.-G.; Li, X.-Y.; Wang, X.; Chian, W.; Liao, Y.-Z.; Li, Y. Zero-order drug release cellulose acetate nanofibers prepared using coaxial electrospinning. *Cellulose* **2013**, *20*, 379–389. [CrossRef]
16. Gizaw, M.; Thompson, J.; Faglie, A.; Lee, S.-Y.; Neuenschwander, P.; Chou, S.-F. Electrospun fibers as a dressing material for drug and biological agent delivery in wound healing applications. *Bioengineering* **2018**, *5*, 9. [CrossRef] [PubMed]
17. Liu, M.; Duan, X.-P.; Li, Y.-M.; Yang, D.-P.; Long, Y.-Z. Electrospun nanofibers for wound healing. *Mater. Sci. Eng. C* **2017**, *76*, 1413–1423. [CrossRef] [PubMed]
18. Pinho, E.; Grootveld, M.; Soares, G.; Henriques, M. Cyclodextrin-based hydrogels toward improved wound dressings. *Crit. Rev. Biotechnol.* **2014**, *34*, 328–337. [CrossRef] [PubMed]
19. Luo, X.; Xie, C.; Wang, H.; Liu, C.; Yan, S.; Li, X. Antitumor activities of emulsion electrospun fibers with core loading of hydroxycamptothecin via intratumoral implantation. *Int. J. Pharm.* **2012**, *425*, 19–28. [CrossRef] [PubMed]
20. Deluzio, T.G.B.; Penev, K.I.; Mequanint, K. Cyclodextrin inclusion complexes as potential oxygen delivery vehicles in tissue engineering. *J. Biomater. Tissue Eng.* **2014**, *4*, 957–966. [CrossRef]
21. Khajavi, R.; Abbasipour, M. Electrospinning as a versatile method for fabricating coreshell, hollow and porous nanofibers. *Sci. Iran.* **2012**, *19*, 2029–2034. [CrossRef]
22. Al-Enizi, A.; Zagho, M.; Elzatahry, A. Polymer-based electrospun nanofibers for biomedical applications. *Nanomaterials* **2018**, *8*, 259. [CrossRef]
23. Dash, T.K.; Konkimalla, V.B. Poly-e-caprolactone based formulations for drug delivery and tissue engineering: A review. *J. Control. Release* **2012**, *158*, 15–33. [CrossRef]
24. Yoon, H.; Kim, G. A three-dimensional polycaprolactone scaffold combined with a drug delivery system consisting of electrospun nanofibers. *J. Pharm. Sci.* **2011**, *100*, 424–430. [CrossRef]
25. Chen, S.C.; Huang, X.B.; Cai, X.M.; Lu, J.; Yuan, J.; Shen, J. The influence of fiber diameter of electrospun poly(lactic acid) on drug delivery. *Fibers Polym.* **2012**, *13*, 1120–1125. [CrossRef]

26. Repanas, A.; Glasmacher, B. Dipyridamole embedded in polycaprolactone fibers prepared by coaxial electrospinning as a novel drug delivery system. *J. Drug Deliv. Sci. Technol.* **2015**, *29*, 132–142. [CrossRef]
27. Schaub, N.J.; Le Beux, C.; Miao, J.; Linhardt, R.J.; Alauzun, J.G.; Laurencin, D.; Gilbert, R.J. The effect of surface modification of aligned poly-L-lactic acid electrospun fibers on fiber degradation and neurite extension. *PLoS ONE* **2015**, *10*, e0136780. [CrossRef] [PubMed]
28. Chou, S.-F.; Carson, D.; Woodrow, K.A. Current strategies for sustaining drug release from electrospun nanofibers. *J. Control. Release* **2015**, *220*, 584–591. [CrossRef]
29. Ulery, B.D.; Nair, L.S.; Laurencin, C.T. Biomedical applications of biodegradable polymers. *J. Polym. Sci. Part B Polym. Phys.* **2011**, *49*, 832–864. [CrossRef]
30. Otero-Espinar, F.J.; Torres-Labandeira, J.J.; Alvarez-Lorenzo, C.; Blanco-Méndez, J. Cyclodextrins in drug delivery systems. *J. Drug Deliv. Sci. Technol.* **2010**, *20*, 289–301. [CrossRef]
31. Loftsson, T.; Vogensen, S.B.; Brewster, M.E.; Konradsdottir, F. Effects of cyclodextrins on drug delivery through biological membranes. *J. Pharm. Sci.* **2007**, *96*, 2532–2546. [CrossRef]
32. Garg, K.; Bowlin, G.L. Electrospinning jets and nanofibrous structures. *Biomicrofluidics* **2011**, *5*, 013403. [CrossRef]
33. Darrell, H.R.; Iksoo, C. Nanometre diameter fibres of polymer, produced by electrospinning. *Nanotechnology* **1996**, *7*, 216.
34. Ziabicki, A. *Fundamentals of Fibre Formation*; Wiley-Interscience: New York, NY, USA, 1976.
35. Fong, H.; Chun, I.; Reneker, D.H. Beaded nanofibers formed during electrospinning. *Polymer* **1999**, *40*, 4585–4592. [CrossRef]
36. Lee, K.H.; Kim, H.Y.; Bang, H.J.; Jung, Y.H.; Lee, S.G. The change of bead morphology formed on electrospun polystyrene fibers. *Polymer* **2003**, *44*, 4029–4034. [CrossRef]
37. Uyar, T.; Besenbacher, F. Electrospinning of uniform polystyrene fibers: The effect of solvent conductivity. *Polymer* **2008**, *49*, 5336–5343. [CrossRef]
38. Li, Z.; Wang, C. Effects of working parameters on electrospinning. In *One-Dimensional Nanostructures: Electrospinning Technique and Unique Nanofibers*; Li, Z., Wang, C., Eds.; Springer: Berlin/Heidelberg, Germany, 2013; pp. 15–28.
39. Qin, X.H.; Yang, E.L.; Li, N.; Wang, S.Y. Effect of different salts on electrospinning of polyacrylonitrile (PAN) polymer solution. *J. Appl. Polym. Sci.* **2006**, *103*, 3865–3870. [CrossRef]
40. Loftsson, T.; Duchene, D. Cyclodextrins and their pharmaceutical applications. *Int. J. Pharm.* **2007**, *329*, 1–11. [CrossRef]
41. Crini, G. Review: A history of cyclodextrins. *Chem. Rev.* **2014**, *114*, 10940–10975. [CrossRef]
42. Morillo, E.; Sánchez-Trujillo, M.A.; Moyano, J.R.; Villaverde, J.; Gómez-Pantoja, M.E.; Pérez-Martínez, J.I. Enhanced solubilisation of six pahs by three synthetic cyclodextrins for remediation applications: Molecular modelling of the inclusion complexes. *PLoS ONE* **2012**, *7*, e44137. [CrossRef]
43. Song, L.X.; Bai, L.; Xu, X.M.; He, J.; Pan, S.Z. Inclusion complexation, encapsulation interaction and inclusion number in cyclodextrin chemistry. *Coord. Chem. Rev.* **2009**, *253*, 1276–1284. [CrossRef]
44. Villiers, A. Sur la fermentation de la fecule par l'action du ferment butyrique. *Compt. Rend. Acad. Sci.* **1891**, *112*, 536–538.
45. Lakkakula, J.R.; Krause, R.W.M. A vision for cyclodextrin nanoparticles in drug delivery systems and pharmaceutical applications. *Nanomedicine* **2014**, *9*, 877–894. [CrossRef] [PubMed]
46. Tiwari, G.; Tiwari, R.; Rai, A.K. Cyclodextrins in delivery systems: Applications. *J. Pharm. Bioallied Sci.* **2010**, *2*, 72–79. [CrossRef] [PubMed]
47. Shieh, W.J.; Hedges, A.R. Properties and applications of cyclodextrins. *J. Macromol. Sci. Part A* **1996**, *33*, 673–683. [CrossRef]
48. Singh, M.; Sharma, R.; Banerjee, U.C. Biotechnological applications of cyclodextrins. *Biotechnol. Adv.* **2002**, *20*, 341–359. [CrossRef]
49. Szejtli, J. Introduction and general overview of cyclodextrin chemistry. *Chem. Rev.* **1998**, *98*, 1743–1754. [CrossRef] [PubMed]
50. Davis, M.E.; Brewster, M.E. Cyclodextrin-based pharmaceutics: Past, present and future. *Nat. Rev. Drug Discov.* **2004**, *3*, 1023. [CrossRef]

51. Wolfram, S.; Mathias, N. Topographie der cyclodextrin-einschlußverbindungen, VII. Röntgenstrukturanalyse des α-cyclodextrin. Krypton-pentahydrats. Zum einschlußmechanismus des modell-enzyms. *Chem. Ber.* **1976**, *109*, 503–517.
52. Harata, K. Structural aspects of stereodifferentiation in the solid state. *Chem. Rev.* **1998**, *98*, 1803–1828. [CrossRef]
53. Sonoda, Y.; Hirayama, F.; Arima, H.; Yamaguchi, Y.; Saenger, W.; Uekama, K. Cyclodextrin-based isolation of ostwald's metastable polymorphs occurring during crystallization. *Chem. Commun.* **2006**, 517–519. [CrossRef] [PubMed]
54. Hapiot, F.; Tilloy, S.; Monflier, E. Cyclodextrins as supramolecular hosts for organometallic complexes. *Chem. Rev.* **2006**, *106*, 767–781. [CrossRef] [PubMed]
55. Loftsson, T.; Jarho, P.; Másson, M.; Järvinen, T. Cyclodextrins in drug delivery. *Expert Opin. Drug Deliv.* **2005**, *2*, 335–351. [CrossRef] [PubMed]
56. Uekama, K.; Hirayama, F.; Irie, T. Cyclodextrin drug carrier systems. *Chem. Rev.* **1998**, *98*, 2045–2076. [CrossRef] [PubMed]
57. Frank, D.W.; Gray, J.E.; Weaver, R.N. Cyclodextrin nephrosis in the rat. *Am. J. Pathol.* **1976**, *83*, 367–382. [PubMed]
58. Matsuda, K.; Mera, Y.; Segawa, Y. Acute toxicity study of γ-cyclodextrin (γ-CD) in mice and rats. *Pharmacometrics* **1983**, *26*, 287–291.
59. Irie, T.; Uekama, K. Pharmaceutical applications of cyclodextrins. Iii. Toxicological issues and safety evaluation. *J. Pharm. Sci.* **1997**, *86*, 147–162. [CrossRef]
60. Ohtani, Y.; Irie, T.; Uekama, K.; Fukunaga, K.; Pitha, J. Differential effects of α-, β- and γ-cyclodextrins on human erythrocytes. *Eur. J. Biochem.* **1989**, *186*, 17–22. [CrossRef]
61. Zimmer, S.; Grebe, A.; Bakke, S.S.; Bode, N.; Halvorsen, B.; Ulas, T.; Skjelland, M.; De Nardo, D.; Labzin, L.I.; Kerksiek, A.; et al. Cyclodextrin promotes atherosclerosis regression via macrophage reprogramming. *Sci. Transl. Med.* **2016**, *8*, 333ra350. [CrossRef]
62. Rajewski, R.A.; Traiger, G.; Bresnahan, J.; Jaberaboansar, P.; Stella, V.J.; Thompson, D.O. Preliminary safety evaluation of parenterally administered sulfoalkyl ether β-cyclodextrin derivatives. *J. Pharm. Sci.* **1995**, *84*, 927–932. [CrossRef]
63. Kantner, I.; Erben, R.G. Long-term parenteral administration of 2-hydroxypropyl-β-cyclodextrin causes bone loss. *Toxicol. Pathol.* **2012**, *40*, 742–750. [CrossRef]
64. Szente, L.; Szejtli, J. Cyclodextrins as food ingredients. *Trends Food Sci. Technol.* **2004**, *15*, 137–142. [CrossRef]
65. Stella, V.J.; He, Q. Cyclodextrins. *Toxicol. Pathol.* **2008**, *36*, 30–42. [CrossRef] [PubMed]
66. Frömming, K.-H.; Szejtli, J. Pharmacokinetics and toxicology of cyclodextrins. In *Cyclodextrins in Pharmacy*; Frömming, K.-H., Szejtli, J., Eds.; Springer: Dordrecht, The Netherlands, 1994; pp. 33–44.
67. Miranda, J.C.D.; Martins, T.E.A.; Veiga, F.; Ferraz, H.G. Cyclodextrins and ternary complexes: Technology to improve solubility of poorly soluble drugs. *Braz. J. Pharm. Sci.* **2011**, *47*, 665–681. [CrossRef]
68. Amiri, S. Introduction. In *Cyclodextrins: Properties and Industrial Applications*; Amiri, S., Ed.; Wiley: Hoboken, NY, USA, 2017; Volume 1, pp. 1–39.
69. Mohanty, J.; Bhasikuttan, A.C.; Nau, W.M.; Pal, H. Host−guest complexation of neutral red with macrocyclic host molecules: Contrasting pka shifts and binding affinities for cucurbit[7]uril and β-cyclodextrin. *J. Phys. Chem. B* **2006**, *110*, 5132–5138. [CrossRef] [PubMed]
70. Kim, H.; Jeong, K.; Park, H.; Jung, S. Preference prediction for the stable inclusion complexes between cyclodextrins and monocyclic insoluble chemicals based on monte carlo docking simulations. *J. Incl. Phenom. Macrocycl. Chem.* **2006**, *54*, 165–170. [CrossRef]
71. Li, S.; Purdy, W.C. Cyclodextrins and their applications in analytical chemistry. *Chem. Rev.* **1992**, *92*, 1457–1470. [CrossRef]
72. Al Omari, M.M.; Zughul, M.B.; Davies, J.E.D.; Badwan, A.A. Effect of buffer species on the complexation of basic drug terfenadine with β-cyclodextrin. *J. Incl. Phenom. Macrocycl. Chem.* **2007**, *58*, 227–235. [CrossRef]
73. Rekharsky, M.V.; Inoue, Y. Complexation thermodynamics of cyclodextrins. *Chem. Rev.* **1998**, *98*, 1875–1918. [CrossRef]
74. Dua, K.; Pabreja, K.; Ramana, M.V.; Lather, V. Dissolution behavior of β-cyclodextrin molecular inclusion complexes of aceclofenac. *J. Pharm. Bioallied Sci.* **2011**, *3*, 417–425. [CrossRef]

75. Shin, K.-M.; Dong, T.; He, Y.; Taguchi, Y.; Oishi, A.; Nishida, H.; Inoue, Y. Inclusion complex formation between α-cyclodextrin and biodegradable aliphatic polyesters. *Macromol. Biosci.* **2004**, *4*, 1075–1083. [CrossRef]
76. Oster, M.; Schlatter, G.; Gallet, S.; Baati, R.; Pollet, E.; Gaillard, C.; Averous, L.; Fajolles, C.; Hebraud, A. The study of the pseudo-polyrotaxane architecture as a route for mild surface functionalization by click chemistry of poly(ε-caprolactone)-based electrospun fibers. *J. Mater. Chem. B* **2017**, *5*, 2181–2189. [CrossRef]
77. Rusa, C.C.; Wei, M.; Bullions, T.A.; Rusa, M.; Gomez, M.A.; Porbeni, F.E.; Wang, X.; Shin, I.D.; Balik, C.M.; White, J.L.; et al. Controlling the polymorphic behaviors of semicrystalline polymers with cyclodextrins. *Cryst. Growth Design* **2004**, *4*, 1431–1441. [CrossRef]
78. Topuz, F.; Uyar, T. Cyclodextrin-functionalized mesostructured silica nanoparticles for removal of polycyclic aromatic hydrocarbons. *J. Colloid Interface Sci.* **2017**, *497*, 233–241. [CrossRef] [PubMed]
79. Topuz, F.; Uyar, T. Poly-cyclodextrin cryogels with aligned porous structure for removal of polycyclic aromatic hydrocarbons (PAHS) from water. *J. Hazard. Mater.* **2017**, *335*, 108–116. [CrossRef] [PubMed]
80. Kotronia, M.; Kavetsou, E.; Loupassaki, S.; Kikionis, S.; Vouyiouka, S.; Detsi, A. Encapsulation of oregano (*Origanum onites* L.) essential oil in β-cyclodextrin (β-CD): Synthesis and characterization of the inclusion complexes. *Bioengineering* **2017**, *4*, 74. [CrossRef] [PubMed]
81. Wadhwa, G.; Kumar, S.; Chhabra, L.; Mahant, S.; Rao, R. *Essential coil*–cyclodextrin complexes: An updated review. *J. Incl. Phenom. Macrocycl. Chem.* **2017**, *89*, 39–58. [CrossRef]
82. Zelikin, A.N.; Ehrhardt, C.; Healy, A.M. Materials and methods for delivery of biological drugs. *Nat. Chem.* **2016**, *8*, 997. [CrossRef] [PubMed]
83. Celebioglu, A.; Uyar, T. Electrospinning of nanofibers from non-polymeric systems: Electrospun nanofibers from native cyclodextrins. *J. Colloid Interface Sci.* **2013**, *404*, 1–7. [CrossRef] [PubMed]
84. Uyar, T.; El-Shafei, A.; Wang, X.; Hacaloglu, J.; Tonelli, A.E. The solid channel structure inclusion complex formed between guest styrene and host γ-cyclodextrin. *J. Incl. Phenom. Macrocycl. Chem.* **2006**, *55*, 109–121. [CrossRef]
85. Kayaci, F.; Ertas, Y.; Uyar, T. Enhanced thermal stability of eugenol by cyclodextrin inclusion complex encapsulated in electrospun polymeric nanofibers. *J. Agric. Food Chem.* **2013**, *61*, 8156–8165. [CrossRef]
86. Kayaci, F.; Sen, H.S.; Durgun, E.; Uyar, T. Functional electrospun polymeric nanofibers incorporating geraniol–cyclodextrin inclusion complexes: High thermal stability and enhanced durability of geraniol. *Food Res. Int.* **2014**, *62*, 424–431. [CrossRef]
87. Liu, L.; Guo, Q.-X. The driving forces in the inclusion complexation of cyclodextrins. *J. Incl. Phenom. Macrocycl. Chem.* **2002**, *42*, 1–14. [CrossRef]
88. Canbolat, M.F.; Celebioglu, A.; Uyar, T. Drug delivery system based on cyclodextrin-naproxen inclusion complex incorporated in electrospun polycaprolactone nanofibers. *Colloids Surf. B Biointerfaces* **2014**, *115*, 15–21. [CrossRef] [PubMed]
89. Sadlej-Sosnowska, N.; Kozerski, L.; Bednarek, E.; Sitkowski, J. Fluorometric and NMR studies of the naproxen–cyclodextrin inclusion complexes in aqueous solutions. *J. Incl. Phenom. Macrocycl. Chem.* **2000**, *37*, 383–394. [CrossRef]
90. Banik, A.; Gogoi, P.; Saikia, M.D. Interaction of naproxen with β-cyclodextrin and its derivatives/polymer: Experimental and molecular modeling studies. *J. Incl. Phenom. Macrocycl. Chem.* **2012**, *72*, 449–458. [CrossRef]
91. Akduman, C.; Ozguney, I.; Kumbasar, E.P. Electrospun thermoplastic polyurethane mats containing naproxen-cyclodextrin inclusion complex. *Autex Res. J.* **2014**, *14*, 239–246. [CrossRef]
92. Aytac, Z.; Sen, H.S.; Durgun, E.; Uyar, T. Sulfisoxazole/cyclodextrin inclusion complex incorporated in electrospun hydroxypropyl cellulose nanofibers as drug delivery system. *Colloids Surf. B. Biointerfaces* **2015**, *128*, 331–338. [CrossRef]
93. Connor, E.E. Sulfonamide antibiotics. *Prim. Care Update Ob Gyns* **1998**, *5*, 32–35. [CrossRef]
94. Tonglairoum, P.; Ngawhirunpat, T.; Rojanarata, T.; Panomsuk, S.; Kaomongkolgit, R.; Opanasopit, P. Fabrication of mucoadhesive chitosan coated polyvinylpyrrolidone/cyclodextrin/clotrimazole sandwich patches for oral candidiasis. *Carbohydr. Polym.* **2015**, *132*, 173–179. [CrossRef]
95. Sun, X.; Yu, Z.; Cai, Z.; Yu, L.; Lv, Y. Voriconazole composited polyvinyl alcohol/hydroxypropyl-β-cyclodextrin nanofibers for ophthalmic delivery. *PLoS ONE* **2016**, *11*, e0167961. [CrossRef]

96. Siafaka, P.I.; Okur, N.U.; Mone, M.; Giannakopoulou, S.; Er, S.; Pavlidou, E.; Karavas, E.; Bikiaris, D.N. Two different approaches for oral administration of voriconazole loaded formulations: Electrospun fibers versus β-cyclodextrin complexes. *Int. J. Mol. Sci.* **2016**, *17*, 282. [CrossRef]
97. Samprasit, W.; Akkaramongkolporn, P.; Ngawhirunpat, T.; Rojanarata, T.; Kaomongkolgit, R.; Opanasopit, P. Fast releasing oral electrospun PVP/CD nanofiber mats of taste-masked meloxicam. *Int. J. Pharm.* **2015**, *487*, 213–222. [CrossRef]
98. Noble, S.; Balfour, J.A. Meloxicam. *Drugs* **1996**, *51*, 424–430. [CrossRef] [PubMed]
99. Samprasit, W.; Akkaramongkolporn, P.; Kaomongkolgit, R.; Opanasopit, P. Cyclodextrin-based oral dissolving films formulation of taste-masked meloxicam. *Pharm. Dev. Technol.* **2018**, *23*, 530–539. [CrossRef]
100. Monteiro, A.P.F.; Rocha, C.M.S.L.; Oliveira, M.F.; Gontijo, S.M.L.; Agudelo, R.R.; Sinisterra, R.D.; Cortés, M.E. Nanofibers containing tetracycline/β-cyclodextrin: Physico-chemical characterization and antimicrobial evaluation. *Carbohydr. Polym.* **2017**, *156*, 417–426. [CrossRef] [PubMed]
101. Prakasam, A.; Elavarasu, S.S.; Natarajan, R.K. Antibiotics in the management of aggressive periodontitis. *J. Pharm. Bioallied Sci.* **2012**, *4*, S252–S255. [CrossRef] [PubMed]
102. Alhusein, N.; Blagbrough, I.S.; Beeton, M.L.; Bolhuis, A.; De Bank, P.A. Electrospun zein/pcl fibrous matrices release tetracycline in a controlled manner, killing staphylococcus aureus both in biofilms and ex vivo on pig skin, and are compatible with human skin cells. *Pharm. Res.* **2016**, *33*, 237–246. [CrossRef] [PubMed]
103. Alhusein, N.; Blagbrough, I.S.; De Bank, P.A. Zein/polycaprolactone electrospun matrices for localised controlled delivery of tetracycline. *Drug Deliv.Transl. Res.* **2013**, *3*, 542–550. [CrossRef] [PubMed]
104. Alhusein, N.; De Bank, P.A.; Blagbrough, I.S.; Bolhuis, A. Killing bacteria within biofilms by sustained release of tetracycline from triple-layered electrospun micro/nanofibre matrices of polycaprolactone and poly(ethylene-co-vinyl acetate). *Drug Deliv. Transl. Res.* **2013**, *3*, 531–541. [CrossRef] [PubMed]
105. Alhusein, N.; Blagbrough, I.S.; De Bank, P.A. Electrospun matrices for localised controlled drug delivery: Release of tetracycline hydrochloride from layers of polycaprolactone and poly(ethylene-co-vinyl acetate). *Drug Deliv. Transl. Res.* **2012**, *2*, 477–488. [CrossRef] [PubMed]
106. Alhusein, N.; De Bank, P.; Blagbrough, I.S. Polycaprolactone electrospun nanofibers for controlled drug delivery. In *The Encyclopedia of Biomedical Polymers and Polymeric Biomaterials*; Mishra, M., Ed.; CRC Press: Boca Raton, FL, USA, 2015; Volume 7, pp. 5239–5249.
107. Liu, W.; Wang, Y.; Yao, J.; Shao, Z.; Chen, X. Tamoxifen-loaded silk fibroin electrospun fibers. *Mater. Lett.* **2016**, *178*, 31–34. [CrossRef]
108. Stygar, D.; Muravitskaya, N.; Eriksson, B.; Eriksson, H.; Sahlin, L. Effects of serm (selective estrogen receptor modulator) treatment on growth and proliferation in the rat uterus. *Reprod. Biol. Endocrinol.* **2003**, *1*, 40. [CrossRef] [PubMed]
109. Osborne, C.K.; Zhao, H.; Fuqua, S.A.W. Selective estrogen receptor modulators: Structure, function, and clinical use. *J. Clin. Oncol.* **2000**, *18*, 3172–3186. [CrossRef] [PubMed]
110. Souza, S.O.L.; Cotrim, M.A.P.; Oréfice, R.L.; Carvalho, S.G.; Dutra, J.A.P.; de Paula Careta, F.; Resende, J.A.; Villanova, J.C.O. Electrospun poly(ε-caprolactone) matrices containing silver sulfadiazine complexed with β-cyclodextrin as a new pharmaceutical dosage form to wound healing: Preliminary physicochemical and biological evaluation. *J. Mater. Sci. Mater. Med.* **2018**, *29*, 67. [CrossRef] [PubMed]
111. Muangman, P.; Pundee, C.; Opasanon, S.; Muangman, S. A prospective, randomized trial of silver containing hydrofiber dressing versus 1% silver sulfadiazine for the treatment of partial thickness burns. *Int. Wound J.* **2010**, *7*, 271–276. [CrossRef] [PubMed]
112. Aytac, Z.; Uyar, T. Core-shell nanofibers of curcumin/cyclodextrin inclusion complex and polylactic acid: Enhanced water solubility and slow release of curcumin. *Int. J. Pharm.* **2017**, *518*, 177–184. [CrossRef] [PubMed]
113. Sun, X.Z.; Williams, G.R.; Hou, X.X.; Zhu, L.M. Electrospun curcumin-loaded fibers with potential biomedical applications. *Carbohydr. Polym.* **2013**, *94*, 147–153. [CrossRef]
114. Sudakaran, S.V.; Venugopal, J.R.; Vijayakumar, G.P.; Abisegapriyan, S.; Grace, A.N.; Ramakrishna, S. Sequel of MgO nanoparticles in PLACL nanofibers for anti-cancer therapy in synergy with curcumin/β-cyclodextrin. *Mater. Sci. Eng. C* **2017**, *71*, 620–628. [CrossRef]
115. Xie, C.; Li, X.; Luo, X.; Yang, Y.; Cui, W.; Zou, J.; Zhou, S. Release modulation and cytotoxicity of hydroxycamptothecin-loaded electrospun fibers with 2-hydroxypropyl-β-cyclodextrin inoculations. *Int. J. Pharm.* **2010**, *391*, 55–64. [CrossRef]

116. Masoumi, S.; Amiri, S.; Bahrami, S.H. Pcl-based nanofibers loaded with ciprofloxacin/cyclodextrin containers. *J. Text. Inst.* **2018**, *109*, 1044–1053. [CrossRef]
117. Sousa, J.; Alves, G.; Oliveira, P.; Fortuna, A.; Falcão, A. Intranasal delivery of ciprofloxacin to rats: A topical approach using a thermoreversible in situ gel. *Eur. J. Pharm. Sci.* **2017**, *97*, 30–37. [CrossRef]
118. Zhou, J.; Wang, Q.; Lu, H.; Zhang, Q.; Lv, P.; Wei, Q. Preparation and characterization of electrospun polyvinyl alcoholstyrylpyridinium/β-cyclodextrin composite nanofibers: Release behavior and potential use for wound dressing. *Fibers Polym.* **2016**, *17*, 1835–1841. [CrossRef]
119. Borbás, E.; Balogh, A.; Bocz, K.; Müller, J.; Kiserdei, É.; Vigh, T.; Sinkó, B.; Marosi, A.; Halász, A.; Dohányos, Z.; et al. In vitro dissolution–permeation evaluation of an electrospun cyclodextrin-based formulation of aripiprazole using μflux™. *Int. J. Pharm.* **2015**, *491*, 180–189. [CrossRef] [PubMed]
120. Panichpakdee, J.; Pavasant, P.; Supaphol, P. Electrospinning of asiaticoside/2-hydroxypropyl-β-cyclodextrin inclusion complex-loaded cellulose acetate fiber mats: Release characteristics and potential for use as wound dressing. *Polymer* **2014**, *38*, 338–350. [CrossRef]
121. Aytac, Z.; Dogan, S.Y.; Tekinay, T.; Uyar, T. Release and antibacterial activity of allyl isothiocyanate/β-cyclodextrin complex encapsulated in electrospun nanofibers. *Colloids Surf. B Biointerfaces* **2014**, *120*, 125–131. [CrossRef] [PubMed]
122. Vega-Lugo, A.C.; Lim, L.T. Controlled release of allyl isothiocyanate using soy protein and poly(lactic acid) electrospun fibers. *Food Res. Int.* **2009**, *42*, 933–940. [CrossRef]
123. Luo, X.; Zhang, H.; Chen, M.; Wei, J.; Zhang, Y.; Li, X. Antimetastasis and antitumor efficacy promoted by sequential release of vascular disrupting and chemotherapeutic agents from electrospun fibers. *Int. J. Pharm.* **2014**, *475*, 438–449. [CrossRef] [PubMed]
124. Vigh, T.; Démuth, B.; Balogh, A.; Galata, D.L.; Van Assche, I.; Mackie, C.; Vialpando, M.; Van Hove, B.; Psathas, P.; Borbás, E.; et al. Oral bioavailability enhancement of flubendazole by developing nanofibrous solid dosage forms. *Drug Dev. Ind. Pharm.* **2017**, *43*, 1126–1133. [CrossRef]
125. Shastri, V.P.; Sy, J.C. Modulation of Drug Release Rate from Electrospun Fibers. U.S. Patent US20080220054A1, 11 September 2008.
126. Kazsoki, A.; Szabó, P.; Domján, A.; Balázs, A.; Bozó, T.; Kellermayer, M.; Farkas, A.; Balogh-Weiser, D.; Pinke, B.; Darcsi, A.; et al. Microstructural distinction of electrospun nanofibrous drug delivery systems formulated with different excipients. *Mol. Pharm.* **2018**. [CrossRef]
127. Filée, P.; Freichels, A.; Jérôme, C.; Aquil, A.; Colige, A.; Tateu, V.T. Chitosan-Based Biomimetic Scaffolds and Methods for Preparing the Same. U.S. Patent WO2011151225A1, 13 February 2011.
128. Puškárová, A.; Bučková, M.; Kraková, L.; Pangallo, D.; Kozics, K. The antibacterial and antifungal activity of six essential oils and their cyto/genotoxicity to human hel 12469 cells. *Sci. Rep.* **2017**, *7*, 8211. [CrossRef]
129. Finnemore, H. The essential oils. *Nature* **1927**, *119*, 920.
130. Toscano-Garibay, J.D.; Arriaga-Alba, M.; Sánchez-Navarrete, J.; Mendoza-García, M.; Flores-Estrada, J.J.; Moreno-Eutimio, M.A.; Espinosa-Aguirre, J.J.; González-Ávila, M.; Ruiz-Pérez, N.J. Antimutagenic and antioxidant activity of the essential oils of citrus sinensis and citrus latifolia. *Sci. Rep.* **2017**, *7*, 11479. [CrossRef] [PubMed]
131. Tonglairoum, P.; Chuchote, T.; Ngawhirunpat, T.; Rojanarata, T.; Opanasopit, P. Encapsulation of plai oil/2-hydroxypropyl-β-cyclodextrin inclusion complexes in polyvinylpyrrolidone (PVP) electrospun nanofibers for topical application. *Pharm. Dev. Technol.* **2014**, *19*, 430–437. [CrossRef] [PubMed]
132. Tonglairoum, P.; Ngawhirunpat, T.; Rojanarata, T.; Kaomongkolgit, R.; Opanasopit, P. Fabrication and evaluation of nanostructured herbal oil/hydroxypropyl-β-cyclodextrin/polyvinylpyrrolidone mats for denture stomatitis prevention and treatment. *AAPS Pharm. Sci. Tech.* **2016**, *17*, 1441–1449. [CrossRef] [PubMed]
133. Lin, L.; Dai, Y.; Cui, H. Antibacterial poly(ethylene oxide) electrospun nanofibers containing cinnamon essential oil/beta-cyclodextrin proteoliposomes. *Carbohydr. Polym.* **2017**, *178*, 131–140. [CrossRef] [PubMed]
134. Wen, P.; Zhu, D.H.; Wu, H.; Zong, M.H.; Jing, Y.R.; Han, S.Y. Encapsulation of cinnamon essential oil in electrospun nanofibrous film for active food packaging. *Food Control* **2016**, *59*, 366–376. [CrossRef]
135. Wen, P.; Zhu, D.H.; Feng, K.; Liu, F.J.; Lou, W.Y.; Li, N.; Zong, M.H.; Wu, H. Fabrication of electrospun polylactic acid nanofilm incorporating cinnamon essential oil/β-cyclodextrin inclusion complex for antimicrobial packaging. *Food Chem.* **2016**, *196*, 996–1004. [CrossRef] [PubMed]

136. Feng, K.; Wen, P.; Yang, H.; Li, N.; Lou, W.Y.; Zong, M.H.; Wu, H. Enhancement of the antimicrobial activity of cinnamon essential oil-loaded electrospun nanofilm by the incorporation of lysozyme. *RSC Adv.* **2017**, *7*, 1572–1580. [CrossRef]
137. Munhuweyi, K.; Caleb, O.J.; van Reenen, A.J.; Opara, U.L. Physical and antifungal properties of β-cyclodextrin microcapsules and nanofibre films containing cinnamon and oregano essential oils. *LWT Food Sci. Technol.* **2018**, *87*, 413–422. [CrossRef]
138. Liu, Y.; Liang, X.; Zhang, R.; Lan, W.; Qin, W. Fabrication of electrospun polylactic acid/cinnamaldehyde/β-cyclodextrin fibers as an antimicrobial wound dressing. *Polymers* **2017**, *9*, 464. [CrossRef]
139. Dhifi, W.; Bellili, S.; Jazi, S.; Bahloul, N.; Mnif, W. Essential oils' chemical characterization and investigation of some biological activities: A critical review. *Medicines* **2016**, *3*, 25. [CrossRef]
140. Dias Antunes, M.; da Silva Dannenberg, G.; Fiorentini, Â.M.; Pinto, V.Z.; Lim, L.T.; da Rosa Zavareze, E.; Dias, A.R.G. Antimicrobial electrospun ultrafine fibers from zein containing eucalyptus essential oil/cyclodextrin inclusion complex. *Int. J. Biol. Macromol.* **2017**, *104*, 874–882. [CrossRef] [PubMed]
141. Aytac, Z.; Kusku, S.I.; Durgun, E.; Uyar, T. Encapsulation of gallic acid/cyclodextrin inclusion complex in electrospun polylactic acid nanofibers: Release behavior and antioxidant activity of gallic acid. *Mater. Sci. Eng. C* **2016**, *63*, 231–239. [CrossRef]
142. Mascheroni, E.; Fuenmayor, C.A.; Cosio, M.S.; Di Silvestro, G.; Piergiovanni, L.; Mannino, S.; Schiraldi, A. Encapsulation of volatiles in nanofibrous polysaccharide membranes for humidity-triggered release. *Carbohydr. Polym.* **2013**, *98*, 17–25. [CrossRef]
143. Uyar, T.; Hacaloglu, J.; Besenbacher, F. Electrospun polystyrene fibers containing high temperature stable volatile fragrance/flavor facilitated by cyclodextrin inclusion complexes. *React. Funct. Polym.* **2009**, *69*, 145–150. [CrossRef]
144. Uyar, T.; Nur, Y.; Hacaloglu, J.; Besenbacher, F. Electrospinning of functional poly(methyl methacrylate) nanofibers containing cyclodextrin-menthol inclusion complexes. *Nanotechnology* **2009**, *20*, 125703. [CrossRef] [PubMed]
145. Uyar, T.; Hacaloglu, J.; Besenbacher, F. Electrospun polyethylene oxide (PEO) nanofibers containing cyclodextrin inclusion complex. *J. Nanosci. Nanotechnol.* **2011**, *11*, 3949–3958. [CrossRef] [PubMed]
146. Kayaci, F.; Uyar, T. Encapsulation of vanillin/cyclodextrin inclusion complex in electrospun polyvinyl alcohol (PVA) nanowebs: Prolonged shelf-life and high temperature stability of vanillin. *Food Chem.* **2012**, *133*, 641–649. [CrossRef]
147. Loong-Tak Lim, S.D.F.M.; Gopinadhan, P.; Jayasankar Subramanian, J. Alan Sullivan Encapsulation and Controlled Release of Volatile Organic Compounds. U.S. Patent US20160330952A1, 17 November 2016.
148. Aytac, Z.; Keskin, N.O.S.; Tekinay, T.; Uyar, T. Antioxidant α-tocopherol/γ-cyclodextrin–inclusion complex encapsulated poly(lactic acid) electrospun nanofibrous web for food packaging. *J. Appl. Polym. Sci.* **2017**, *134*, 44858. [CrossRef]
149. Aytac, Z.; Kusku, S.I.; Durgun, E.; Uyar, T. Quercetin/β-cyclodextrin inclusion complex embedded nanofibres: Slow release and high solubility. *Food Chem.* **2016**, *197*, 864–871. [CrossRef]
150. Lemma, S.M.; Scampicchio, M.; Mahon, P.J.; Sbarski, I.; Wang, J.; Kingshott, P. Controlled release of retinyl acetate from β-cyclodextrin functionalized poly(vinyl alcohol) electrospun nanofibers. *J. Agric. Food Chem.* **2015**, *63*, 3481–3488. [CrossRef]
151. Oliveira, M.F.; Suarez, D.; Rocha, J.C.B.; de Carvalho Teixeira, A.V.N.; Cortés, M.E.; De Sousa, F.B.; Sinisterra, R.D. Electrospun nanofibers of polycd/PMAA polymers and their potential application as drug delivery system. *Mater. Sci. Eng. C* **2015**, *54*, 252–261. [CrossRef] [PubMed]
152. Costoya, A.; Ballarin, F.M.; Llovo, J.; Concheiro, A.; Abraham, G.A.; Alvarez-Lorenzo, C. Hmdso-plasma coated electrospun fibers of poly(cyclodextrin)s for antifungal dressings. *Int. J. Pharm.* **2016**, *513*, 518–527. [CrossRef] [PubMed]
153. Ouerghemmi, S.; Degoutin, S.; Tabary, N.; Cazaux, F.; Maton, M.; Gaucher, V.; Janus, L.; Neut, C.; Chai, F.; Blanchemain, N.; et al. Triclosan loaded electrospun nanofibers based on a cyclodextrin polymer and chitosan polyelectrolyte complex. *Int. J. Pharm.* **2016**, *513*, 483–495. [CrossRef] [PubMed]
154. Heydari, A.; Mehrabi, F.; Shamspur, T.; Sheibani, H.; Mostafavi, A. Encapsulation and controlled release of vitamin b2 using peracetyl-β-cyclodextrin polymer-based electrospun nanofiber scaffold. *Pharm. Chem. J.* **2018**, *52*, 19–25. [CrossRef]

155. Nada, A.A.; Montaser, A.S.; Abdel Azeem, R.A.; Mounier, M.M. Eco-friendly gelatin-based electrospun fibers to control the release of chloramphenicol. *Fibers Polym.* **2016**, *17*, 1985–1994. [CrossRef]
156. Gross, B.J.; Branchflower, R.V.; Burke, T.R.; Lees, D.E.; Pohl, L.R. Bone marrow toxicity in vitro of chloramphenicol and its metabolites. *Toxicol. Appl. Pharmacol.* **1982**, *64*, 557–565. [CrossRef]
157. Schwinté, P.; Mariotte, A.; Anand, P.; Keller, L.; Idoux-Gillet, Y.; Huck, O.; Fioretti, F.; Tenenbaum, H.; Georgel, P.; Wenzel, W.; et al. Anti-inflammatory effect of active nanofibrous polymeric membrane bearing nanocontainers of atorvastatin complexes. *Nanomedicine* **2017**, *12*, 2651–2674. [CrossRef]
158. Bazhban, M.; Nouri, M.; Mokhtari, J. Electrospinning of cyclodextrin functionalized chitosan/pva nanofibers as a drug delivery system. *Chin. J. Polym. Sci.* **2013**, *31*, 1343–1351. [CrossRef]
159. Horst, A.; von Recum, T.T.; Julius, N.K.; Travis, S.; Iryna, M. Therapeutic Agent Delivery System and Method. U.S. Patent US20150010608A1, 8 January 2015.
160. Cecone, C.; Caldera, F.; Trotta, F.; Bracco, P.; Zanetti, M. Controlled release of deet loaded on fibrous mats from electrospun pmda/cyclodextrin polymer. *Molecules* **2018**, *23*, 1694. [CrossRef]
161. Celebioglu, A.; Uyar, T. Cyclodextrin nanofibers by electrospinning. *Chem. Commun.* **2010**, *46*, 6903–6905. [CrossRef]
162. Celebioglu, A.; Uyar, T. Electrospinning of nanofibers from non-polymeric systems: Polymer-free nanofibers from cyclodextrin derivatives. *Nanoscale* **2012**, *4*, 621–631. [CrossRef] [PubMed]
163. Celebioglu, A.; Uyar, T. Electrospun gamma-cyclodextrin ([gamma]-CD) nanofibers for the entrapment of volatile organic compounds. *RSC Adv.* **2013**, *3*, 22891–22895. [CrossRef]
164. Celebioglu, A.; Uyar, T. Electrospinning of polymer-free nanofibers from cyclodextrin inclusion complexes. *Langmuir* **2011**, *27*, 6218–6226. [CrossRef] [PubMed]
165. Celebioglu, A.; Umu, O.C.O.; Tekinay, T.; Uyar, T. Antibacterial electrospun nanofibers from triclosan/cyclodextrin inclusion complexes. *Colloids Surf. B Biointerfaces* **2014**, *116*, 612–619. [CrossRef] [PubMed]
166. Celebioglu, A.; Aytac, Z.; Kilic, M.E.; Durgun, E.; Uyar, T. Encapsulation of camphor in cyclodextrin inclusion complex nanofibers via polymer-free electrospinning: Enhanced water solubility, high temperature stability, and slow release of camphor. *J. Mater. Sci.* **2018**, *53*, 5436–5449. [CrossRef]
167. Celebioglu, A.; Yildiz, Z.I.; Uyar, T. Fabrication of electrospun eugenol/cyclodextrin inclusion complex nanofibrous webs for enhanced antioxidant property, water solubility, and high temperature stability. *J. Agric. Food Chem.* **2018**, *66*, 457–466. [CrossRef] [PubMed]
168. Celebioglu, A.; Yildiz, Z.I.; Uyar, T. Electrospun nanofibers from cyclodextrin inclusion complexes with cineole and p-cymene: Enhanced water solubility and thermal stability. *Int. J. Food Sci. Technol.* **2018**, *53*, 112–120. [CrossRef]
169. Aytac, Z.; Yildiz, Z.I.; Kayaci-Senirmak, F.; Tekinay, T.; Uyar, T. Electrospinning of cyclodextrin/linalool-inclusion complex nanofibers: Fast-dissolving nanofibrous web with prolonged release and antibacterial activity. *Food Chem.* **2017**, *231*, 192–201. [CrossRef]
170. Aytac, Z.; Yildiz, Z.I.; Kayaci-Senirmak, F.; San Keskin, N.O.; Kusku, S.I.; Durgun, E.; Tekinay, T.; Uyar, T. Fast-dissolving, prolonged release, and antibacterial cyclodextrin/limonene-inclusion complex nanofibrous webs via polymer-free electrospinning. *J. Agric. Food Chem.* **2016**, *64*, 7325–7334. [CrossRef]
171. Aytac, Z.; Yildiz, Z.I.; Kayaci-Senirmak, F.; San Keskin, N.O.; Tekinay, T.; Uyar, T. Electrospinning of polymer-free cyclodextrin/geraniol-inclusion complex nanofibers: Enhanced shelf-life of geraniol with antibacterial and antioxidant properties. *RSC Adv.* **2016**, *6*, 46089–46099. [CrossRef]
172. Celebioglu, A.; Yildiz, Z.I.; Uyar, T. Thymol/cyclodextrin inclusion complex nanofibrous webs: Enhanced water solubility, high thermal stability and antioxidant property of thymol. *Food Res. Int.* **2018**, *106*, 280–290. [CrossRef] [PubMed]
173. Yildiz, Z.I.; Celebioglu, A.; Kilic, M.E.; Durgun, E.; Uyar, T. Menthol/cyclodextrin inclusion complex nanofibers: Enhanced water-solubility and high-temperature stability of menthol. *J. Food Eng.* **2018**, *224*, 27–36. [CrossRef]
174. Celebioglu, A.; Kayaci-Senirmak, F.; Ipek, S.; Durgun, E.; Uyar, T. Polymer-free nanofibers from vanillin/cyclodextrin inclusion complexes: High thermal stability, enhanced solubility and antioxidant property. *Food Funct.* **2016**, *7*, 3141–3153. [CrossRef]

175. Celebioglu, A.; Uyar, T. Antioxidant vitamin e/cyclodextrin inclusion complex electrospun nanofibers: Enhanced water solubility, prolonged shelf life, and photostability of vitamin E. *J. Agric. Food Chem.* **2017**, *65*, 5404–5412. [CrossRef]
176. Yildiz, Z.I.; Celebioglu, A.; Kilic, M.E.; Durgun, E.; Uyar, T. Fast-dissolving carvacrol/cyclodextrin inclusion complex electrospun fibers with enhanced thermal stability, water solubility, and antioxidant activity. *J. Mater. Sci.* **2018**. [CrossRef]
177. Ultee, A.; Bennik, M.H.J.; Moezelaar, R. The phenolic hydroxyl group of carvacrol is essential for action against the food-borne pathogen bacillus cereus. *Appl. Environ. Microbiol.* **2002**, *68*, 1561–1568. [CrossRef] [PubMed]
178. Beena; Kumar, D.; Rawat, D.S. Synthesis and antioxidant activity of thymol and carvacrol based schiff bases. *Bioorg. Med. Chem. Lett.* **2013**, *23*, 641–645. [CrossRef]
179. Yildiz, Z.I.; Celebioglu, A.; Uyar, T. Polymer-free electrospun nanofibers from sulfobutyl ether7-beta-cyclodextrin (SBE7-β-CD) inclusion complex with sulfisoxazole: Fast-dissolving and enhanced water-solubility of sulfisoxazole. *Int. J. Pharm.* **2017**, *531*, 550–558. [CrossRef]
180. Balogh, A.; Horváthová, T.; Fülöp, Z.; Loftsson, T.; Harasztos, A.H.; Marosi, G.; Nagy, Z.K. Electroblowing and electrospinning of fibrous diclofenac sodium-cyclodextrin complex-based reconstitution injection. *J. Drug Deliv. Sci. Technol.* **2015**, *26*, 28–34. [CrossRef]
181. Vigh, T.; Horváthová, T.; Balogh, A.; Sóti, P.L.; Drávavölgyi, G.; Nagy, Z.K.; Marosi, G. Polymer-free and polyvinylpirrolidone-based electrospun solid dosage forms for drug dissolution enhancement. *Eur. J. Pharm. Sci.* **2013**, *49*, 595–602. [CrossRef]
182. Yu, H.S.; Lee, J.M.; Youn, Y.S.; Oh, K.T.; Na, K.; Lee, E.S. γ-cyclodextrin-phenylacetic acid mesh as a drug trap. *Carbohydr. Polym.* **2018**, *184*, 390–400. [CrossRef] [PubMed]
183. Celebioglu, A.; Yildiz, Z.I.; Uyar, T. Electrospun crosslinked poly-cyclodextrin nanofibers: Highly efficient molecular filtration thru host-guest inclusion complexation. *Sci. Rep.* **2017**, *7*, 7369. [CrossRef] [PubMed]
184. Ma, M.; Li, D. New organic nanoporous polymers and their inclusion complexes. *Chem. Mater.* **1999**, *11*, 872–874. [CrossRef]

7

A Tailored Thermosensitive PLGA-PEG-PLGA/Emulsomes Composite for Enhanced Oxcarbazepine Brain Delivery via the Nasal Route

Ghada M. El-Zaafarany [1], Mahmoud E. Soliman [1], Samar Mansour [1,2], Marco Cespi [3], Giovanni Filippo Palmieri [3], Lisbeth Illum [4], Luca Casettari [5,*] and Gehanne A. S. Awad [1]

1 Department of Pharmaceutics and Industrial Pharmacy, Faculty of Pharmacy, Ain Shams University, Monazzamet Elwehda Elafrikeya Street, Abbaseyya, Cairo 11566, Egypt; ghada@pharma.asu.edu.eg (G.M.E.-Z.); mahmoud.e.soliman@pharma.asu.edu.eg (M.E.S.); samar.mansour@guc.edu.eg (S.M.); gawad@pharma.asu.edu.eg (G.A.S.A.)

2 Department of Pharmaceutical Technology, Faculty of Pharmacy and Biotechnology, German University in Cairo, Al-Tagmoaa Alkhames, Cairo 11835, Egypt

3 School of Pharmacy, University of Camerino, Via S. Agostino 1, 62032 Camerino (MC), Italy; marco.cespi@unicam.it (M.C.); gianfilippo.palmieri@unicam.it (G.F.P.)

4 IDentity, 19 Cavendish Crescent North, The Park, Nottingham NG7 1BA, UK; lisbeth.illum@illumdavis.com

5 Department of Biomolecular Sciences, School of Pharmacy, University of Urbino, Piazza del Rinascimento 6, 61029 Urbino (PU), Italy

* Correspondence: luca.casettari@uniurb.it

Abstract: The use of nanocarrier delivery systems for direct nose to brain drug delivery shows promise for achieving increased brain drug levels as compared to simple solution systems. An example of such nanocarriers is emulsomes formed from lipid cores surrounded and stabilised by a corona of phospholipids (PC) and a coating of Tween 80, which combines the properties of both liposomes and emulsions. Oxcarbazepine (OX), an antiepileptic drug, was entrapped in emulsomes and then localized in a poly(lactic acid-*co*-glycolic acid)-poly(ethylene glycol)-poly(lactic acid-*co*-glycolic acid) (PLGA-PEG-PLGA) triblock copolymer thermogel. The incorporation of OX emulsomes in thermogels retarded drug release and increased its residence time (MRT) in rats. The OX-emulsome and the OX-emulsome-thermogel formulations showed in vitro sustained drug release of 81.1 and 53.5%, respectively, over a period of 24 h. The pharmacokinetic studies in rats showed transport of OX to the systemic circulation after nasal administration with a higher uptake in the brain tissue in case of OX-emulsomes and highest MRT for OX-emulsomal-thermogels as compared to the IN OX-emulsomes, OX-solution and Trileptal® suspension. Histopathological examination of nasal tissues showed a mild vascular congestion and moderate inflammatory changes around congested vessels compared to saline control, but lower toxic effect than that reported in case of the drug solution.

Keywords: nose to brain delivery; antiepileptic drug; drug delivery; block copolymers; thermogel system

1. Introduction

Hydrogels that are prepared from "intelligent" or "smart" polymers and capable of exhibiting a physicochemical response in a nonlinear manner to an external stimuli, such as temperature [1,2], pH [3], light [4], counter-ion changes [5] and biological molecules [6] have been extensively investigated in the literature. These polymers have great potential in drug delivery and tissue engineering [7–9], in addition to sensors and valves [10].

Thermosensitive polymers are a subcategory of smart polymers that undergo temperature-induced reversible sol-gel transition upon heating/cooling of the aqueous polymer solution. Drugs/formulations sequestered within these copolymers by simple mixing are administered as a solution that gels at body temperature at the desired site of application [11], and are used particularly in the field of controlled drug release.

Thermosensitive di-block copolymers that are composed of hydrophilic polyethylene glycol (PEG) as block A and hydrophobic biodegradable polyesters as block B e.g., poly(lactic acid) (PLA); poly(glycolic acid) (PGA); polyethylene terephthalate (PET); and polycaprolactone (PCL), have been studied as controlled release drug carriers [12–14]. Particularly, the di-block copolymer PEG/PLGA hydrogels are attractive polymers for the delivery of drugs since they are biodegradable with a good safety profile and their compositions can be tailored to provide sustained drug delivery [15–17].

Tri-block thermosensitive copolymers are used in either ABA or BAB configuration, with the poloxamers (ABA) (PEG-PPO-PEG) being of interest due to their commercial availability in a wide range of molecular weights and block ratios [18]. However, they show slow biodegradation kinetics and the inability to provide sustained drug delivery over more than just a few days [19,20]. Therefore, triblock copolymers consisting of PEG and PLGA copolymer moieties are regarded as good alternatives, being non-toxic, water-soluble biocompatible, biodegradable according to copolymer ratio used, and thus, can have tailor-made properties [21].

The gelation mechanisms of thermosensitive hydrogels based on PLGA-PEG-PLGA are illustrated in Figure 1. The cited copolymer self-assembles in micellar formations in aqueous media. A rise in temperature results in the dehydration of the PEG chains, causing the micelle formations to shrink, thus enhancing the interaction between the PEG and PLGA blocks [22]. At temperatures below the critical gelation temperature (CGT), the bridging between micelles are usually unstable due to the low hydrophobicity of PLGA [23]. With increasing temperatures that approach CGT and exceed it, a firm bridged micellar network forms because of the increase in hydrophobic interaction between the chains, thus enhancing inter micellar interaction and aggregation, leading to subsequent gelation [24,25].

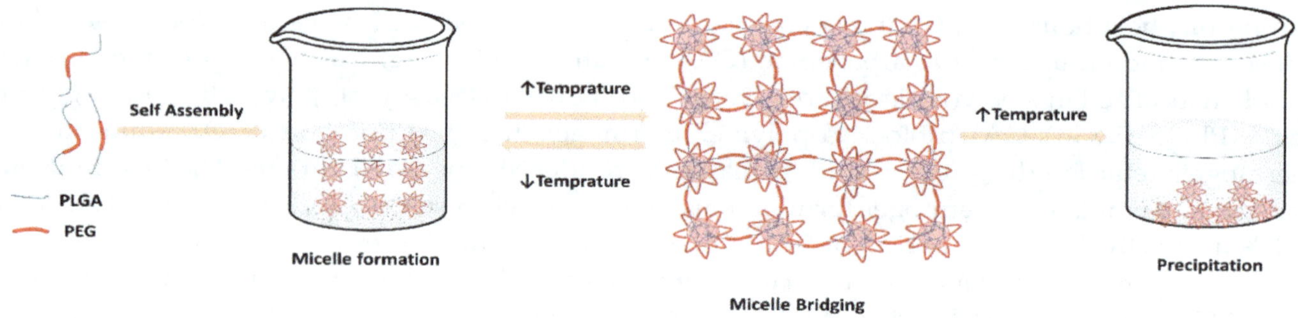

Figure 1. Schematic diagram of the sol-gel transition of BAB type poly(lactic acid-*co*-glycolic acid)-poly(ethylene glycol)-poly(lactic acid-*co*-glycolic acid) (PLGA-PEG-PLGA) tri-block copolymer aqueous solution in response to temperature.

In the present study we adopted a PLGA-PEG-PLGA tri-block copolymer (PLGA (3:1) M_W 1.88 kDa and PEG M_W 1.5 kDa) that was first synthesized by Zentner et al., 2001. Gelling of an aqueous solution of a PLGA-PEG-PLGA copolymer is initiated at around 32 °C, while at 37 °C, the flow of the copolymer solution decreases dramatically as the gel state is established, maintaining the gel in situ for prolonged periods of time. Hence, it is an excellent candidate for prolonging residence time of the sequestered drug/formulation on the nasal mucosa after IN application [26].

Oxcarbazepine (OX), which is used as a model drug in this study, is employed for the treatment of partial and generalized seizures that are associated with epilepsy. OX is usually administered via the oral route exhibiting distribution to non-targeted tissues, a high first pass metabolism, with potential drug-drug interactions as well as undesirable side effects [27]. OX is a microsomal enzyme inducer that necessitates the use of high therapeutic doses which support the interest in a direct transport of the drug to the brain such as what may be achieved by nose to brain delivery [28].

Emulsomes are nanocarriers prepared with lipid cores either in the solid or liquid crystalline state at 25 °C, coated with a phospholipid bilayer. These nanocarriers combine the characteristics of lipid spheres (apolar core) and liposomes (hydrophilic surface) [29]. Due to the apolar solid core, emulsomes can entrap higher amounts of lipophilic drugs [30]. Being composed of triglycerides that are surrounded by phospholipids, emulsomes form particles similar to micelles, hence, vastly increasing the solubility, as well as the bioavailability of poorly soluble drugs [31]. Previous studies from our laboratories optimised the emulsomes in terms of physicochemical characteristics, especially in terms of a prolonged release profile and nose to brain delivery of OX. It was found that the emulsomes delivery system showed a significantly higher brain C_{max} and a higher brain $AUC_{0-1440min}$ than an IV injection of OX and the oral administration of the marketed OX product.

The aim of this study was to investigate whether a combination of the thermo-responsive hydrogel and lipid-based nanoparticles (emulsomes) would enhance the promising results obtained previously for the OX emulsomes alone in delivery of the drug from nose to brain.

In the first instance the thermogelling PLGA-PEG-PLGA copolymer was synthesized and characterized using NMR, GPC, DSC, DLS, and its rheological behaviour investigated. Oxcarbazepine (OX)-loaded emulsomes was than mixed with PLGA-PEG-PLGA tri-block copolymer to develop a 2-phase drug depot system and the formed thermogel was characterized in terms of sol-gel transition temperature, viscosity, drug release and mucoadhesion.

Finally, the delivery system was evaluated in rats for the transport of OX from the nasal cavity to the systemic circulation and the brain tissue, and the histopathology of the OX-emulsome-thermogel delivery system in the nasal cavity investigated.

2. Materials and Methods

2.1. Materials

Oxcarbazepine (OX) was a gift from Novartis Pharmaceutical Co. (Cairo, Egypt). Triolein (TO) (Captex GTO) was generously supplied by Abitec Corp. (Janesville, WI, USA). Soya phosphatidylcholine (PC) and Tween 80 (Tw) were purchased from Sigma Chemical Co. (St. Louis, MO, USA). Chloroform and methanol were purchased from ADWIC, El Nasr Pharmaceutical Co. (Cairo, Egypt). The dialysis membrane made from standard grade regenerated cellulose (molecular weight cut off 12–14 Da) was purchased from Spectrum Laboratories Inc. (Rancho Dominguez, CA, USA). Di-hydroxyl-terminated polyethylene glycol (M_w 1.5 kDa) (PEG 1.5 kDa) and stannous-2-ethyl-hexanoate were purchased from Sigma-Aldrich (Steinheim, Germany). 3,6-dimethyl-1,4-dioxane-2,5-dione (D,L-lactide) and 1,4-dioxane-2,5-dione (glycolide) were kindly supplied by PURAC Biochem (Gorinchem, Netherlands). All other chemical used were of analytical grade.

2.2. Synthesis of PLGA-PEG-PLGA Tri-Block Copolymers

The composition and choice of molecular weights of the PEG and the PLGA components of the PLGA-PEG-PLGA copolymer was designed to have similar sol-gel forming properties as those that were previously synthesized by Chen et al. [32]. They found that the gel-to-sol and sol-to-gel transition only occurred with appropriate molecular weight and molar mass dispersity of the copolymer.

The PLGA-PEG-PLGA copolymer was produced by the method described by Zentner et al. [7]. Briefly, PEG 1.5 kDa was initially dried by azeotropic distillation in toluene under an atmosphere of nitrogen, followed by drying at 130 °C under vacuum, then allowed to melt by placing 6 g in a three-neck flask under vacuum with continuous agitation at150 °C for 3 h, thus generating a viscous liquid mass [33]. D,L-lactide and glycolide were then added with respective amounts of 6 and 1.5 g to maintain a fixed molar ratio of 3:1.

The reaction mixture was maintained at 150 °C under vacuum for another 30 min with constant mixing to allow the fusion of D,L-lactide and glycolide. Stannous-2-ethyl-hexanoate was subsequently added and the reaction mixture was further heated for 1 h [7].

In order to remove the unreacted monomers at the end of the reaction, the raw copolymer was dissolved in dichloromethane and poured dropwise into ethyl ether kept in an ice bath. The pure copolymer was precipitated, then separated by filtration, dried under vacuum and kept refrigerated [34].

2.3. *Characterization of PLGA-PEG-PLGA Copolymers*

In order to verify polymer formation and determine its chemical structure and molecular weight, the following characterisation methods were utilized on PLGA-PEG-PLGA copolymer solutions:

2.3.1. Nuclear Magnetic Resonance (^{1}H-NMR)

Structural analysis of the PLGA-PEG-PLGA copolymer, initial determination of its molecular weight and estimation of the lactide:glycolide ratio, was carried out via NMR spectroscopy. The copolymer was dissolved in deuterated acetone and analysis was done using NMR spectroscopy (Varian Mercury 400 MHz spectrometer, Varian Inc., Palo-Alto, CA, USA) operating at 400 MHz [35]. Subsequently, the molecular weight was calculated by comparing the integral of the signal for PEG protons chemical shift at 3.6 ppm with the integrals of glycolide at 4.8 ppm and those of lactide at 1.6 and 5.2 ppm.

2.3.2. Gel Permeation Chromatography (GPC)

7.5 mg of the PLGA-PEG-PLGA copolymer was dissolved in tetrahydrofuran and acetonitrile and then placed in a water bath at 40 °C for one hour. Vial contents were filtered through a regenerated cellulose syringe filter (diameter 13 mm and 0.45 μm pore size) then analyzed by a high performance liquid chromatography system (HPLC, Agilent Series 1100 LCsystem (Agilent Technologies, Waldbronn, Germany), equipped with a Gel permeation column (TSKGel 2500HHR from Tosoh Bioscience LLC, Montgomeryville, PA, USA) maintained at 37 °C, with tetrahydrofuran as the eluent at a flow rate of 1 mL/min [36].

The molecular weight was quantified by use of a calibration curve resulting from a series of PEG standards with low polydispersity and known molecular weights ranging from 106 Da to 21.3 kDa (PEG Calibration Kit PL 2070-0100, Varian Inc., Palo-Alto, CA, USA). Data were analyzed using the software DATAAPEX (DataApex Ltd., Prague, Czech Republic). Accordingly, the molecular weights of the copolymer were computed, expressed as number average molecular weight, M_n, and weight average molecular weight, M_w.

2.3.3. Differential Scanning Calorimetry (DSC)

Thermal analysis of the PLGA-PEG-PLGA copolymer was carried out in a DSC apparatus (PerkinElmer 8500, Perkin Elmer, Waltham, MA, USA) equipped with an intracooler in inert nitrogen atmosphere. A sample of the copolymer was placed in a closed aluminium pan and heated with a two-stage program at a rate of 10 °C/min. The 1st heating run was conducted from ambient temperature to 150 °C to remove the thermal history of the polymer (i.e., remaining solvent and humidity) and the 2nd run from −40 to 210 °C to determine the sample specific data. Both heating cycles were separated by a cooling run that was conducted at a rate of 10 °C/min [37].

2.3.4. Size Measurement of Copolymer Solution by Dynamic Light Scattering (DLS)

The DLS equipment (Zetasizer Nano ZS, Malvern Instrument, Malvern, UK) was adopted to measure the hydrodynamic diameter and size distribution of the PLGA-PEG-PLGA copolymer micelles, using a detector laser beam fixed at an angle of 90° [38]. To investigate the formation of micelles and the variation in micellar size in relation to temperature, a copolymer solution of 20% *w/w* in deionized water was prepared. 1 mL of the sample was analyzed at increasing temperatures from 10 to 40 °C. The experiment was performed in triplicate.

2.4. *Preparation and Characterization of PLGA-PEG-PLGA Thermogel Solutions Loaded with Emulsomes*

2.4.1. Sample Preparation

An optimised emulsome formulation (TO17-TW) was chosen from previous studies comprising a 3:1 ratio of PC:TG (TG ~Triolein), a total lipid content of 30 mg and coated with Tween 80 [36,37]. The emulsomes were prepared and characterized as a lipid mixture of PC and TO, as previously described [39,40]. Briefly, 10 mgs OX were introduced into a clean, dry round bottom flask, dissolved in chloroform, and then mixed with 30 mg lipid mixture composed of PC:TG (3:1). The organic solvent was removed using a rotary evaporator (Model RVO5, Janke and Kunkel, IKA Laboratories, Staufen, Germany). The formed thin film was hydrated by agitation for 1 h at room temperature with phosphate buffer (pH 6.8) containing 5% tween 80. The formed dispersion was sonicated for 1 min (Bath sonicator model 275T, Crest Ultrasonics Carp, Trenton, NJ, USA), then extruded through 450 nm cellulose nitrate membranes, and stored at 4 °C. The size of the emulsomes has previously been found to be in the order of 101.5 ± 2.9 nm [40].

For characterization of the final thermogel, different formulation concentrations (5, 10, 20, and 30% *w/w*) of aqueous PLGA-PEG-PLGA copolymer solutions were investigated. The solutions were prepared by dissolving pre-cooled PLGA-PEG-PLGA copolymer in deionized water via continuous magnetic stirring of the mixture in an ice bath until complete dissolution. This was followed by the addition of emulsomes in different loading concentrations (0, 10, 25, and 50% *v/v*) by physical mixing. Table 1 shows the coding, compositions and gelation temperature of all prepared thermogel formulations with G1-G16 indicating the individual compositions.

Table 1. Coding, compositions and gelation temperatures of prepared thermogels.

Emulsome Concentration % *v/v*	**Gelation Temperature (°C ± SD)**			
	PLGA-PEG-PLGA Copolymer (% *w/w*)			
	5%	**10%**	**20%**	**30%**
0%	G1 No gelation	G2 Opaque solution	G3 30.2 ± 0.05 °C	G4 28.5 ± 0.1 °C
10%	G5 No gelation	G6 Opaque solution	G7 31.5 ± 0.1 °C *	G8 29.0 ± 0.06 °C *
25%	G9 No gelation	G10 Opaque solution	G11 32.0 ± 0.06 °C *	G12 30.1 ± 0.05 °C *
50%	G13 No gelation	G14 Opaque solution	G15 33.4 ± 0.05 °C *	G16 31.0 ± 0.0 °C *

* Significantly different ($p < 0.05$) from emulsome free gel.

2.4.2. Macroscopic Phase Behaviour of Aqueous Copolymer Solutions and Determination of Gelation Temperature

The sol-gel transition temperatures of the aqueous copolymer solutions with the addition of 0–50% emulsomes were investigated by a tube inversion method [38]. Briefly, 0.5 mL of each solution (G1-G16) was placed in a thermoset circulating water bath where the temperature increased stepwise (0.5 °C) from 20 to 52 °C, with an equilibrium time of 3 min. At each temperature setting, tubes were inverted to check the flow properties. Solutions were considered to be in the gel state if the appearance changed from transparent to opaque with no observed flow for 30 s following the tube inversion [41].

2.4.3. Viscosity Measurement

The viscosities of the copolymer solutions that completely gelled at a temperature ranging between room (25 °C) and body temperatures (37 °C) were measured using a programmable Brookfield viscometer (Brookfield engineering laboratories Inc. model HADV-II, Middleboro, MA, USA) connected to a digital thermostatically controlled water bath (Polyscience Inc. model 9101, Niles, IL, USA). A sample of 0.5 g thermogel was applied onto the lower plate of the viscometer, adjusted at 37 °C. Rheological measurements were conducted at rpm range of 1–100 (shear rate 2–200 s^{-1}), using CPE-52 spindle.

2.5. *In Vitro Drug Release*

Franz type diffusion cells (Variomag Telesystem, H+P Labortechnik, Oberschleißheim, Germany) were used to compare the release and transport of OX from OX-emulsomes [40] to that from OX-emulsomal gel (G16) through a dialysis membrane in. An amount of the OX-emulsomes or the OX-emulsomal gel equivalent to 3 mg OX was introduced to the donor compartment of the diffusion cell. The detailed methodology was as described elsewhere [40].

2.6. *Mucoadhesion Studies*

The mucoadhesive strengths of the G16 emulsomal thermogel in comparison to its corresponding plain thermogel G4 and 0.5% Carbopol 980 gel as a positive control were determined by measuring the force that is required to detach the formulation from freshly excised sheep nasal mucosa, using a texture analyser CT3 (Brookfield Engineering Laboratories, Inc., Middleboro, MA, USA) in tension mode. The sheep nasal mucosa was obtained from the local slaughter house. The mucosal membrane was separated from underlying fat and loose tissues, then washed with distilled water followed by phosphate buffer (pH 6.8) at 37 °C and cut into pieces that fit the stainless-steel cylindrical probe of the device of 10 mm in diameter (3.14 cm^2).

A cut sample of the nasal mucosa was glued to the upper probe using a cyanoacrylate adhesive, keeping the mucosal side exposed. Fixed amounts of the appropriate thermogel were attached to the lower probe of the instrument with double-sided adhesive tape. The upper probe with the nasal tissue was lowered until the tissue contacted the surface of the gelled sample with a downward trigger force of 4 N for a contact time of 5 min to ensure intimate contact between the tissues and the samples [42]. The probe was then moved vertically upwards at a constant speed of 3 mm/s [43]. Work of adhesion, mJ, peak detachment force, N, deformation peak, mm, and final load, N, were all calculated from force-distance plots using the built-in Texture Exponent software.

2.7. *In Vivo Studies*

2.7.1. Pharmacokinetic Study

- Administration of OX containing formulations to rats

Male Wister albino rats weighing 200–250 g were divided into two groups, each containing forty eight rats. Group 1 received OX IN in phosphate buffer solution (pH 6.8) intranasally (IN), Group 2 received IN OX-emulsomes dispersion, Group 3 received IN G16 emulsomal thermogel and Group 4 received Oral Trileptal suspension. The drug dose was adjusted to be 0.32 mg/kg.

Results obtained from Group 2 and Group 4 were taken from identical experiments reported in El-Zaafarany et al. [40] for comparative reasons.

Conscious, non-anaesthetised rats were fixed in a prostrate position and 80 μL/kg of the formulations were administered into each of the two nostrils using a microinjector [44]. Blood samples were collected from the retro-orbital vein of four rats at predetermined time intervals and introduced into heparinized tubes. Plasma was separated from blood samples by centrifugation at 4000 rpm for 10 min and OX was analysed using a LC-MS/MS technique [40]. At each time interval, the animals were sacrificed and the brain tissues (not including the olfactory bulb) were separated, homogenized with saline and stored at −80°C until further assay. Ethical approval of this protocol was given by the "Experiments and Advanced Pharmaceutical Research Unit" of the Faculty of Pharmacy, Ain Shams University, Cairo, Egypt and National Institutes of Health guidelines for the use and care of Laboratory animals were followed in the course of this study (Project No.: 6 10 2016 approved on December 2016).

- Assay of OX content in plasma and brain samples

Chromatographic conditions (LC–MS/MS analysis parameters) and pharmacokinetic analysis of OX in plasma and brain (Peak plasma and brain concentrations (C_{max}), the time to reach these peaks (t_{max}) were determined, area under OX concentration-time curve ($AUC_{0–2880min}$), time to reach half the maximum plasma concentration ($t_{1/2}$), and the mean residence time (MRT)), as reported in our previous publication [40].

2.7.2. Histopathological Study

20 µL of the Ox loaded G16 emulsomal thermogel was applied daily to one nostril of male Wister rats (group size $n = 3$) weighing 180–220 g for 14 consecutive days, while the other nostril was used as control and treated with normal saline. Rats were then sacrificed and the nasal septa with their covering membranes were separated, formalin-fixed for one day, decalcified, washed with tap water, and then dehydrated by sequential exposure to methyl, ethyl and absolute alcohol).

Specimens were cleared by xylene, embedded in paraffin blocks, sectioned by slide microtome. Sections were deparaffinized and stained with hematoxylin and eosin and examined with a light microscope (Olympus optical microscope, Tokyo, Japan).

2.8. Statistical Analysis

Experiments were done in triplicates and all data that are shown in this study are expressed as a mean ± standard deviation (SD). Comparison of means was undertaken using Student *t*-test for dual comparisons and ANOVA test followed by Tukey-Kramer post-Hoc test for multiple comparisons using a statistical software program (GraphPad Instat, La Jolla, CA, USA). $p < 0.05$ were considered to be statistically significant.

3. Results

3.1. Preparation and Characterization of PLGA-PEG-PLGA Triblock Copolymers

PLGA-PEG-PLGA triblock copolymers were synthesized via ring-opening polymerization of D,L-lactide and glycolide initiated with PEG. The copolymer formed appeared as a sticky yellowish-brown semisolid. PLGA-PEG-PLGA is a non-ionic triblock copolymer consisting of hydrophilic PEG segments and hydrophobic PLGA segments. The process of polymer synthesis is shown in the supplementary part Figure S1.

3.1.1. NMR Spectroscopy

A typical NMR spectrum of PLGA-PEG-PLGA triblock copolymer is shown in the supplementary part Figure S2, showing the same characteristic signals as those reported in the literature [37]. Respective methyl (–CH_3) and methine (–CH–) proton peaks pertaining to lactide monomer were observed at 1.6 and 5.2 ppm. A peak at 4.8 ppm, corresponding to methene protons (–CH_2–) of glycolide monomer was obtained, as well as a peak at 3.6 ppm relative to methene in PEG monomer which was used for the calculation of the PEG:PLGA ratio.

By comparing the peak areas of specific types of prominent protons at corresponding chemical shifts or by the total number of these protons, the molecular weight of the polymer was calculated [36,37,45]. By analyzing the value of the integrals of peaks that are related to lactide and glycolide, the chain number molecular weight (M_n) of the tri-block copolymer was determined to be 5.2 kDa

3.1.2. GPC

Figure S3 in the supplementary part shows the GPC chromatograms of PEG and the prepared PLGA-PEG-PLGA block copolymer. It is obvious that the copolymer was eluted at a shorter time (at 6.76 min) than PEG, indicating that polymerization was successful and products of lower retention time have been formed. In addition, the unimodal GPC curve reflects that the purity of the prepared copolymer is sufficiently high. The number average molecular weight (M_n) was found to be 4.4 kDa, which corresponds to that obtained by NMR. Also, the weight average molecular weight (M_w) was determined to be 7.6 kDa, with a calculated PDI of 1.69.

3.1.3. DSC

DSC thermograms shown in Figure S4 of the supplementary part illustrate that PEG had a melting point at 49.2 °C with a melting enthalpy of 160.5 J/g. On the other hand, PLGA-PEG-PLGA exhibited glass transition at a temperature of −13.3 °C, which is comparable to what has been reported in the literature of PEG containing copolymers that show crystallization in the range of −25 to 0 °C [46].

3.1.4. DLS

Copolymers composed of hydrophilic and hydrophobic portions can when in solution be present both as individual hydrated molecules or as spherical aggregates (micelles) [37]. When these copolymers are exposed to aqueous conditions, the hydrophilic PEG and glycol portions will be oriented on the outside of the micelle in contact with water, and the hydrophobic PLGA parts will be located in the inner part of the micelle due to their hydrophobic intermolecular interactions. Thus, self-assembled micelles are formed [47]. Hence, DLS can be used as a method to highlight the transition of non-hydrated molecules to micelles i.e., copolymer association.

Figure S5 of the supplementary part shows the average micellar sizes of PLGA-PEG-PLGA copolymer samples that were prepared at 20% *w/v* and measured by DLS at temperatures ranging from 10–40 °C. No significant differences were encountered in the micellar sizes of the copolymer samples measured in the tested temperature range, as indicated by nearly overlapping peaks, always achieving results comparable to those relating to micellar systems (in the range of 4–20 nm). The observed larger size of samples measured at temperatures between 35–40 °C may be regarded as indication of system aggregation due to thermogelation [48,49].

3.2. Preparation and Characterization of Plain and Emulsome-Loaded PLGA-PEG-PLGA Thermogel Solutions

In order to study the physicochemical characteristics of PLGA-PEG-PLGA triblock copolymer solutions, either plain or emulsome-loaded, the solutions were prepared in different concentrations of the copolymer (5, 10, 20, and 30% *w/w*). Likewise, emulsomes were loaded into the copolymer solutions in concentrations of 0, 10, 25, and 50% *v/v*. For all of the prepared thermogel solutions, sol-gel transition temperature and viscosity were measured. Rheological properties of plain thermogels were studied as shown in the supplementary part (Figure S6).

3.2.1. Thermogelation of the Copolymer Solutions

The phase transition temperatures of thermogel solutions G1 to G16 were evaluated using the inverted tube method by increasing temperatures from 20 to 52 °C while checking phase changes.

Before insertion of the copolymer solution in the water bath, and below its transition temperature, the copolymer solution was clear (Figure 2A). Upon heating, the copolymer solutions became opaque without gelation (Figure 2B) or they formed a gel with an absence of flowability upon inversion (Figure 2C). Subsequent temperature decrease transforms the gel into its initial liquid state.

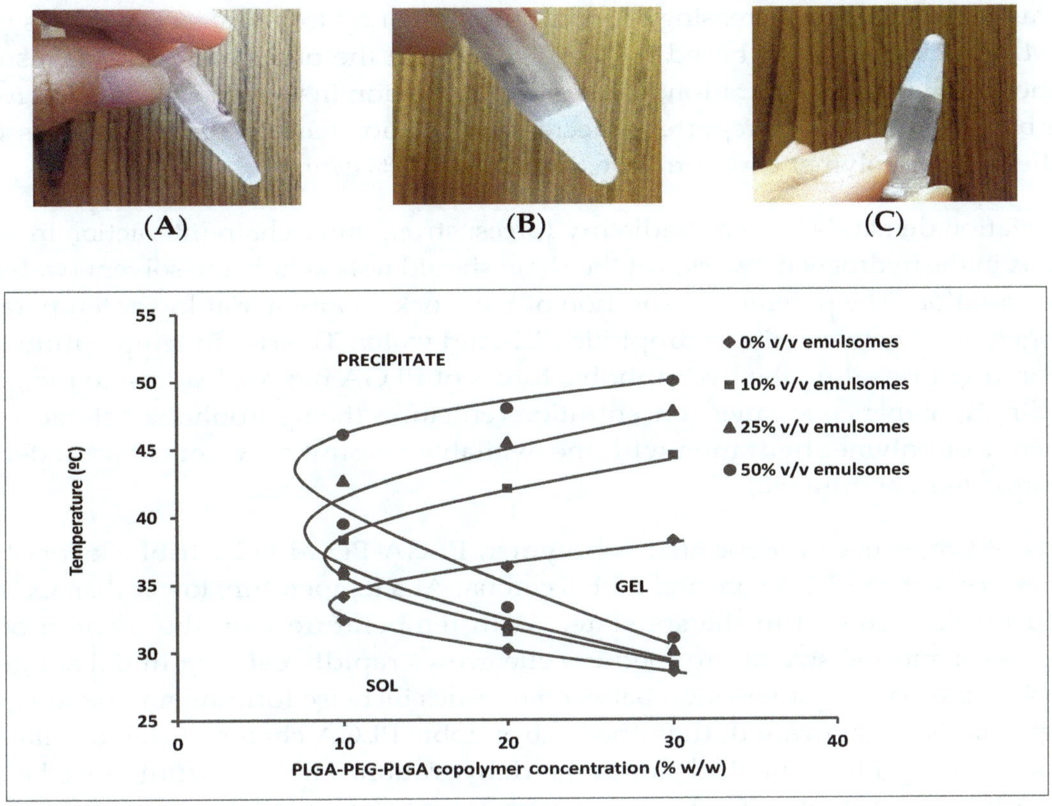

(D)

Figure 2. (**A**,**B**) are the photographs of a PLGA-PEG-PLGA copolymer solution prior to sol-gel transition (**A**) and formation of opaque solution (**B**), thermogels produced after sol-gel transition retain their position (**C**). (**D**) is the phase diagrams of polymers prepared from different PLGA-PEG-PLGA copolymer concentrations with different emulsomes loading, showing sol-gel and gel-precipitate transitions).

The sol-gel transition temperatures of all the prepared polymer solutions (G1-G16) are given in Table 1. Plain or drug loaded polymer solutions that were prepared from 5 and 10% *w/w* PLGA-PEG-PLGA copolymer (formulations G1, G5, G9, and G13) and (formulations G2, G6, G10, and G14), respectively, remained either clear or they formed turbid solutions showing no gelation till 52°C. Non-gelling opaque solutions were formed. However, formulations with higher concentrations of PLGA-PEG-PLGA (20 and 30% *w/w*) gelled, completely, at temperatures ranging between 28.50 and 33.37 °C. With temperature rise, up to 52 °C, copolymers prepared from 10, 20, and 30% *w/w* PLGA-PEG-PLGA underwent gel-precipitate transition in which the polymers reverted to a sol state (resol) but as a turbid suspension in which the polymer eventually precipitated. This thermo-reversible behavior of PLGA-PEG-PLGA copolymers has been reported in the literature [23,24,50,51]. Similar to our results, Duvvuri et al., (2005) reported the sol-gel transition temperature of 20–25% *w/v* aqueous polymer solution to be 32 °C [34]. The phase diagram of the copolymer with different emulsome loads is shown in Figure 2D.

The effect of varying PLGA-PEG-PLGA and emulsomes concentrations on the thermogelation temperatures of the copolymer solutions is shown in Table 1. At the same polymer concentration, increasing the emulsomes concentration resulted in a statistically significant increase in the transition temperatures from 30.2 ± 0.05 to 33.4 ± 0.05 °C at 20% *w/w* polymer and from 28.5 ± 0.1 to 31 ± 0.0 °C at 30% *w/w* polymer ($p > 0.05$). The increase in emulsomes concentration hinders PLGA interaction leading to retardation in gelation. The hydrophilic Tween 80 coated emulsomes with their polyoxyethylene chains are expected to render the interaction of hydrophobic blocks of PLGA-PEG-PLGA more difficult and they increase transition temperature of the composite. Similar behaviour was recorded upon increasing the concentration of hydrophilic nanoparticles incorporated in PDEGMMA block copolymer based hydrogels [51]. On the other hand, it was also found that increasing the copolymer concentration resulted in a reduction in the phase transition temperatures. On a similar basis, Qiao et al. [45] reported a decrease in gelation temperature that was associated with increasing the same copolymer concentrations from 15 to 25% *w/w*.

Hydrogelation demands two contradictory forces: strong inter-chain interaction in order to form junction points in the hydrogel network, yet the chain should not exclude the solvent (water) to prevent polymer precipitation. The polymer dissolution of the block copolymer at lower temperatures is due to the hydrogen bond between the hydrophilic PEG and water. The rise in temperature weakens the hydrogen bonding prevailing the hydrophobic forces of PLGA blocks, leading to the gel transition state. Accordingly, higher copolymer concentrations enhances the hydrophobic interactions and with the insufficiency of polymer hydration with the available amount of water causes a decrease in the sol-gel transition temperature [52].

In terms of properties of associated copolymer, PLGA-PEG-PLGA triblock copolymers form micellar structures, with a PLGA core and a PEG corona. At a temperature lower than CGT, individual and grouped micelles coexist in the sol state. With temperature rise, the fraction of individual micelles decreases and the size of grouped micelle grows rapidly causing initial sol-gel transition. The aggregation and packing interaction between micelles increase forming an opaque gel (Figure 2). If the temperature is further raised, then the hydrophobic PLGA chains of the micellar core shrink tightly and the hydrophilic PEG blocks undergo dehydration. Highly shrunk micellar groups will eventually precipitate in water, and the system becomes separated into two phases, water and polymer (Figure 1) [24].

3.2.2. Viscosity Measurement

The viscosities of all polymer solutions, post gelation at 37 °C, prepared using 20 and 30% *w/w* PLGA-PEG-PLGA copolymer and 0, 10, 25, and 50% *v/v* emulsomes, and measured at rpms ranging from 1 to 100 are shown in Figure 3. The figure shows that the rheological behavior of both plain and emulsome-loaded thermogels was concentration-dependent. Generally, an increase in viscosity accompanied the increase in copolymer and emulsome concentrations, especially when measured at the lowest rpm due to the preservation of the gel network structure.

Figure 3A shows that at 20% *w/w* copolymer concentration the viscosities were in the order: G15 > G11 > G7 > G3, at lower rpms ($p < 0.05$), directly correlated to with increasing emulsome concentration. However, G15 showed the absolute highest viscosity at all rpm values due to its 50% emulsomal content ($p < 0.01$). A similar trend was observed for G16 containing 30% *w/w* copolymer Figure 3B.

The incorporation of emulsomes will contribute to the formation of a stronger gel matrix. The presence of emulsomes caused a delay in PLGA interaction and micellar formation. Better polymer hydration occurred with the formation of highly viscous gel. A suggestion confirmed by the increase in gelation temperature by the incorporation of emulsomes. Likewise, Guo et al. [53] reported a concentration dependent rheological behavior of methoxyestradiol solid lipid nanoparticles loaded into a PLGA-PEG-PLGA thermosensitive hydrogel accompanied with viscosity increase.

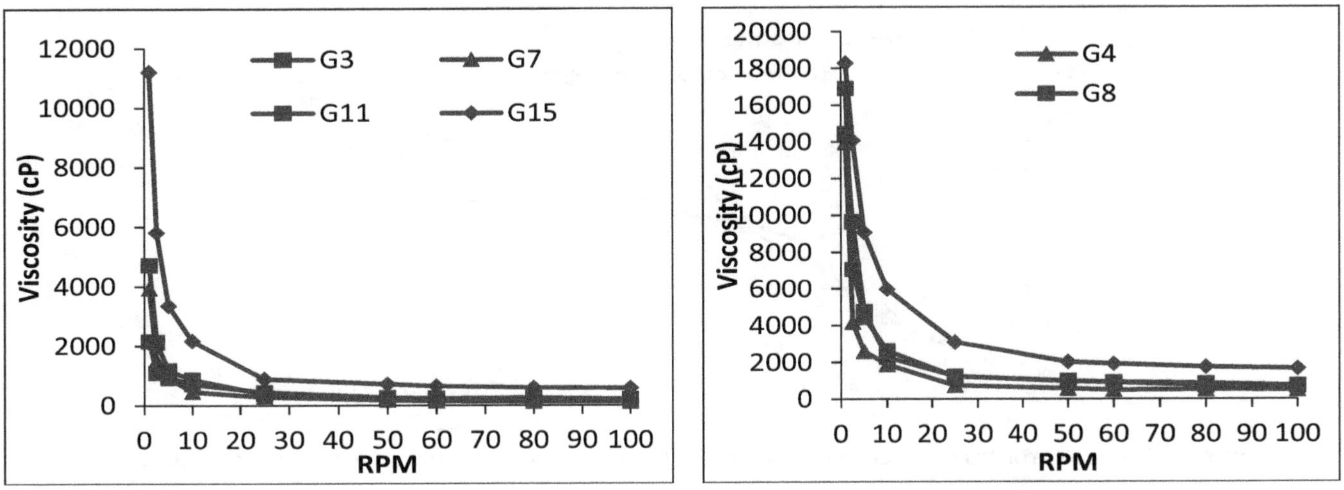

(A) (B)

Figure 3. Rheograms of thermogels G3, G7, G11 and G15 prepared from 20% *w/w* PLGA-PEG-PLGA copolymer solution (**A**) and thermogels G4, G8, G12 and G16 prepared from 30% *w/w* PLGA-PEG-PLGA copolymer solution (**B**) in combination with 0, 10, 25, and 50% *v/v* emulsomes measured at 37 °C.

The study also revealed that significantly higher viscosities were encountered ($p < 0.01$) for 30% *w/w* copolymer (formulations: G4, G8, G12, and G16), at all emulsomal concentrations, than for 20% (formulations: G3, G7, G11, and G15). This was an expected behavior because higher copolymer concentration is translated into a denser thermogel matrix, and hence, higher viscosity [38,54]. Due to its high viscosity, G16 emulsomal thermogel was selected for further studies. The G16 emulsomal thermogel showed viscosity values of 3090 cp and 1656 cp at shear rate of 50 and 200 s^{-1} (sneezing produce a maximum shear rate of only >180 s^{-1} [55]). Knowing that IN formulations may leave the nasal cavity by gravity when their viscosity is less than about 2500 centipoise [56], G16 emulsomal thermogel represents a good candidate for IN delivery of OX.

3.3. *In Vitro* Release Study

Three mechanisms for controlling drug release from PLGA based matrices have previously been described, namely (i) Fickian diffusion through the polymer matrix, (ii) diffusion through water-filled pores (aqueous channels) formed by water penetration into the matrix, and (iii) liberation by erosion of the polymer matrix [57]. The actual drug release from these polymer matrices may be controlled by a combination of these three mechanisms [58].

Figure 4 shows the cumulative average amounts of OX released from emulsomes in comparison with G16 emulsomal thermogel for up to 24 h. Both formulations showed similar release profiles with no significant difference ($p < 0.05$) during the first 8 h. However, after 24 h, the OX release was reduced significantly from 81.1 to 53.5% ($p < 0.01$) in the G16 emulsomal thermogel as compared to the OX-emulsomes. The lack of initial difference in release profile between emulsomes and emulsomal thermogel may be due to the low solubility of OX, which would enhance its retention in both emulsomes and emulsomal thermogel up to 8 h of release. However, after 24 h more OX dissolved from the emulsomal core, and was released directly to the medium in case of emulsomes in comparison with emulsomes dispersed in hydrogel which showed a retarded OX release. Similar behaviour has been shown in situ with emulsomal thermosensitive gel, which was loaded with sparfloxacin for ocular delivery. A release profile that depended on drug solubility for up to 8–10 h was shown, however, when drug release was assessed at longer times it increased dramatically [59].

Moreover, drug release from hydrogel depots can be influenced by many factors, including pore size, rate of degradability of the hydrogel, size and morphology of the matrix, concentration of drug, interactions between the hydrogel and the loaded drug delivery system, polymer molecular weight, lactide/glycolide copolymer ratio, as well as matrix fabrication method [60].

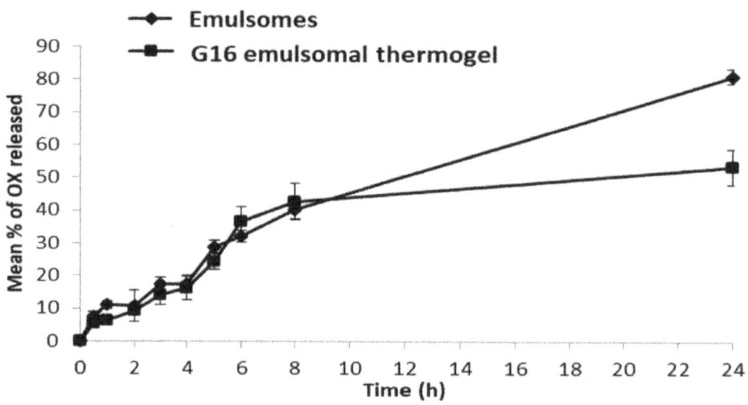

Figure 4. Release profiles of Oxcarbazepine (OX) from emulsomes and G16 emulsomal thermogel.

3.4. Mucoadhesion Study

One important design feature of formulations designed for IN administration is the ability to exhibit retention within the nasal cavity with the constant exposure to mucocilliary clearance and enzymatic degradation. Table 2 shows the mucoadhesion parameters (peak detachment, deformation peak, work of adhesion, final load) measured for plain (thermogel G4) and emulsome-loaded PLGA-PEG-PLGA copolymer (G16 emulsomal thermogel), as compared with a 0.5% carbopol gel as a positive standard.

Table 2. Mucoadhesion parameters measured for plain (G4) and G16 emulsome-loaded PLGA-PEG-PLGA thermogel compared with a standard Carbopol 980 gel.

Parameter	Plain G4 Thermogel (Mean ± SD)	G16 Emulsomal Thermogel (Mean ± SD)	Carbopol 980 Gel (Mean ± SD)
Peak detachment force (N)	21.9 ± 1.7 *	18.7 ± 2.3 *	10.52 ± 0.1
Deformation peak (mm)	10.5 ± 2 *	8.2 ± 1.3	5.4 ± 0.8
Work of adhesion (mJ)	788.3 ± 23.7 *	746.6 ± 52.2 *	304.8 ± 35
Final load (N)	20.2 ± 1.7	17.84 ± 2.9	15.41 ± 1.9

* Significantly different from Carbopol 980 gel ($p < 0.05$).

The "work of adhesion", also termed "adhesiveness", describes the work that is required to overcome the attractive forces between the surface of the sample and the surface of the probe [61]. This infers that probe removal occurs due to cleavage of both internal bonds within the sample (cohesive bonds), as well as, bonds occurring between the sample and the surface of the probe (adhesive bonds) [62].

The G4 and G16 gels both showed statistically significant higher adhesive properties for all mucoadhesive parameters, when compared to the Carbopol980 gel standard ($p < 0.05$). During optimal contact time between formulation and mucosa that ensures maximal adhesion, gel hydration occurs, which allows for exposure of its adhesive sites. This facilitates interpenetration of the gel adhesive moieties and entanglement with mucus glycoproteins of the nasal mucosa, to a sufficient depth that enables the creation of adhesive bonds [63], thus creating mucoadhesion. On a similar basis, Yu and co-workers proved that PLGA-PEG nanoparticles can penetrate human mucus secretions due to strong interactions with mucin [64]. Besides the results show that the increase in viscosity might help, but it is not crucial for mucoadhesion [65]. Thus, G16 emulsomal thermogel would be expected to show prolonged retention in the nasal cavity through the formation of adhesive bonds with the tissues lining the nasal mucosa. Since the half-life of clearance from the nasal cavity in humans, even for bioadhesive materials is in the order of 1–2 h [66], the differences in OX release after 8 h between the OX-emulsomes and the G16 emulsomal thermogel will likely not affect the nasal absorption of the OX in humans.

It is worthy to note that emulsomes had no influence on the mucoadhesive characters of PLGA-PEG-PLGA copolymer, probably because the binding with mucin occurs via hydrophilic interaction with the PEG chains of the polymer while emulsomes only interact with hydrophobic PLGA domains.

3.5. Pharmacokinetic Study

3.5.1. Plasma Pharmacokinetic Parameters

Nose-to-brain drug delivery represents a potential route for targeting drugs to the CNS and avoiding large systemic losses after drug administration. Figure 5A shows plasma concentration-time profiles of OX after the administration of Trileptal® suspension, IN solution, IN emulsomes, and IN G16 emulsomal thermogel loaded with the drug, with the corresponding PK parameters given in Table 3. Data of OX-emulsomes and Trileptal® suspension were incorporated into the paper for comparative purposes.

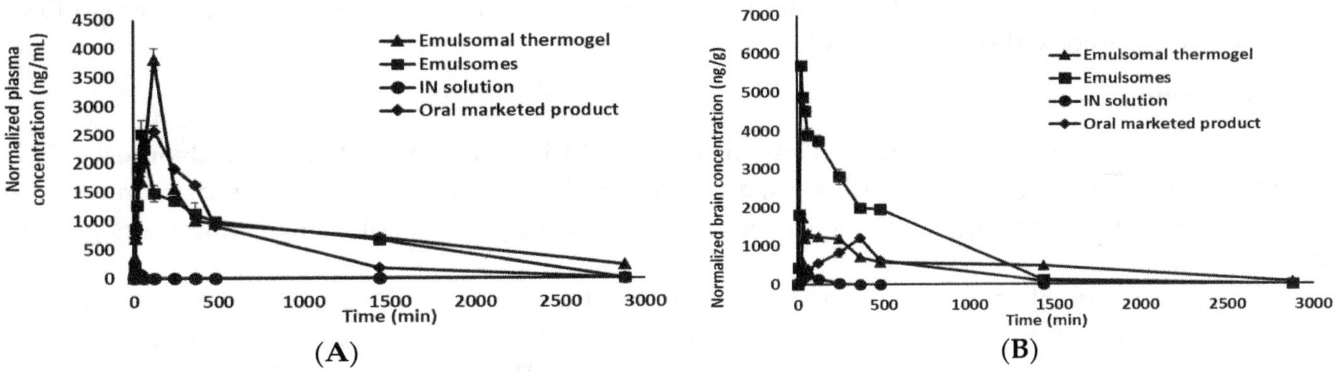

Figure 5. Mean OX concentrations in plasma (**A**) in brain (**B**) of rat groups receiving IN administration of emulsomes, G16 emulsomal thermogel, OX solution and Oral Trileptal® suspension. Data of IN administration of emulsomes, and Oral Trileptal® suspension reproduced with permission from El-Zaafarany et al. [40], Elsevier, 2016.

Table 3. Pharmacokinetic parameters for OX in rat plasma/brain following the IN administration of emulsomes, G16 emulsomal thermogel, OX solution and Oral Trileptal® suspension.

Parameter	Plasma				Brain			
	IN Emulsomes *	IN Emulsomal Thermogel	IN OX Solutions	Trileptal® Suspension *	IN Emulsomes *	IN Emulsomal Thermogel	IN OX Solutions	Trileptal® Suspension *
C_{max} (ng/mL)/(ng/g)	2514.4	3818.8	80.9	2567.6	5699.9	1733.2	249.1	1198.9
T_{max} (min)	45	120	20	120	20	30	60	360
$AUC_{0-2880min}$ (μg/mL·min)/(μg/g·min)	1943.4	2757.7	111.2	1524.6	2445.1	1440.5	57.7	742.8
$T_{1/2}$ (min)	1581.8	1919.6	302.1	364	250.9	734	197.4	285.6
MRT (min)	2024.3	2638.1	34.5	465.4	378	1007.8	95.4	504.5

* Data reproduced with permission from El-Zaafarany et al. [40], Elsevier, 2016.

In terms of plasma concentrations, the results revealed that the highest C_{max} of 3818.8 ng/mL ($p < 0.01$) was encountered after the instillation of IN G16 emulsomal thermogel at a T_{max} of 120 min, followed by Trileptal® suspension and IN emulsomes, which reached C_{max} value of 2567.6 and 2514.4 ng/mL at T_{max} value of 45 and 120 min, respectively, and finally the IN OX solution had the lowest C_{max} of 80.9 ng/mL after 20 min. The largest AUC $_{0-2880min}$ was obtained after administration of the IN G16 thermogel, followed by the IN OX emulsomes, Trileptal® suspension then IN OX solution ($p < 0.05$).

Furthermore, emulsomes and G16 thermogel formulations showed an MRT in plasma 58.7 and 76.5 times that of the IN OX solution respectively. Significantly larger residual amounts of OX after

2880 min were found in the plasma for G16 thermogel than for the OX emulsomes and IN OX solution ($p < 0.01$) (Figure 6). On the other hand, the OX administered IN in emulsomes and G16 thermogel resided in the plasma for up to 34 and 44 h, respectively. The plasma half-life of the G16 thermogel was found to be 1.2 times that of the IN OX emulsomes and significantly higher i.e., 6.4 and 5.3 times that of the IN OX solution and Trileptal® suspension, respectively ($p < 0.05$).

The long residence in plasma of OX when administered in combination with emulsomes (as opposed to the OX solution) might be explained by the lipophilic nature of the emulsomes that may allow for the partitioning of the OX in the emulsome particles (and/or the free OX) into the nasal epithelial cell membranes and further into the systemic circulation. The high absorption of OX, as shown by the $AUC_{0\text{–}2880min}$ and long mean residence time from the IN G16 emulsomal thermogel compared to IN OX-solution could be partly attributed to the high viscosity of the gel formulation which prolonged the contact time with nasal mucosa, thus enhancing the penetration of OX-emulsomes and/or free OX through the nasal mucosa into the systemic circulation [67]. The pharmacokinetic results suggest that the encapsulation of OX in emulsomes slowed its elimination, retained a high concentration in the bloodstream for a longer time period, and increased the circulation time of OX in rats, when compared to the free drug [68].

3.5.2. Brain Pharmacokinetic Parameters

OX concentrations in the brains of rats after the administration of IN OX-emulsomes, IN G16 OX-emulsomal thermogel, IN OX solution, and Trileptal® suspension of OX at predetermined time intervals are depicted in Figure 5B, with the corresponding pharmacokinetic parameters given in Table 3.

The OX concentration in the brain after administration in an IN OX solution was detected after 10 min of administration, showed a low C_{max} and reached baseline in 6 h. This observation and the low C_{max} in the plasma support the reported low ability of OX to cross mucosal membranes [69–71].

OX released from emulsomes and G16 thermogel was detected in the brain only 5 min after administration, but with significantly ($p < 0.01$) higher brain concentration (5 times) for the OX- emulsome formulation, as compared with that of the G16 OX-emulsomal thermogel formulation. Furthermore, the nasal administration of OX-emulsomes resulted in the highest OX brain C_{max} which was nearly 3.3, 22.9, and 4.8 times that of G16 OX-emulsomal thermogel, IN solution and Trileptal® suspension, respectively, with earlier T_{max} for emulsomes than all tested formulations. In contrast to the plasma data, the OX-emulsomes showed higher brain $AUC_{0\text{–}2880min}$ than G16 OX-emulsomal thermogel, IN OX solution and Trileptal® suspension. This could be attributed to the structure of emulsomes that comprises its lipidic phospholipid sheath, the Tween 80 coat and the small size (100–200 nm), all which are contributing factors to enable transcellular diffusion of OX (free or encapsulated) through the blood brain barrier [72]. Detection of OX in the brain within a time frame of 10–20 min after IN administration of emulsomes indicates that direct nose-to-brain transport was a main route for brain uptake from the nasal mucosa [73], in addition to its systemic absorption.

On the other hand, G16 OX-emulsomal thermogel had longer mean residence times in the brain, which exceeded that of the OX-emulsomes, IN OX solution and Trileptal® suspension. Also, the G16 emulsomal thermogel was the only tested formulation in which OX was detected in the brain after 48 h of its IN instillation (data not shown) which could result in a better control of seizures in patients for a longer time period. These results are in accordance with previously reported studies in animals that proved that formulations with a prolonged residence in the nasal cavity using either mucoadhesive systems or gels with very high viscosity can enhance the nose to brain delivery of drugs due to reduced mucociliary clearance and increased residence which ensure higher absorption. Furthermore, it has also been reported that some mucoadhesive polymer-containing systems may directly change epithelial tight junctions and thus, increase drug absorption [74,75].

Although the IN adminstration of emulsomal thermogel showed a lower C_{max} in the brain, it showed higher MRT values. It was previously reported that it is more advisable to use extended-action formulations for antiepileptic drugs with short half-lives (OX $t_{1/2}$ = 1–5 h) for a more efficient way of treating epilepsy [76].

When compared with formulations that rapidly release antiepileptic drugs, products with extended residence in the brain not only allow for a long dosing interval, which improve patient compliance but also decrease the risk of seizure breakthrough after missing a dose. Furthermore it was found that the use of sustained OX formulations for the treatment of focal epilepsy showed better tolerability and higher maintenance dosages to be reached than immediate action formulations [77].

3.6. Histopathological Examination

Nasal histopathology studies on rats were done to check the probable changes in the nasal mucosa caused by G16 emulsomal thermogel, in comparison to normal saline treated nasal epithelium. The control group showed normal, well defined histological structures without any signs of vascular or inflammatory changes (Figure 6A). The histopathology of the treated group revealed some signs of very low toxicity after administration of the G16 OX-emulsome thermogel (Figure 6B). This toxicity was lower than that reported for the drug alone and it is seen here as mild vascular congestion and moderate inflammatory changes around congested vessels.

The safety of PLGA-PEG-PLGA thermogels for a variety of biological applications has been previously reported [32,78–80]. Hence, this mild inflammation probably pertains to the effect of the drug on the nasal mucosa due to its controlled release throughout the study, since OX has been reported to have an irritant effect on cells by NADPH dependant DNA intercalation [81].

This observation of mild cell toxicity induced by OX is in agreement with previous finding [40,82] that showed OX as an agent that can cause anatomic and organizational disruption in cell layers, nuclear shrinkage, and cell atrophy. Conclusively, these findings would add to our previous finding that emulsomes can shield OX cell damaging effects [40] the ability of G16 emulsomal thermogel composite to further protect nasal cells from the severe effect of OX. Thus, adopted PLGA-PEG-PLGA thermogel matrices could be used to enhance safety and reduce the nasal damage of many other cell membrane damaging drugs.

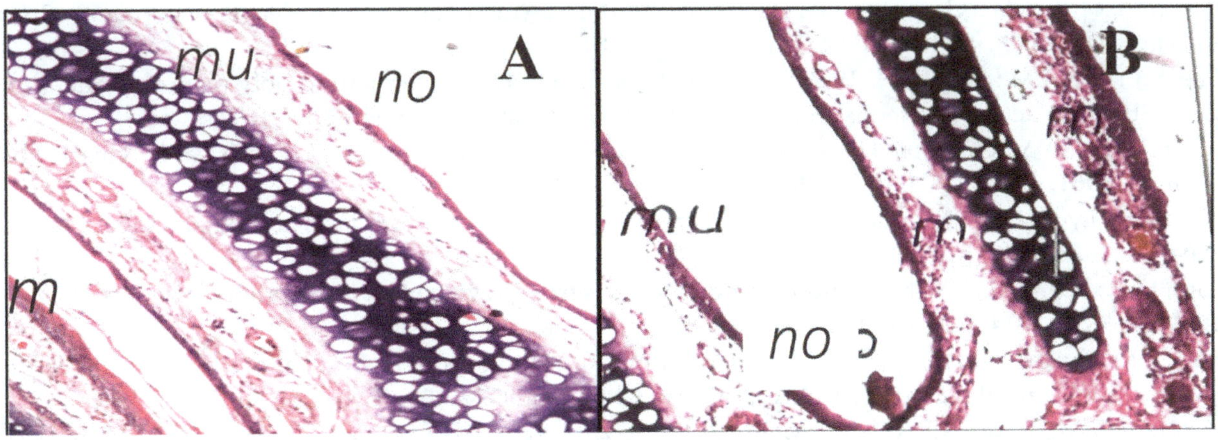

Figure 6. Light micrograph of (**A**) untreated nasal rat epithelium (with saline only) showing normal structure of the nose (no) with intact mucosal epithelium (mu). (**B**) nasal rat epithelium treated with OX-loaded G16 emulsomal thermogel showing intact mucosal epithelium (mu) with minimal focal inflammatory cells infiltration (m). (Maginifcation 16×).

4. Conclusions

A successful PEG-initiated ring opening polymerization of lactide and glycolide to prepare PLGA-PEG-PLGA triblock copolymer was confirmed by NMR, GPC, DSC, and DLS. The copolymer was mixed with emulsomes to form thermoresponsive gels for the nasal delivery of OX. All of the prepared thermoresponsive gels exhibited a reversible thermogelling behavior with visible precipitation of the copolymer at elevated temperatures. Both copolymer and emulsome concentrations contributed, to the formation of thermogels with high viscosities. Sequestration of emulsomes in 30% thermogel resulted in retardation of OX release, increased gel matrix viscosity, but did not affect mucoadhesive properties as compared to thermogel alone. The OX-emulsome thermogel dramatically increased the systemic OX absorption but did not improve the OX brain concentration in terms of C_{max} and AUC as compared to the OX-emulsomes alone. However, the emulsomal thermogel, extended the presence of OX in the brain to up to 48 h, which could offer a better control of seizures for a longer time period. A fact that needs to be investigated further.

Supplementary Materials:
Figure S1. Synthesis of PLGA-PEG-PLGA triblock copolymer by ring opening polymerization of glycolide, D,L-lactide and polyethylene glycol (PEG); Figure S2. ^{1}H-NMR spectrum of PLGA-PEG-PLGA tri-block copolymer with (a) and (d) pertaining to lactide methyl and methane protons, (b) pertaining to ethylene oxide methene protons and (c) pertaining to glycolide methene protons; Figure S3. GPC chromatograms of PEG and PLGA-PEG-PLGA copolymer; Figure S4. DSC thermograms of PEG polymer and the synthesized PLGA-PEG-PLGA tri-block copolymer; Figure S5. Size distribution of PLGA-PEG-PLGA micellar solution (20% *w/v* in deionized water) measured at temperatures in the range of 10 to 45 °C; Figure S6. (A)Temperature sweep data that shows variation in viscosity and phase angle with temperature for PLGA-PEG-PLGA copolymer samples prepared in concentrations of 15, 20, and 25% *w/v* in deionized water (B) Time sweep data that shows variation in elastic modulus, viscous modulus and viscosity of PLGA-PEG-PLGA copolymer sample with time (C) Frequency sweep data that shows variation in elastic and viscous modulus with frequency for PLGA-PEG-PLGA copolymer samples prepared in concentrations of 15, 20, and 25% *w/v* in deionized water.

Author Contributions: Conceptualization, L.C., M.E.S and G.A.S.A.; methodology, L.C., M.E.S., G.M.E.-Z. and M.C.; formal analysis and investigation L.C., G.M.E.-Z., S.M., M.C. and M.E.S.; resources, L.C., G.F.P. and G.A.S.A.; writing—original draft preparation, L.C., S.M., M.E.S. and M.C.; writing—review and editing, L.C., M.E.S., L.I. and G.A.S.A.; funding acquisition, L.C., G.F.P. and G.A.S.A.

Acknowledgments: The authors wish to thank Fabio De Belvis for the design and realization of the graphical abstract.

References

1. Yan, H.; Fujiwara, H.; Sasaki, K.; Tsujii, K. Rapid Swelling/Collapsing Behavior of Thermoresponsive Poly(*N*-isopropylacrylamide) Gel Containing Poly(2-(methacryloyloxy)decyl phosphate) Surfactant. *Angew. Chem.* **2005**, *44*, 1951–1954. [CrossRef] [PubMed]
2. Bae, S.J.; Suh, J.M.; Sohn, Y.S.; Bae, Y.H.; Kim, S.W.; Jeong, B. Thermogelling poly (caprolactone-b-ethylene glycol-b-caprolactone) aqueous solutions. *Macromolecules* **2005**, *38*, 5260–5265. [CrossRef]
3. Ji, S.; Ding, J. A Macroscopic Helix Formation Induced by the Shrinking of a Cylindrical Polymeric Hydrogel. *Polym. J.* **2001**, *33*, 701–703. [CrossRef]
4. Nayak, S.; Lyon, L.A. Photoinduced phase transitions in poly(*N*-isopropylacrylamide) microgels. *Chem. Mater.* **2004**, *16*, 2623–2627. [CrossRef]
5. Kim, H.-J.; Lee, J.-H.; Lee, M. Stimuli-Responsive Gels from Reversible Coordination Polymers. *Angew. Chem.* **2005**, *44*, 5810–5814. [CrossRef] [PubMed]
6. Suri, J.T.; Cordes, D.B.; Cappuccio, F.E.; Wessling, R.A.; Singaram, B. Continuous Glucose Sensing with a Fluorescent Thin-Film Hydrogel. *Angew. Chem.* **2003**, *42*, 5857–5859. [CrossRef] [PubMed]
7. Zentner, G.M.; Rathi, R.; Shih, C.; McRea, J.C.; Seo, M.-H.; Oh, H.; Rhee, B.; Mestecky, J.; Moldoveanu, Z.; Morgan, M. Biodegradable block copolymers for delivery of proteins and water-insoluble drugs. *J. Control. Release* **2001**, *72*, 203–215. [CrossRef]
8. Tiller, J.C. Increasing the Local Concentration of Drugs by Hydrogel Formation. *Angew. Chem.* **2003**, *42*, 3072–3075. [CrossRef] [PubMed]
9. Zhang, Y.; Zhu, W.; Wang, B.; Ding, J. A novel microgel and associated post-fabrication encapsulation technique of proteins. *J. Control. Release* **2005**, *105*, 260–268. [CrossRef] [PubMed]
10. Beebe, D.J.; Moore, J.S.; Bauer, J.M.; Yu, Q.; Liu, R.H.; Devadoss, C.; Jo, B.-H. Functional hydrogel structures for autonomous flow control inside microfluidic channels. *Nature* **2000** *404*, 588–590. [CrossRef] [PubMed]
11. Eeckman, F.; Moës, A.J.; Amighi, K. Synthesis and characterization of thermosensitive copolymers for oral controlled drug delivery. *Eur. Polym. J.* **2004**, *40*, 873–881. [CrossRef]

12. Casey, D.J.; Jarrett, P.K.; Rosati, L. Diblock and Triblock Copolymers. Patents US4716203A, 29 December 1987.
13. Cerrai, P.; Tricoli, M.; Andruzzi, F.; Paci, M.; Paci, M. Polyether-polyester block copolymers by non-catalysed polymerization of ϵ-caprolactone with poly (ethylene glycol). *Polymer* **1989**, *30*, 338–343. [CrossRef]
14. Youxin, L.; Kissel, T. Synthesis and properties of biodegradable ABA triblock copolymers consisting of poly (L-lactic acid) or poly (L-lactic-*co*-glycolic acid) A-blocks attached to central poly (oxyethylene) B-blocks. *J. Control. Release* **1993**, *27*, 247–257. [CrossRef]
15. Jeong, B.; Bae, Y.H.; Kim, S.W. Drug release from biodegradable injectable thermosensitive hydrogel of PEG–PLGA–PEG triblock copolymers. *J. Control. Release* **2000**, *63*, 155–163. [CrossRef]
16. Jeong, B.; Lee, K.M.; Gutowska, A.; An, Y.H. % Thermogelling Biodegradable Copolymer Aqueous Solutions for Injectable Protein Delivery and Tissue Engineering. *Biomacromolecules* **2002**, *3*, 865–868. [CrossRef] [PubMed]
17. Kim, H.-J.; Lee, J.-H.; Lee, M. Stimuli-responsive gels from reversible coordination polymers. *Angew. Chem.* **2005**, *117*, 5960–5964. [CrossRef]
18. Ruel-Gariepy, E.; Leroux, J.-C. In situ-forming hydrogels—Review of temperature-sensitive systems. *Eur. J. Pharm. Biopharm.* **2004**, *58*, 409–426. [CrossRef] [PubMed]
19. Katakam, M.; Ravis, W.R.; Banga, A.K. Controlled release of human growth hormone in rats following parenteral administration of poloxamer gels. *J. Control. Release* **1997**, *49*, 21–26. [CrossRef]
20. Wenzel, J.G.; Balaji, K.S.; Koushik, K.; Navarre, C.; Duran, S.H.; Rahe, C.H.; Kompella, U.B. Pluronic® F127 gel formulations of Deslorelin and GnRH reduce drug degradation and sustain drug release and effect in cattle. *J. Control. Release* **2002**, *85*, 51–59. [CrossRef]
21. Huh, K.M.; Cho, Y.W.; Park, K. PLGA-PEG block copolymers for drug formulations. *Drug Dev. Deliv.* **2003**, *3*, 1–11.
22. Zhang, J. *Switchable and Responsive Surfaces and Materials for Biomedical Applications*; Elsevier: New York, NY, USA, 2014.
23. Nguyen, M.K.; Lee, D.S. Injectable biodegradable hydrogels. *Macromol. Biosci.* **2010**, *10*, 563–579. [CrossRef] [PubMed]
24. Shim, M.S.; Lee, H.T.; Shim, W.S.; Park, I.; Lee, H.; Chang, T.; Kim, S.W.; Lee, D.S. Poly (D,L-lactic acid-*co*-glycolic acid)-*b*-poly (ethylene glycol)-*b*-poly (D,L-lactic acid-*co*-glycolic acid) triblock copolymer and thermoreversible phase transition in water. *J. Biomed. Mater. Res. A* **2002**, *61*, 188–196. [CrossRef] [PubMed]
25. Lee, A.L.; Venkataraman, S.; Fox, C.H.; Coady, D.J.; Frank, C.W.; Hedrick, J.L.; Yang, Y.Y. Modular composite hydrogels from cholesterol-functionalized polycarbonates for antimicrobial applications. *J. Mater. Chem. B* **2015**, *3*, 6953–6963. [CrossRef]
26. Karavasili, C.; Fatouros, D.G. Smart materials: In situ gel-forming systems for nasal delivery. *Drug Discov. Today* **2016**, *21*, 157–166. [CrossRef] [PubMed]
27. Toledano, R.; Gil-Nagel, A. Adverse effects of antiepileptic drugs. *Semin. Neurol.* **2008**, *28*, 317–327. [CrossRef] [PubMed]
28. Minn, A.; Leclerc, S.; Heydel, J.-M.; Minn, A.-L.; Denizot, C.; Cattarelli, M.; Netter, P.; Gradinaru, D. Drug transport into the mammalian brain: The nasal pathway and its specific metabolic barrier. *J. Drug Target.* **2002**, *10*, 285–296. [CrossRef] [PubMed]
29. Chandrika, M.V.; Babu, M.K. Design and development of Candesartan cilexetil emulsomal drug delivery systems for the effective management of cardiovascular diseases. *Indian J. Res. Pharm. Biotechnol.* **2014**, *2*, 1283.
30. Ucisik, M.H.; Küpcü, S.; Schuster, B.; Sleytr, U.B. Characterization of CurcuEmulsomes: Nanoformulation for enhanced solubility anddelivery of curcumin. *J. Nanobiotechnol.* **2013**, *11*, 37. [CrossRef] [PubMed]
31. Kumar, D.; Sharma, D.; Singh, G.; Singh, M.; Rathore, M.S. Lipoidal soft hybrid biocarriers of supramolecular construction for drug delivery. *ISRN Pharm.* **2012**, *2012*, 474830. [CrossRef] [PubMed]
32. Chen, Y.-C.; Hsieh, W.-Y.; Lee, W.-F.; Zeng, D.-T. Effects of surface modification of PLGA-PEG-PLGA nanoparticles on loperamide delivery efficiency across the blood–brain barrier. *J. Biomater. Appl.* **2013**, *27*, 909–922. [CrossRef] [PubMed]
33. Ding, M.; Li, J.; Tan, H.; Fu, Q. Self-assembly of biodegradable polyurethanes for controlled delivery applications. *Soft Matter* **2012**, *8*, 5414–5428. [CrossRef]

34. Duvvuri, S.; Janoria, K.G.; Mitra, A.K. Development of a novel formulation containing poly (D, L-lactide-*co*-glycolide) microspheres dispersed in PLGA–PEG–PLGA gel for sustained delivery of ganciclovir. *J. Control. Release* **2005**, *108*, 282–293. [CrossRef] [PubMed]
35. Senesi, A. *Analysis of Rheological Properties of Thermogel Copolymers Based PLGA-PEG1500-PLGA: Effect of the Molecular Weight of the Side Chains*; University of Camerino: Camerino, Italy, 2013.
36. Ghahremankhani, A.A.; Dorkoosh, F.; Dinarvand, R. PLGA-PEG-PLGA tri-block copolymers as an in-situ gel forming system for calcitonin delivery. *Polym. Bull.* **2007**, *59*, 637–646. [CrossRef]
37. Song, Z.; Feng, R.; Sun, M.; Guo, C.; Gao, Y.; Li, L.; Zhai, G. Curcumin-loaded PLGA-PEG-PLGA triblock copolymeric micelles: Preparation, pharmacokinetics and distribution in vivo. *J. Colloid Interface Sci.* **2011**, *354*, 116–123. [CrossRef] [PubMed]
38. Gao, Y.; Ren, F.; Ding, B.; Sun, N.; Liu, X.; Ding, X.; Gao, S. A thermo-sensitive PLGA-PEG-PLGA hydrogel for sustained release of docetaxel. *J. Drug Target.* **2011**, *19*, 516–527. [CrossRef] [PubMed]
39. Paliwal, R.; Paliwal, S.R.; Mishra, N.; Mehta, A.; Vyas, S.P. Engineered chylomicron mimicking carrier emulsome for lymph targeted oral delivery of methotrexate. *Int. J. Pharm.* **2009**, *380*, 181–188. [CrossRef] [PubMed]
40. El-Zaafarany, G.M.; Soliman, M.E.; Mansour, S.; Awad, G.A.S. Identifying lipidic emulsomes for improved oxcarbazepine brain targeting: In vitro and rat in vivo studies. *Int. J. Pharm.* **2016**, *503*, 127–140. [CrossRef] [PubMed]
41. Khodaverdi, E.; Hadizadeh, F.; Tekie, F.S.M.; Jalali, A.; Mohajeri, S.A.; Ganji, F. Preparation and analysis of a sustained drug delivery system by PLGA–PEG–PLGA triblock copolymers. *Polym. Bull.* **2012**, *69*, 429–438. [CrossRef]
42. Basu, S.; Bandyopadhyay, A.K. Development and characterization of mucoadhesive in situ nasal gel of midazolam prepared with Ficus carica mucilage. *AAPS PharmSciTech* **2010**, *11*, 1223–1231. [CrossRef] [PubMed]
43. Patel, V.M.; Prajapati, B.G.; Patel, M.M. Formulation, evaluation, and comparison of bilayered and multilayered mucoadhesive buccal devices of propranolol hydrochloride. *AAPS PharmSciTech* **2007**, *8*, E147–E154. [CrossRef] [PubMed]
44. Gabal, Y.M.; Kamel, A.O.; Sammour, O.A.; Elshafeey, A.H. Effect of surface charge on the brain delivery of nanostructured lipid carriers in situ gels via the nasal route. *Int. J. Pharm.* **2014**, *473*, 442–457. [CrossRef] [PubMed]
45. Qiao, M.; Chen, D.; Ma, X.; Liu, Y. Injectable biodegradable temperature-responsive PLGA–PEG–PLGA copolymers: Synthesis and effect of copolymer composition on the drug release from the copolymer-based hydrogels. *Int. J. Pharm.* **2005**, *294*, 103–112. [CrossRef] [PubMed]
46. Shit, S.C.; Maiti, S. Application of NMR spectroscopy in molecular weight determination of polymers. *Eur. Polym. J.* **1986**, *22*, 1001–1008. [CrossRef]
47. Perinelli, D.; Bonacucina, G.; Cespi, M.; Naylor, A.; Whitaker, M.; Palmieri, G.; Giorgioni, G.; Casettari, L. Evaluation of P (L) LA-PEG-P (L) LA as processing aid for biodegradable particles from gas saturated solutions (PGSS) process. *Int. J. Pharm.* **2014**, *468*, 250–257. [CrossRef] [PubMed]
48. Kwon, G.S.; Cho, H. Thermogel Formulation for Combination Drug Delivery. Patents US20150025106, 22 July 2014.
49. Chen, Y.; Li, Y.; Shen, W.; Li, K.; Yu, L.; Chen, Q.; Ding, J. Controlled release of liraglutide using thermogelling polymers in treatment of diabetes. *Sci. Rep.* **2016**, *6*, 31593. [CrossRef] [PubMed]
50. Yu, L.; Zhang, Z.; Ding, J. Influence of LA and GA sequence in the PLGA block on the properties of thermogelling PLGA-PEG-PLGA block copolymers. *Biomacromolecules* **2011**, *12*, 1290–1297. [CrossRef] [PubMed]
51. Chen, L.; Ci, T.; Yu, L.; Ding, J. Effects of molecular weight and its distribution of peg block on micellization and thermogellability of plga–peg–plga copolymer aqueous solutions. *Macromolecules* **2015**, *48*, 3662–3671. [CrossRef]
52. Jeong, B.; Kim, S.W.; Bae, Y.H. Thermosensitive sol–gel reversible hydrogels. *Adv. Drug Deliv. Rev.* **2012**, *64*, 154–162. [CrossRef]
53. Guo, X.; Cui, F.; Xing, Y.; Mei, Q.; Zhang, Z. Investigation of a new injectable thermosensitive hydrogel loading solid lipid nanoparticles. *Die Pharmazie* **2011**, *66*, 948–952. [PubMed]

54. Yang, Y.; Wang, J.; Zhang, X.; Lu, W.; Zhang, Q. A novel mixed micelle gel with thermo-sensitive property for the local delivery of docetaxel. *J. Control. Release* **2009**, *135*, 175–182. [CrossRef] [PubMed]
55. Gwaltney, J.J.M.; Hendley, J.O.; Phillips, C.D.; Bass, C.R.; Mygind, N.; Winther, B. Nose blowing propels nasal fluid into the paranasal sinuses. *Clin. Infect. Dis.* **2000**, *30*, 387–391. [CrossRef] [PubMed]
56. Clarot, T.; Hensley, C. System for Delivering a Composition to the Nasal Membrane and Method of Using Same. U.S. Patent US20060275343A1, 7 December 2006.
57. Hsu, Y.Y.; Gresser, J.D.; Stewart, R.R.; Trantolo, D.J.; Lyons, C.M.; Simons, G.A.; Gangadharam, P.R.; Wise, D.L. Mechanisms of isoniazid release from poly (*d*, *l*-lactide-*co*-glycolide) matrices prepared by dry-mixing and low density polymeric foam methods. *J. Pharm. Sci.* **1996**, *85*, 706–713. [CrossRef] [PubMed]
58. Athanasiou, K.A.; Niederauer, G.G.; Agrawal, C.M. Sterilization, toxicity, biocompatibility and clinical applications of polylactic acid/polyglycolic acid copolymers. *Biomaterials* **1996**, *17*, 93–102. [CrossRef]
59. Sawant, D.; Dandagi, P.M.; Gadad, A.P. Formulation and evaluation of sparfloxacin emulsomes-loaded thermosensitive in situ gel for ophthalmic delivery. *J. Sol-Gel Sci. Technol.* **2016**, *77*, 654–665. [CrossRef]
60. Khodaverdi, E.; Tekie, F.S.M.; Mohajeri, S.A.; Ganji, F.; Zohuri, G.; Hadizadeh, F. Preparation and investigation of sustained drug delivery systems using an injectable, thermosensitive, in situ forming hydrogel composed of PLGA–PEG–PLGA. *AAPS PharmSciTech* **2012**, *13*, 590–600. [CrossRef] [PubMed]
61. Jones, D.S.; Woolfson, A.D.; Djokic, J.; Coulter, W. Development and mechanical characterization of bioadhesive semi-solid, polymeric systems containing tetracycline for the treatment of periodontal diseases. *Pharm. Res.* **1996**, *13*, 1734–1738. [CrossRef] [PubMed]
62. Jones, D.S.; Woolfson, A.D.; Brown, A.F.; Coulter, W.A.; McClelland, C.; Irwin, C.R. Design, characterisation and preliminary clinical evaluation of a novel mucoadhesive topical formulation containing tetracycline for the treatment of periodontal disease. *J. Control. Release* **2000**, *67*, 357–368. [CrossRef]
63. Eouani, C.; Piccerelle, P.; Prinderre, P.; Bourret, E.; Joachim, J. In-vitro comparative study of buccal mucoadhesive performance of different polymeric films. *Eur. J. Pharm. Biopharm.* **2001**, *52*, 45–55. [CrossRef]
64. Yu, T.; Wang, Y.-Y.; Yang, M.; Schneider, C.; Zhong, W.; Pulicare, S.; Choi, W.-J.; Mert, O.; Fu, J.; Lai, S.K. Biodegradable mucus-penetrating nanoparticles composed of diblock copolymers of polyethylene glycol and poly (lactic-*co*-glycolic acid). *Drug Deliv. Transl. Res* **2012**, *2*, 124–128. [CrossRef] [PubMed]
65. Carvalho, F.C.; Bruschi, M.L.; Evangelista, R.C.; Gremião, M.P.D. Mucoadhesive drug delivery systems. *Braz. J. Pharm. Sci.* **2010**, *46*, 1–17. [CrossRef]
66. Soane, R.; Frier, M.; Perkins, A.; Jones, N.; Davis, S.; Illum, L. Evaluation of the clearance characteristics of bioadhesive systems in humans. *Int. J. Pharm.* **1999**, *178*, 55–65. [CrossRef]
67. Gao, K.; Jiang, X. Influence of particle size on transport of methotrexate across blood brain barrier by polysorbate 80-coated polybutylcyanoacrylate nanoparticles. *Int. J. Pharm.* **2006**, *310*, 213–219. [CrossRef] [PubMed]
68. Zhou, X.; Chen, Z. Preparation and performance evaluation of emulsomes as a drug delivery system for silybin. *Arch. Pharm. Res.* **2015**, *38*, 2193–2200. [CrossRef] [PubMed]
69. Shorvon, S. Oxcarbazepine: A review. *Seizure* **2000**, *9*, 75–79. [CrossRef] [PubMed]
70. Hellewell, J.S. Oxcarbazepine (Trileptal) in the treatment of bipolar disorders: A review of efficacy and tolerability. *J. Affect. Disord.* **2002**, *72*, S23–S34. [CrossRef]
71. Martinez, W.; Ingenito, A.; Blakeslee, M.; Barkley, G.L.; McCague, K.; D'Souza, J. Efficacy, safety, and tolerability of oxcarbazepine monotherapy. *Epilepsy Behav.* **2006**, *9*, 448–456. [CrossRef] [PubMed]
72. Kaur, I.P.; Bhandari, R.; Bhandari, S.; Kakkar, V. Potential of solid lipid nanoparticles in brain targeting. *J. Control. Release* **2008**, *127*, 97–109. [CrossRef] [PubMed]
73. Jin, K.; Xie, L.; Childs, J.; Sun, Y.; Mao, X.O.; Logvinova, A.; Greenberg, D.A. Cerebral neurogenesis is induced by intranasal administration of growth factors. *Ann. Neurol.* **2003**, *53*, 405–409. [CrossRef] [PubMed]
74. Kumar, M.; Misra, A.; Mishra, A.; Mishra, P.; Pathak, K. Mucoadhesive nanoemulsion-based intranasal drug delivery system of olanzapine for brain targeting. *J. Drug Target.* **2008**, *16*, 806–814. [CrossRef] [PubMed]
75. Jain, N.; Akhter, S.; Jain, G.K.; Khan, Z.I.; Khar, R.K.; Ahmad, F.J. Antiepileptic intranasal Amiloride loaded mucoadhesive nanoemulsion: Development and safety assessment. *J. Biomed. Nanotechnol.* **2011**, *7*, 142–143. [CrossRef] [PubMed]
76. Perucca, E. Extended-release formulations of antiepileptic drugs: Rationale and comparative value. *Epilepsy Curr.* **2009**, *9*, 153–157. [CrossRef] [PubMed]

77. Steinhoff, B.; Stefan, H.; Schulze-Bonhage, A.; Hueber, R.; Paulus, W.; Wangemann, M.; Elger, C. Retardiertes vs. schnell freisetzendes Oxcarbazepin bei therapierefraktärer fokaler Epilepsie. *Der Nervenarzt* **2012**, *83*, 1292–1299. [CrossRef] [PubMed]
78. Moffatt, S.; Cristiano, R.J. Uptake characteristics of NGR-coupled stealth PEI/pDNA nanoparticles loaded with PLGA-PEG-PLGA tri-block copolymer for targeted delivery to human monocyte-derived dendritic cells. *Int. J. Pharm.* **2006**, *321*, 143–154. [CrossRef] [PubMed]
79. Chang, C.-W.; Choi, D.; Kim, W.J.; Yockman, J.W.; Christensen, L.V.; Kim, Y.-H.; Kim, S.W. Non-ionic amphiphilic biodegradable PEG–PLGA–PEG copolymer enhances gene delivery efficiency in rat skeletal muscle. *J. Control. Release* **2007**, *118*, 245–253. [CrossRef] [PubMed]
80. Chang, G.; Li, C.; Lu, W.; Ding, J. N-Boc-Histidine-Capped PLGA-PEG-PLGA as a Smart Polymer for Drug Delivery Sensitive to Tumor Extracellular pH. *Macromol. Biosci.* **2010**, *10*, 1248–1256. [CrossRef] [PubMed]
81. Castrén, K.; Pienimäki, P.; Arvela, P.; Vähäkangas, K. Metabolites and DNA-binding of carbamazepine and oxcarbazepine in vitro by rat liver microsomes. *Hum. Exp. Toxicol.* **1996**, *15*, 577–582. [CrossRef] [PubMed]
82. Aktaş, Z.; Cansu, A.; Erdoğan, D.; Take, G.; Goktas, G.; Ozdek, S.; Serdaroglu, A. Retinal ganglion cell toxicity due to oxcarbazepine and valproic acid treatment in rat. *Seizure* **2009**, *18*, 396–399. [CrossRef] [PubMed]

8

Engineering of Nanofibrous Amorphous and Crystalline Solid Dispersions for Oral Drug Delivery

Laura Modica de Mohac [1,2], Alison Veronica Keating [2], Maria de Fátima Pina [3] and Bahijja Tolulope Raimi-Abraham [2,*]

1 DIBIMIS Department, University of Study of Palermo, 90128 Palermo, Italy; laura.modicademohac@unipa.it
2 Drug Delivery Group, Institute of Pharmaceutical Science Faculty of Life Sciences and Medicine, King's College London, London SE1 9NH, UK; Alison.Keating@kcl.ac.uk
3 Department of Pharmaceutics, University College London School of Pharmacy, London WC1N 1AX, UK; mariafatima.gpina@gmail.com
* Correspondence: bahijja.raimi-abraham@kcl.ac.uk

Abstract: Poor aqueous solubility (<0.1 mg/mL) affects a significant number of drugs currently on the market or under development. Several formulation strategies including salt formation, particle size reduction, and solid dispersion approaches have been employed with varied success. In this review, we focus primarily on the emerging trends in the generation of amorphous and micro/nano-crystalline solid dispersions using electrospinning to improve the dissolution rate and in turn the bioavailability of poorly water-soluble drugs. Electrospinning is a simple but versatile process that utilizes electrostatic forces to generate polymeric fibers and has been used for over 100 years to generate synthetic fibers. We discuss the various electrospinning studies and spinneret types that have been used to generate amorphous and crystalline solid dispersions.

Keywords: solid dispersion; aqueous solubility enhancement; amorphous; crystalline; oral drug delivery; electrospinning

---

1. Introduction

Approximately 40% of marketed oral drugs are categorized as having poor aqueous solubility (i.e., <0.1 mg/mL) [1] resulting in a significant challenge in drug development. Several formulation strategies such as co-crystals [2], salt formation [3], particle size reduction [4], and more commonly, solid dispersion (SD) approaches [5–7] have been employed to increase aqueous solubility (and in turn enhance the oral bioavailability) of Biopharmaceutics Classification System (BCS) II (i.e., low solubility and high permeability) and IV (i.e., low solubility and permeability) drugs.

SDs have been redefined several times over time. For example, in 1961, Sekiguchi and Obi suggested that when the drug was formulated as a SD, it was present in a microcrystalline state as a eutectic mixture i.e., a combination of crystalline components (drug and a carrier) that are miscible in the molten liquid state, but show little to no miscibility in the solid state and on cooling would crystallize as two components [8]. Later, Chiou and Riegelman (1971) referred to SDs as a dispersion of one or more active ingredients present within an inert carrier or matrix in the solid state prepared by the melting (fusion), solvent-based, or melting-solvent method [9]. This was further defined by Lerner et al. (2000) as a dispersion in which the drug is only partially molecularly dispersed and is generated from physical mixtures of the carrier and drug [10]. In 2002, Craig described SDs as a delivery system whereby the drug is dispersed in a biologically inert matrix, to enhance oral bioavailability [11]. A range of materials are used as the inert matrix or carrier in a SD ranging from sugars [12,13], wax based systems [14] and, more commonly, polymers.

There are several hypotheses regarding the mechanism of drug release from SD systems amorphous and crystalline alike. The most agreed hypothesis is the existence of two different mechanisms of drug release, carrier-controlled or drug-controlled (Figure 1). This hypothesis is based on key findings by Corrigan et al. [15] in their drug release study of a phenobarbitone-(poly)ethylene glycol (PEG) SD where the rate of phenobarbitone release from the SD was the same as that of PEG on its own. Craig [11] further suggested that, if a system underwentcarrier-controlled dissolution then the physical properties such as initial particle size of the drug or crystallinity should be largely irrelevant. In comparison with drug-controlled dissolution, the physical property of the drug as well as its solubility is of greater relevance [11], highlighting the potential of SDs to enhance drug dissolution rate through a preferential selection of the appropriate carrier (in this case polymer) or a combination of carrier and carrier types (e.g., wax and polymers polymer blends [14]).

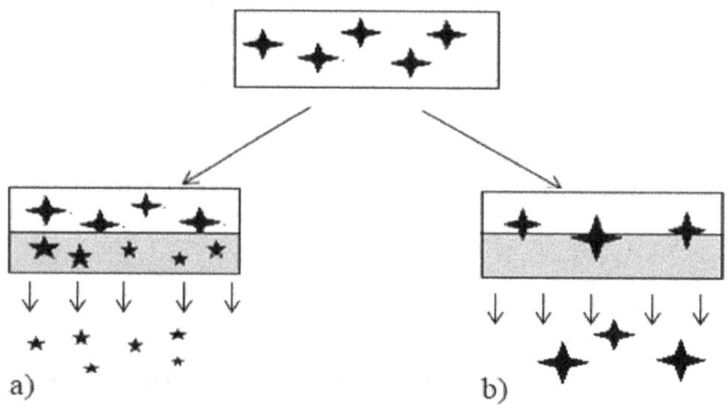

Figure 1. Schematic diagram shows (**a**) Carrier-controlled dissolution and (**b**) drug-controlled dissolution (Adapted with permission from [11], copyright Elsevier, 2002). *The larger ✦ represents dissolved drug, the smaller ✦ represent the partially dissolved drug. Grey box represents an aqueous environment.*

In most cases where SDs are generated, a comparison is made with the physical mixture (PM). The PM is essentially where the drug and carrier are not chemically combined through a process but prepared through gentle or mild mixing. To ensure drug release compared to SD is not influenced by additional factors such as particle size, it is good practice for both drug and carrier to be passed through a dry sieve of known aperture so any effects observed are due entirely to the properties of the PM. Examples in the literature exist that demonstrate enhanced drug release of a PM compared to its SD counterpart. For example Leonardi and Salomon (2013) PM of benznidazole and PEG 6000 offered greater dissolution compared to it a SD prepared by a solvent method [16].

SDs have been characterized into two main classifications, firstly in accordance to carrier type and secondly taking into account the correlation to stability and solubility, preparation, and characterization techniques [17].

When classifying SDs by carrier type, there are four generations that have been discussed and explored in the literature. The first generation SDs were introduced by Sekiguchi and Obi as eutectic mixtures where both drug and carrier were present in the crystalline state [18]. Second generation SDs were carriers are generally polymeric and present in the amorphous state with the drug dispersed molecularly within the inert matrix. The drug is generally supersaturated to ensure its solubilization in the carriers in second generation SDs [19]. Third generation SDs were the carriers can be a co-polymer system or a mixture of surfactants and polymers and improvement of the drug release profile is due to the carrier's surface activity or self-emulsifying properties which in addition could reduce drug re-crystallization and improve SD stability [20]. Finally, fourth generation SDs are the carriers are bifunctional in nature and have solubilizing as well as surfactant properties [21]. The carriers are non-ionic and so the solubility is independent of pH changes making these carriers more suited for SD development. Soluplus®, a polyvinyl caprolactam-polyvinyl acetate-polyethylene glycol graft co-polymer solubilizer with an amphiphilic chemical structure has been highlighted as a fourth generation SD carrier [22].

When classifying SDs in accordance to their correlation to stability and solubility, preparation and characterization techniques, six classes have been identified [23]. Class C–C and Class C–A where the Active Pharmaceutical Ingredient (API) is present in the crystalline state are dispersed in either a crystalline or amorphous carrier respectively. Class C–C and C–A SDs are deemed stable, however, less soluble due to the crystalline nature of the API. Class A–C and Class A-A were the API is present in the amorphous state dispersed in either a crystalline or amorphous carrier. Class A–C and CC SDs are considered to increase API solubility enhancement, however, low miscibility is observed between the API and carrier has been highlighted as an issue. Class M–C and Class M–A are where the drug is molecularly dispersed within either a crystalline or amorphous carrier. These systems have been shown to greatly improve drug dissolution behavior with great physical stability due to the high miscibility and strong molecular interaction between the two components with the API being molecularly dispersed [23].

In this review, we discuss amorphous and crystalline SDs which we define as a system where the drug is molecularly dispersed with an amorphous polymer matrix and as a system where the micronized or nanosized crystalline drug is dispersed within an amorphous polymer matrix with or without the use of stabilizing agents respectively.

SD stability has been studied at length over the years and factors influencing can be summarized as follows: physical stability, crystallization tendency, amorphization, drug-polymer miscibility, dissolution enhancement, and method of preparation. Electrospinning is a rapid solvent evaporation method and is well suited for drugs with thermal instability and can avoid drug re-crystallization or amorphization during processing [24]. Many polymers have been used to prepare SDs such as poly(*N*-vinvylpyrrolidone) (PVP) [25], polyethylene glycol (PEG) [26], zein [27], hydroxypropyl methylcellulose (HPMC) [28,29], polycaprolactone [30], and polyacrylic acid [31], expanding the potential of processes used to make SDs from the traditional solvent-based methods [32,33], hot melt extrusion (HME) [34–36], spray-drying [22,37], to polymer-based nanofabrication methods such as electrospinning [38–40] and other centrifugal spinning based methods [12,13,41,42].

In this review, we focus primarily on the emerging trends in the generation of amorphous and crystalline SDs using nanofabrication techniques namely electrospinning to improve the dissolution rate and in turn bioavailability of poorly water-soluble drugs. It is important to note that there are more studies investigating the generation of electrospun nanofibrous amorphous solid dispersions than crystalline SDs suggesting that electrospun nanofibrous crystalline SDs are still a relatively under-investigated formulation strategy.

2. Nanofibrous Amorphous Solid Dispersions

Amorphous materials have higher enthalpy, entropy, and free energy compared to their crystalline counterparts, leading to higher apparent solubility. The weaker attractive intermolecular forces of amorphous materials are more easily broken, allowing molecules to move from the material's surface into the medium greater ease compared to crystalline counterparts. As a result, amorphous materials are more soluble and have a faster dissolution rate. Unfortunately, even with such advantages the success and usefulness of amorphous materials in drug development is greatly dependent on their long stability within a dosage form [3,43,44]. Given the high solubility of amorphous compounds (compared to their crystalline counterparts), amorphous solid dispersions (ASDs) are an important strategy to improve the apparent solubility, dissolution rate, and in turn bioavailability of poorly water-soluble drugs [45].

Nanofibers possess a high surface area to volume ratio and have gained increased interest in drug delivery beyond their known application in areas such as tissue engineering scaffolds [46] or wound dressing for example [47]. Due to their high drug-loading capacity, internal architecture, porosity, and malleability the addition of therapeutically relevant molecules has several benefits. For further information on recent developments in the application of micro and nanofabrication techniques in drug delivery and on nanofibres in drug delivery, the reader is directed to a recent review by Qi and Craig [26].

2.1. Electrospinning

Electrospinning is a simple but versatile process that utilizes electrostatic forces to generate polymeric fibers and has been used for over 100 years to generate synthetic fibers [48–50]. Typically, electrospinning involves pushing a viscous polymer or polymer/drug solution through a spinneret (narrow gauge syringe needle) at a constant flow rate. A voltage is applied to the polymer solution, creating repulsive forces between the like charges in the solution and attractive forces between the charged solution and the grounded collector. When the electrostatic forces equal the surface tension of the liquid, a Taylor cone is formed. If the electric field is increased beyond this point, the electrostatic repulsion will exceed the surface tension and result in the ejection of a fiber jet from the apex of the cone which accelerates towards the grounded collector [51,52]. As the fiber jet accelerates towards the collector it undergoes chaotic whipping instability which increases the transit time and path length to the collector, allowing the solvent to evaporate leaving solid, thin fibers. Cheng et al. presented electrospinning as a novel processing method to generate functional nanomaterials with many applications ranging from wound healing and medical textiles, to production of oral-dispersible film SD and controlled delivery systems [27,53–55]. Electrospinning is a rapid solvent evaporation process well suited to amorphous materials as by this process the drug does not have time to form a crystal lattice within the nanofiber and remains distributed in its amorphous form at a molecular scale [56]. Additionally, the internal structure of the fibers themselves can be altered to be hollow or biphasic by using specific electrospinning approaches [57].

2.1.1. Mono-Axial Electrospinning

Mono-axial electrospinning is the simplest and as a result of this the most common electrospinning experiment. The polymer (and API) in solution or suspension is dispensed through a single-bore blunt-end needle resulting in a monolithic product, with the API and polymer typically evenly and homogeneously blended throughout the fibers [58].

In Verreck et al.'s study, Itraconazole-HPMC SDs were generated by electrospinning and properties of the resultant nanofibres were compared relative to other SD techniques namely HME and solvent casting with regards their dissolution behavior [59]. Though the dissolution methods varied for the different presentations, several apparent trends were observed. PMs of itraconazole and HPMC generated little (<1–3%) drug release in any of the dissolution approaches assessed. Interestingly, electrospun ASDs samples resulted in complete in vitroitraconazole release over but however, the dissolution rate was slower compared to the cast thin films, melt extruded and milled powders [59]. The authors concluded that for this drug-polymer system, there could be potential as a controlled drug delivery system. Nagy et al. compared the drug dissolution behavior of spironolactone-soluplus SDs generated by electrospinning to those prepared by HME with key findings confirming the generation of ASDs with the electrospun nanofibers showing enhanced drug dissolution behavior compared to the HME SDs [60,61].

PVP-acetaminophen SDs prepared by electrospinning generating non-woven nanofibrous meshes were compared to traditional SD preparation processes namely freeze drying, vacuum drying, and heat drying with an advantage of the electrospinning process over the traditional processes being the unique microstructural characteristics of the electrospun nanofibres generated. Freeze dried samples and electrospun fibers did not show any evidence of phase separation phenomenon which was evident in heat-dried and vacuum-dried samples which led to visible (in scanning electron microscopy studies) microparticles on the sample surfaces. The in vitro dissolution tests illustrated that the electrospun SDs nanofibers released 93.8% acetaminophen in the first 2 min and the dissolution rates of acetaminophen from the different SDs had the following order: electrospun > vacuum-dried ≈ freeze-dried > heating-dried [62]. They also highlighted [62] the advantage of third generation SDs (where the state the carrier has surface activity or self-emulsifying properties) and the potential for these to be generated using mono-axial electrospinning. Third generation SDs of ferulic acid in composite nanofibers with three-dimensional continuous web structure were generated by electrospinning co-dissolving solutions of ferulic acid, PVP with the surfactant sodium dodecyl sulfate (SDS) and sucralose. In vitro dissolution and permeation tests showed that the nanofiber-based SDs rapidly released all of the ferulic acid within in 1 min and had a 13-fold greater permeation rate across sublingual mucosa compared to crude ferulic acid particles [63,64].

2.1.2. Coaxial and Multi-Axial Electrospinning

Coaxial electrospinning (also known as co-electrospinning) involves the use of a two-needle spinneret, with one needle nested inside another in a concentric fashion. Fires generated tend to have greater versatility in terms of the range of materials used, therapeutic agents incorporated (ranging from small molecules to biological molecules), size (e.g., from 100 nm to 300 μm), and can offer complete drug encapsulation and higher drug stability compared to mono-axial fibers [58]. The use of coaxial and multi-axial electrospinning approaches has been applied in drug delivery with great success to generate biphasic [65], targeted release [66,67] and multifunctional materials [68] as well as SDs. Yang et al. [69] explored three types of electrospinning namely coaxial, modified coaxial, and tri-axial (characterized by the use of un-spinnable liquids as the sheath working fluids) electrospinning to generate nanofibrous ferulic acid-cellulose acetate ASDs depot systems [69]. In vitro dissolution tests revealed that the fibers were able to provide close to zero-order release over 36 h, with no initial burst release and minimal tailing-off. The release properties of the depot systems generated showed improved properties over the monolithic fibers, which exhibited a significant burst release and also considerable tailing-off at the end of the drug release studies [69]. Tri-axial electrospinning has also been successfully used to fabricate nanofibres of lecithin (known to be un-spinnable), diclofenac sodium with Eudragit S100 a methacrylic acid/methyl methacrylate copolymer (which only dissolves at pH > 7.0) as the carrier matrix for oral colon targeting [70].

2.1.3. Others

Several other electrospinning systems exist which have been used to generate ASDs. The core-cut nozzle system where the exit pipe of the core nozzle is removed so that the core fluid can form an envelope inside the shell solution [71] has been shown to improve spinnability of two fluids by reducing jet instability. This system is also suitable for the production of multi-layered nanofibers where the drug is in the internal layer. Due to this, drug release is shown to start from the core then moving through to the external environment with applications as a controlled drug delivery system as the thickness of each layer can be tailored to vary the drug release [71]. Side-by-side electrospinning is a two-liquid process and the structure of the spinneret is propagated into the solid products creating Janus fibers with two different sides [72]. The different sides could hold two different polymers with two different drugs loaded resulting in concomitant drug release [73].

Unfortunately, in spite of the enormous research efforts both in academia and in industry very few ASDs products let alone nanofibrous ASDs have reached the market so far [74]. Works by Démuth et al. have successfully turned ASDs nanofibers into a viable nanofibrous ASDs solid dosage forms by compressing them into tablets with enhanced drug dissolution rates [75,76]. With promising work on-going in the field, there is the potential to have a commercially available nanofibrous ASD based dosage form.

3. Nanofibrous Micro/Nano-Crystalline Solid Dispersions

Due to the challenges associated with the stability of ASDs, there is a push to reconsider the crystalline state in the micron or nanoscale as an alternative method for SD production. It is well-known that the dissolution rate of smaller particles is greater due to the increased surface area in accordance with Noyes–Whitney equation and Nernst–Brunner theory [66–68]. Several investigations into drug particle size reduction [77–79] have shown that particle size reduction leads to increased drug solubility. It has also been demonstrated that a further increase in drug bioavailability is observed when the particle size of a drug is reduced from micrometer to nanometer [80].

Nanosuspensions are sub-micron colloidal dispersions of the drug, which are stabilized by surfactants [81]. This technology has shown great promise as a strategy to improve the dissolution rate of poorly soluble drugs by maintaining the drug in its preferred crystalline state of a size sufficiently small for pharmaceutical acceptability [82,83]. Major advantages of this technology are its general applicability to most drugs and its simplicity [80]. Solid micro/nano-crystalline dispersions have been generated using techniques such as film making [82,84], solvent casting method [32], spray drying [84,85], hot melt extrusion [25], and electrospinning [86].

4. Conclusions

In this review, we focused on the emerging trends in the generation of amorphous and micro/nano-crystalline solid dispersions using electrospinning to improve the dissolution rate and in turn the bioavailability of poorly water-soluble drugs. With electrospinning being a simple but versatile process, various studies have successfully generated mainly amorphous solid dispersions with few studies exploring the generation of crystalline solid dispersions. The scalability of electrospinning and its products for commercial drug delivery applications is a topic of great discussion and debate. The industrial upscaling of electrospinning and application of resultant fibers is discussed by Taylor et al. [86]. The electrospinning equipment market for laboratory research and industrial production is expected to grow significantly in the future due to the continuous development of new electrospinning technologies influenced by demand.

References

1. Vo, C.L.N.; Park, C.; Lee, B.J. Current trends and future perspectives of solid dispersions containing poorly water-soluble drugs. *Eur. J. Pharm. Biopharm.* **2013**, *85*, 799–813. [CrossRef] [PubMed]
2. Demetzos, C. *Pharmaceutical Nanotechnology*; Springer Singapore: Singapore, 2016; ISBN 978-981-10-0790-3.
3. Serajuddln, A.T.M. Solid dispersion of poorly water-soluble drugs: Early promises, subsequent problems, and recent breakthroughs. *J. Pharm. Sci.* **1999**, *88*, 1058–1066. [CrossRef]
4. Loh, Z.H.; Samanta, A.K.; Sia Heng, P.W. Overview of milling techniques for improving the solubility of poorly water-soluble drugs. *Asian J. Pharm. Sci.* **2015**, *10*, 255–274. [CrossRef]
5. Paudel, A.; Worku, Z.A.; Meeus, J.; Guns, S.; Van den Mooter, G. Manufacturing of solid dispersions of poorly water soluble drugs by spray drying: Formulation and process considerations. *Int. J. Pharm.* **2013**, *453*, 253–284. [CrossRef] [PubMed]
6. Shah, N.; Iyer, R.M.; Mair, H.-J.; Choi, D.; Tian, H.; Diodone, R.; Fahnrich, K.; Pabst-Ravot, A.; Tang, K.; Scheubel, E.; et al. Improved human bioavailability of vemurafenib, a practically insoluble drug, using an amorphous polymer-stabilized solid dispersion prepared by a solvent-controlled coprecipitation process. *J. Pharm. Sci.* **2013**, *102*, 967–981. [CrossRef] [PubMed]
7. Huang, Y.; Dai, W.-G. Fundamental aspects of solid dispersion technology for poorly soluble drugs. *Acta Pharm. Sin. B.* **2014**, *4*, 18–25. [CrossRef]
8. Sekiguchi, K.; Obi, N. Studies on absorption of eutectic mixture I. A comparison of the behaviour of eutectic mixture of sulfathiazole and that of ordinary sulfathiazole in man. *Chem. Pharm. Bull.* **1961**, *9*, 866–872. [CrossRef]
9. Chiou, W.L.; Riegelman, S. Pharmaceutical applications of solid dispersion systems. *J. Pharm. Sci.* **1971**, *60*, 1281–1302. [CrossRef]

10. Leuner, C.; Dressman, J. Improving drug solubility for oral delivery using solid dispersions. *Eur. J. Pharm. Biopharm.* **2000**, *50*, 47–60. [CrossRef]
11. Craig, D.Q.M. The mechanisms of drug release from solid dispersions in water-soluble polymers. *Int. J. Pharm.* **2002**, *231*, 131–144. [CrossRef]
12. Marano, S.; Barker, S.A.; Raimi-Abraham, B.T.; Missaghi, S.; Rajabi-Siahboomi, A.; Aliev, A.E.; Craig, D.Q.M. Microfibrous solid dispersions of poorly water-soluble drugs produced via centrifugal spinning: unexpected dissolution behavior on recrystallization. *Mol. Pharm.* **2017**, *14*, 1666–1680. [CrossRef] [PubMed]
13. Marano, S.; Barker, S.A.; Raimi-Abraham, B.T.; Missaghi, S.; Rajabi-Siahboomi, A.; Craig, D.Q.M. Development of micro-fibrous solid dispersions of poorly water-soluble drugs in sucrose using temperature-controlled centrifugal spinning. *Eur. J. Pharm. Biopharm.* **2016**, *103*, 84–94. [CrossRef]
14. Yan, H.-X.; Zhang, S.-S.; He, J.-H.; Liu, J.-P. Application of ethyl cellulose, microcrystalline cellulose and octadecanol for wax based floating solid dispersion pellets. *Carbohydr. Polym.* **2016**, *148*, 143–152. [CrossRef] [PubMed]
15. Corrigan, O.I. Retardation of polymeric carrier dissolution by dispersed drugs: factors influencing the dissolution of solid dispersions containing polyethlene glycols. *Drug Dev. Ind. Pharm.* **1986**, *12*, 1777–1793. [CrossRef]
16. Leonardi, D.; Salomon, C.J. Unexpected performance of physical mixtures over solid dispersions on the dissolution behavior of benznidazole from tablets. *J. Pharm. Sci.* **2013**, *102*, 1016–1023. [CrossRef] [PubMed]
17. Sharma, P.K.; Panda, A.; Pradhan, A.; Zhang, J.; Thakkar, R.; Whang, C.-H.; Repka, M.A.; Murthy, S.N. Solid-state stability issues of drugs in transdermal patch formulations. *AAPS PharmSciTech* **2017**, *19*. [CrossRef] [PubMed]
18. Vasconcelos, T.; Sarmento, B.; Costa, P. Solid dispersions as strategy to improve oral bioavailability of poor water soluble drugs. *Drug Discov. Today* **2007**, *12*, 1068–1075. [CrossRef]
19. van Drooge, D.J.; Braeckmans, K.; Hinrichs, W.L.J.; Remaut, K.; De Smedt, S.C.; Frijlink, H.W. Characterization of the mode of incorporation of lipophilic compounds in solid dispersions at the nanoscale using fluorescence resonance energy transfer (FRET). *Macromol. Rapid Commun.* **2006**, *27*, 1149–1155. [CrossRef]
20. Pouton, C.W. Formulation of poorly water-soluble drugs for oral administration: Physicochemical and physiological issues and the lipid formulation classification system. *Eur. J. Pharm. Sci.* **2006**, *29*, 278–287. [CrossRef] [PubMed]
21. Khan, A.W.; Kotta, S.; Ansari, S.H.; Sharma, R.K.; Ali, J. Enhanced dissolution and bioavailability of grapefruit flavonoid Naringenin by solid dispersion utilizing fourth generation carrier. *Drug Dev. Ind. Pharm.* **2015**, *41*, 772–779. [CrossRef]
22. Shamma, R.N.; Basha, M. Soluplus: A novel polymeric solubilizer for optimization of Carvedilol solid dispersions: Formulation design and effect of method of preparation. *Powder Technol.* **2013**, *237*, 406–414. [CrossRef]
23. Meng, F.; Gala, U.; Chauhan, H. Classification of solid dispersions: correlation to (i) stability and solubility (ii) preparation and characterization techniques. *Drug Dev. Ind. Pharm.* **2015**, *41*, 1401–1415. [CrossRef] [PubMed]
24. Kumar, B. Solid Dispersion—A Review. *PharmaTutor* **2017**, *5*, 24–29.
25. Pina, M.F.; Zhao, M.; Pinto, J.F.; Sousa, J.J.; Craig, D.Q.M. The influence of drug physical state on the dissolution enhancement of solid dispersions prepared via hot-melt extrusion: A case study using olanzapine. *J. Pharm. Sci.* **2014**, *103*, 1214–1223. [CrossRef] [PubMed]
26. Qi, S.; Craig, D. Recent developments in micro- and nanofabrication techniques for the preparation of amorphous pharmaceutical dosage forms. *Adv. Drug Deliv. Rev.* **2016**, *100*, 67–84. [CrossRef] [PubMed]
27. Alhusein, N.; Blagbrough, I.S.; Beeton, M.L.; Bolhuis, A.; De Bank, P.A. Electrospun Zein/PCL fibrous matrices release tetracycline in a controlled manner, killing *Staphylococcus aureus* both in biofilms and *ex vivo* on pig skin, and are compatible with human skin cells. *Pharm. Res.* **2016**, *33*, 237–246. [CrossRef] [PubMed]
28. Li, B.; Konecke, S.; Harich, K.; Wegiel, L.; Taylor, L.S.; Edgar, K.J. Solid dispersion of quercetin in cellulose derivative matrices influences both solubility and stability. *Carbohydr. Polym.* **2013**, *92*, 2033–2040. [CrossRef]
29. Zidan, A.S.; Rahman, Z.; Sayeed, V.; Raw, A.; Yu, L.; Khan, M.A. Crystallinity evaluation of tacrolimus solid dispersions by chemometric analysis. *Int. J. Pharm.* **2012**, *423*, 341–350. [CrossRef]

30. Alhusein, N.; De Bank, P.A.; Blagbrough, I.S.; Bolhuis, A. Killing bacteria within biofilms by sustained release of tetracycline from triple-layered electrospun micro/nanofibre matrices of polycaprolactone and poly (ethylene-co-vinyl acetate). *Drug Deliv. Transl Res.* **2013**, *3*, 531–541. [CrossRef]
31. Alshahrani, S.M.; Lu, W.; Park, J.-B.; Morott, J.T.; Alsulays, B.B.; Majumdar, S.; Langley, N.; Kolter, K.; Gryczke, A.; Repka, M.A. Stability-enhanced hot-melt extruded amorphous solid dispersions via combinations of soluplus®and hpmcas-hf. *AAPS PharmSciTech* **2015**, *16*, 824–834. [CrossRef]
32. Modica de Mohac, L.; de Fátima Pina, M.; Raimi-Abraham, B.T. Solid microcrystalline dispersion films as a new strategy to improve the dissolution rate of poorly water soluble drugs: A case study using olanzapine. *Int. J. Pharm.* **2016**, *508*, 42–50. [CrossRef] [PubMed]
33. De Caro, V.; Ajovalasit, A.; Sutera, F.M.; Murgia, D.; Sabatino, M.A.; Dispenza, C. Development and characterization of an amorphous solid dispersion of furosemide in the form of a sublingual bioadhesive film to enhance bioavailability. *Pharmaceutics* **2017**, *9*, 22. [CrossRef] [PubMed]
34. Li, Y.; Pang, H.; Guo, Z.; Lin, L.; Dong, Y.; Li, G.; Lu, M.; Wu, C. Interactions between drugs and polymers influencing hot melt extrusion. *J. Pharm. Pharmacol.* **2014**, *66*, 148–166. [CrossRef] [PubMed]
35. Zhang, K.; Yu, H.; Luo, Q.; Yang, S.; Lin, X.; Zhang, Y.; Tian, B.; Tang, X. Increased dissolution and oral absorption of itraconazole/Soluplus extrudate compared with itraconazole nanosuspension. *Eur. J. Pharm. Biopharm.* **2013**, *85*, 1285–1292. [CrossRef] [PubMed]
36. Keating, A.V.; Soto, J.; Tuleu, C.; Forbes, C.; Zhao, M.; Craig, D.Q.M. Solid state characterisation and taste masking efficiency evaluation of polymer based extrudates of isoniazid for paediatric administration. *Int. J. Pharm.* **2018**, *536*, 536–546. [CrossRef] [PubMed]
37. Davis, M.T.; Potter, C.B.; Mohammadpour, M.; Albadarin, A.B.; Walker, G.M. Design of spray dried ternary solid dispersions comprising itraconazole, soluplus and HPMCP: Effect of constituent compositions. *Int. J. Pharm.* **2017**, *519*, 365–372. [CrossRef] [PubMed]
38. Qi, S.; Moffat, J.G.; Yang, Z. Early stage phase separation in pharmaceutical solid dispersion thin films under high humidity: improved spatial understanding using probe based thermal and spectroscopic nano-characterisation methods. *Mol. Pharm.* **2013**, *10*, 918–930. [CrossRef]
39. Ng, Y.C.; Yang, Z.; McAuley, W.J.; Qi, S. Stabilisation of amorphous drugs under high humidity using pharmaceutical thin films. *Eur. J. Pharm. Biopharm.* **2013**, *84*, 555–565. [CrossRef]
40. Luo, C.J.; Stoyanov, S.D.; Stride, E.; Pelan, E.; Edirisinghe, M. Electrospinning versus fibre production methods: from specifics to technological convergence. *Chem. Soc. Rev.* **2012**, *41*, 4708–4735. [CrossRef]
41. Illangakoon, U.E.; Nazir, T.; Williams, G.R.; Chatterton, N.P. Mebeverine-loaded electrospun nanofibers: physicochemical characterization and dissolution studies. *J. Pharm. Sci.* **2014**, *103*, 283–292. [CrossRef]
42. Raimi-Abraham, B.T.; Mahalingam, S.; Davies, P.J.; Edirisinghe, M.; Craig, D.Q.M. Development and characterization of amorphous nanofiber drug dispersions prepared using pressurized gyration. *Mol. Pharm.* **2015**, *12*, 3851–3861. [CrossRef] [PubMed]
43. Bhut, V.Z.; Prajapati, A.B.; Patel, K.N.; Patel, B.A.; Patel, P.A. Solid dispersion as a strategy to enhance solubility: A review article. *IJPRS* **2012**, *5*, 490–498.
44. Thakral, S.; Thakral, N.K. Prediction of drug–polymer miscibility through the use of solubility parameter based flory–huggins interaction parameter and the experimental validation: PEG as model polymer. *J. Pharm. Sci.* **2013**, *102*, 2254–2263. [CrossRef] [PubMed]
45. Son, Y.J.; Kim, W.J.; Yoo, H.S. Therapeutic applications of electrospun nanofibers for drug delivery systems. *Arch. Pharm. Res.* **2013**, *37*, 69–78. [CrossRef]
46. Liu, M.; Duan, X.-P.; Li, Y.-M.; Yang, D.-P.; Long, Y.-Z. Electrospun nanofibers for wound healing. *Mater. Sci. Eng. C* **2017**, *76*, 1413–1423. [CrossRef] [PubMed]
47. Jun, I.; Han, H.S.; Edwards, J.R.; Jeon, H. Electrospun Fibrous Scaffolds for Tissue Engineering: Viewpoints on Architecture and Fabrication. *Int. J. Mol. Sci.* **2018**, *19*, 745. [CrossRef] [PubMed]
48. Cooley, J.F. Improved methods of and apparatus for electrically separating the relatively volatile liquid component from the component of relatively fixed substances of composite fluids. *United Kingdom Patent* **1900**, *6385*, 19.
49. Cooley, J.F. Apparatus for Electrically Dispersing Fluids. U.S. Patent Application No. 692,631, 4 February 1902.
50. Morton, W.J. Method of Dispersing Fluids. U.S. Patent US705691A, 29 July 1902.
51. Sill, T.J.; von Recum, H.A. Electrospinning: applications in drug delivery and tissue engineering. *Biomaterials* **2008**, *29*, 1989–2006. [CrossRef] [PubMed]

52. Williams, G.R.; Chatterton, N.P.; Nazir, T.; Yu, D.G.; Zhu, L.M.; Branford-White, C.J. Electrospun nanofibers in drug delivery: recent developments and perspectives. *Ther. Deliv.* **2012**, *3*, 515–533. [CrossRef]
53. Cheng, H.; Yang, X.; Che, X.; Yang, M.; Zhai, G. Biomedical application and controlled drug release of electrospun fibrous materials. *Mater. Sci. Eng. C* **2018**, *90*, 750–763. [CrossRef]
54. Vogt, L.; Liverani, L.; Roether, J.; Boccaccini, A. Electrospun Zein Fibers Incorporating Poly(glycerol sebacate) for Soft Tissue Engineering. *Nanomaterials* **2018**, *8*, 150. [CrossRef]
55. Alhusein, N.; Blagbrough, I.S.; De Bank, P.A. Zein/polycaprolactone electrospun matrices for localised controlled delivery of tetracycline. *Drug Deliv. Transl. Res.* **2013**, *3*, 542–550. [CrossRef] [PubMed]
56. Zhang, H.; Lou, S.; Williams, G.R.; Branford-White, C.; Nie, H.; Quan, J.; Zhu, L.-M. A systematic study of captopril-loaded polyester fiber mats prepared by electrospinning. *Int. J. Pharm.* **2012**, *439*, 100–108. [CrossRef] [PubMed]
57. Qu, H.; Wei, S.; Guo, Z. Coaxial electrospun nanostructures and their applications. *J. Mater. Chem. A.* **2013**, *1*, 11513–11518. [CrossRef]
58. Williams, G.R.; Raimi-Abraham, B.T.; Luo, C.J. *Nanofibres in Drug Delivery*; UCL Press: London, UK, 2018; ISBN 9781787350182.
59. Verreck, G.; Chun, I.; Peeters, J.; Rosenblatt, J.; Brewster, M.E. Preparation and characterization of nanofibers containing amorphous drug dispersions generated by electrostatic spinning. *Pharm. Res.* **2003**, *20*, 810–817. [CrossRef] [PubMed]
60. Nagy, Z.K.; Balogh, A.; Vajna, B.; Farkas, A.; Patyi, G.; Kramarics, Á.; Marosi, G. Comparison of electrospun and extruded soluplus®-based solid dosage forms of improved dissolution. *J. Pharm. Sci.* **2012**, *101*, 322–332. [CrossRef] [PubMed]
61. Nagy, Z.K.; Balogh, A.; Démuth, B.; Pataki, H.; Vigh, T.; Szabó, B.; Molnár, K.; Schmidt, B.T.; Horák, P.; Marosi, G.; et al. High speed electrospinning for scaled-up production of amorphous solid dispersion of itraconazole. *Int. J. Pharm.* **2015**, *480*, 137–142. [CrossRef] [PubMed]
62. Yu, D.-G.; Branford-White, C.; White, K.; Li, X.-L.; Zhu, L.-M. dissolution improvement of electrospun nanofiber-based solid dispersions for acetaminophen. *AAPS PharmSciTech* **2010**, *11*, 809–817. [CrossRef]
63. Huang, Z.-M.; Zhang, Y.-Z.; Kotaki, M.; Ramakrishna, S. A review on polymer nanofibers by electrospinning and their applications in nanocomposites. *Compos. Sci. Technol.* **2003**, *63*, 2223–2253. [CrossRef]
64. Li, D.; Xia, Y. Electrospinning of nanofibers: reinventing the wheel? *Adv. Mater.* **2004**, *16*, 1151–1170. [CrossRef]
65. Yu, D.G.; Wang, X.; Li, X.Y.; Chian, W.; Li, Y.; Liao, Y.Z. Electrospun biphasic drug release polyvinylpyrrolidone/ethyl cellulose core/sheath nanofibers. *Acta Biomater.* **2013**, *9*, 5665–5672. [CrossRef]
66. Maincent, J.; Williams, R.O. Sustained-release amorphous solid dispersions. *Drug Deliv. Transl. Res.* **2018**, *8*, 1–12. [CrossRef] [PubMed]
67. Lin, W.C.; Yeh, I.T.; Niyama, E.; Huang, W.R.; Ebara, M.; Wu, C.S. Electrospun poly(ε-caprolactone) nanofibrous mesh for imiquimod delivery in melanoma therapy. *Polymers* **2018**, *10*, 231. [CrossRef]
68. Wei, Q.; Xu, F.; Xu, X.; Geng, X.; Ye, L.; Zhang, A.; Feng, Z. The multifunctional wound dressing with core–shell structured fibers prepared by coaxial electrospinning. *Front. Mater. Sci.* **2016**, *10*, 113–121. [CrossRef]
69. Yang, G.; Li, J.; Yu, D.; He, M.; Yang, J.; Williams, G.R. Nanosized sustained-release drug depots fabricated using modified tri-axial electrospinning. *Acta Biomater.* **2017**, *53*, 233–241. [CrossRef] [PubMed]
70. Yang, C.; Yu, D.-G.; Pan, D.; Liu, X.-K.; Wang, X.; Bligh, S.W.A.; Williams, G.R. Electrospun pH-sensitive core–shell polymer nanocomposites fabricated using a tri-axial process. *Acta Biomater.* **2016**, *35*, 77–86. [CrossRef]
71. Lee, B.S.; Jeon, S.Y.; Park, H.; Lee, G.; Yang, H.S.; Yu, W.R. New electrospinning nozzle to reduce jet instability and its application to manufacture of multi-layered nanofibers. *Sci. Rep.* **2014**, *4*, 6758. [CrossRef] [PubMed]
72. Yu, D.-G.; Yang, C.; Jin, M.; Williams, G.R.; Zou, H.; Wang, X.; Bligh, S.W.A. Medicated Janus fibers fabricated using a Teflon-coated side-by-side spinneret. *Colloids Surf B Biointerfaces* **2016**, *138*, 110–116. [CrossRef]
73. Geng, Y.; Zhang, P.; Wang, Q.; Liu, Y.; Pan, K. Novel PAN/PVP Janus ultrafine fiber membrane and its application for biphasic drug release. *J. Mater. Chem. B* **2017**, *5*, 5390–5396. [CrossRef]
74. Van Den Mooter, G. The use of amorphous solid dispersions: A formulation strategy to overcome poor solubility and dissolution rate. *Drug Discov. Today Technol.* **2012**, *9*, 79–86. [CrossRef]

75. Démuth, B.; Farkas, A.; Balogh, A.; Bartosiewicz, K.; Kállai-Szabó, B.; Bertels, J.; Vigh, T.; Mensch, J.; Verreck, G.; Van Assche, I.; et al. Lubricant-induced crystallization of itraconazole from tablets made of electrospun amorphous solid dispersion. *J. Pharm. Sci.* **2016**, *105*, 2982–2988. [CrossRef]
76. Démuth, B.; Farkas, A.; Szabó, B.; Balogh, A.; Nagy, B.; Vágó, E.; Vigh, T.; Tinke, A.P.; Kazsu, Z.; Demeter, Á.; et al. Development and tableting of directly compressible powder from electrospun nanofibrous amorphous solid dispersion. *Adv. Powder Technol.* **2017**, *28*, 1554–1563. [CrossRef]
77. Li, M.; Gogos, C.G.; Ioannidis, N. Improving the API dissolution rate during pharmaceutical hot-melt extrusion I: Effect of the API particle size, and the co-rotating, twin-screw extruder screw configuration on the API dissolution rate. *Int. J. Pharm.* **2015**, *478*, 103–112. [CrossRef] [PubMed]
78. Ige, P.P.; Baria, R.K.; Gattani, S.G. Fabrication of fenofibrate nanocrystals by probe sonication method for enhancement of dissolution rate and oral bioavailability. *Colloids Surf. B Biointerfaces* **2013**, *108*, 366–373. [CrossRef] [PubMed]
79. Frizon, F.; de Oliveira Eloy, J.; Donaduzzi, C.M.; Mitsui, M.L.; Marchetti, J.M. Dissolution rate enhancement of loratadine in polyvinylpyrrolidone K-30 solid dispersions by solvent methods. *Powder Technol.* **2013**, *235*, 532–539. [CrossRef]
80. Gao, L.; Liu, G.; Wang, X.; Liu, F.; Xu, Y.; Ma, J. Preparation of a chemically stable quercetin formulation using nanosuspension technology. *Int. J. Pharm.* **2011**, *404*, 231–237. [CrossRef] [PubMed]
81. Rabinow, B.E. Nanosuspensions in drug delivery. *Drug Deliv.* **2004**, *3*, 785–796. [CrossRef] [PubMed]
82. Bodmeier, R.; Oh, K.H.; Chen, H. The effect of the addition of low molecular weight poly(DL-lactide) on drug release from biodegradable poly(DL-lactide) drug delivery systems. *Int. J. Pharm.* **1989**, *51*, 1–8. [CrossRef]
83. Tinke, A.P.; Carnicer, A.; Govoreanu, R.; Scheltjens, G.; Lauwerysen, L.; Mertens, N.; Vanhoutte, K.; Brewster, M.E. Particle shape and orientation in laser diffraction and static image analysis size distribution analysis of micrometer sized rectangular particles. *Powder Technol.* **2008**, *186*, 154–167. [CrossRef]
84. Choi, H.J.; Kim, S.G.; Hyun, Y.H.; Jhon, M.S. Preparation and rheological characteristics of solvent-cast poly (ethylene oxide)/ montmorillonite nanocomposites. *Macromol. Rapid Commun.* **2001**, *22*, 320–325. [CrossRef]
85. Singh, A.; Van den Mooter, G. Spray drying formulation of amorphous solid dispersions. *Adv. Drug Deliv. Rev.* **2016**, *100*, 27–50. [CrossRef]
86. Taylor, M.J.; Tanna, S.; Sahota, T. In vivo study of a polymeric glucose-sensitive insulin delivery system using a rat model. *J. Pharm. Sci.* **2010**, *99*, 4215–4227. [CrossRef] [PubMed]

9

Strategies to Enhance Drug Absorption via Nasal and Pulmonary Routes

Maliheh Ghadiri *, Paul M. Young and Daniela Traini

Respiratory Technology, Woolcock Institute of Medical Research and Discipline of Pharmacology, Faculty of Medicine and Health, The University of Sydney, Camperdown, NSW 2006, Australia; paul.young@sydney.edu.au (P.M.Y.); daniela.traini@sydney.edu.au (D.T.)

* Correspondence: Maliheh.ghadiri@sydney.edu.au

Abstract: New therapeutic agents such as proteins, peptides, and nucleic acid-based agents are being developed every year, making it vital to find a non-invasive route such as nasal or pulmonary for their administration. However, a major concern for some of these newly developed therapeutic agents is their poor absorption. Therefore, absorption enhancers have been investigated to address this major administration problem. This paper describes the basic concepts of transmucosal administration of drugs, and in particular the use of the pulmonary or nasal routes for administration of drugs with poor absorption. Strategies for the exploitation of absorption enhancers for the improvement of pulmonary or nasal administration are discussed, including use of surfactants, cyclodextrins, protease inhibitors, and tight junction modulators, as well as application of carriers such as liposomes and nanoparticles.

Keywords: nasal; pulmonary; drug administration; absorption enhancers; nanoparticle; and liposome

---

1. Background

Absorption enhancers are functional excipients included in formulations to improve the absorption of drugs across biological barriers. They have been investigated for many years, particularly to enhance the efficacy of peptides, proteins, and other pharmacologically active compounds that have poor barrier permeability [1]. The ideal absorption enhancer should be one that protects biological agents against enzymatic degradation and causes a rapid opening of the relevant barrier while enhancing absorption transiently.

As a portal for non-invasive delivery, nasal and pulmonary administration has several advantages over traditional oral medication or injection. Nasal and pulmonary delivery are non-invasive routes of administration that target the delivered dose directly to the site of drug action [2,3]. Moreover, drug delivery to the respiratory area can also be used for systemic delivery of peptides and proteins due to the large surface area for drug absorption. Pulmonary and nasal administration bypasses first-pass metabolism that is observed in oral administration and the lung and nasal cavity have a low drug metabolizing environment [4]. Despite all these advantages, there is a significant challenge to enhance the absorption of the active agent via these routes. In nasal and pulmonary administration, absorption enhancers have been investigated over the last two decades, to increase the rate of absorption by targeting different mechanisms [5,6]. These mechanisms are either to improve the permeation of materials across the epithelial barrier via intracellular or paracellular mechanisms (Figure 1) or to enhance stability and mucus solubility of the drugs regionally. However, to date, no safe absorption enhancer for pulmonary administration of drugs has translated into commercial products. Their use has generated safety concerns due to potential irreversible alteration of the epithelial cell membrane, which could potentially make the lung susceptible to the entry of exogenous allergens. While there are no absorption enhancers for pulmonary drug administration on the market, quite a few appear to be at the threshold of becoming products for nasal administration.

This review critically assesses advances in the field of absorption enhancers for nasal and pulmonary drug administration. The various agents used to increase the absorption of poorly permeable drugs, their mechanisms of action, safety, and effectiveness are also presented.

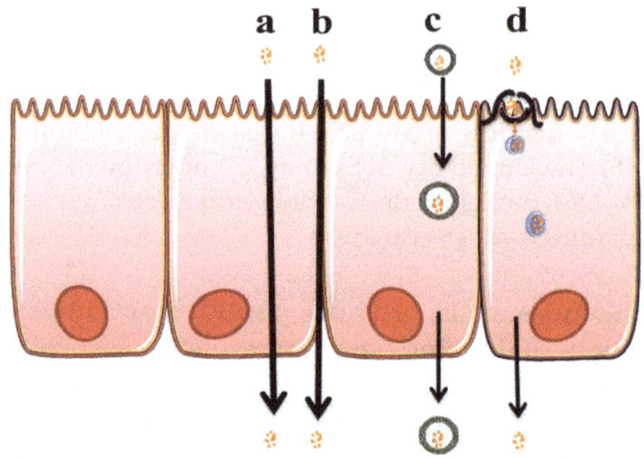

Figure 1. Mechanisms of absorption includes; (a) Transcellular diffusion, (b) Para cellular transport, (c) Vesicle mediated transport, and (d) Carrier mediated transport.

2. The Barriers

The first requirement for drug absorption is for the active pharmaceutical ingredient (API, or drug) to reach the absorbing barrier. For the respiratory system, the drug has to be deposited on the luminal surface of the epithelial membrane and be absorbed before being cleared or degraded. Furthermore, adequate absorption of the API may also require controlling its release profile as it passes through multiple biological barriers. These barriers include: (1) the surfactant layer, mucus layer, (2) epithelial layer, (3) interstitium and basement membrane, and (4) capillary endothelium (Figure 2).

The mucus layer is the first barrier. The deposited drug needs to be dissolved or transverse the mucus layer before degradation due to the enzymatic activity or clearance by mucociliary activity. Because the ciliary action is relatively fast in removing the drug from the absorption site, permeation enhancers must act rapidly to increase bioavailability. The understanding of mucus layer thickness and clearance rate is important to develop drug delivery strategies to overcome mucosal clearance mechanisms. In the lung, the thickness of the luminal mucus gel has been reported to be ~5–10 μm [7]. The underlying, less viscoelastic sol layer, also known as the periciliary liquid, covers the cilia and has an additional 5–10 μm thickness [7]. However, other studies based on confocal fluorescence microscopy suggest that airway mucus may range in thickness from 5 to 55 μm [8,9]. The nasal tract has a thin mucus layer which is readily accessible and considered highly permeable compared to other mucosal surfaces [10]. In the nasal tract, the ciliary motion transports mucus with the flow rate of about 5 mm per minute, and the mucus layer is renewed approximately every 20 min [11,12]. Similarly, the luminal gel layer of respiratory tract mucus is replaced every 10 to 20 min, [11]. While, the sol layer of respiratory mucus has a slower rate of clearance than the more solid-like luminal gel layer. Drug absorption via the nose is dependent on drug clearance from the nasal cavity, which is determined by nasal mucociliary clearance (MC). In a study by Inoue et al., the effect of nasal MC on in vivo absorption of norfloxacin after intranasal administration to rats was estimated quantitatively. This study resulted in a model to precisely estimate nasal drug absorption [13].

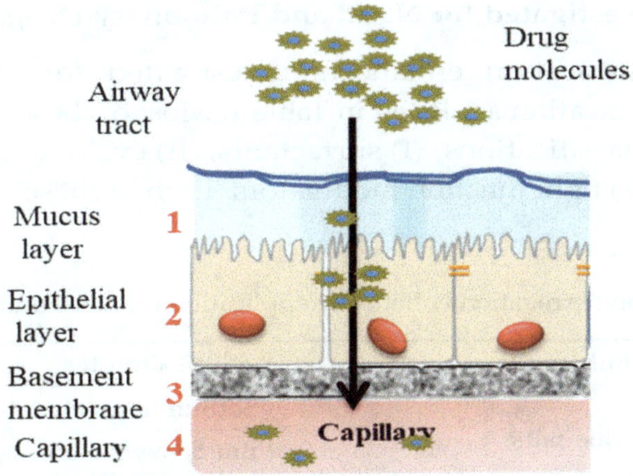

Figure 2. Barriers against drug absorption in pulmonary drug administration including; (1) mucus layer, (2) epithelial layer, (3) interstitium and basement membrane, and (4) capillary endothelium.

The second barrier is the epithelial cell membrane. It is comprised of a layer of pseudostratified columnar cells interconnected via tight junctions. Most drugs are primarily absorbed via transcellular diffusion, permeating through the epithelial cell membrane. Small hydrophobic molecules can partition across biological membranes via a concentration gradient. Hydrophilic molecules generally require some sort of selective transport system to cross the lipid bilayer. Large and polar drugs may be absorbed by a paracellular mechanism, and the tight junction structure represents the barrier to paracellular absorption.

Once a drug molecule has passed through to the basolateral side of the epithelium, the next barrier is the capillary endothelium for absorption into the blood. While this is not critical for locally acting drugs, it is important for systemically targeting APIs.

Strategies used to overcome these barriers to absorption include: A. Preventing degradation/ metabolism; B. Enhancing barrier permeability via transient opening of tight junctions, C. Disruption of lipid bilayer packing/complexation/carrier/ion pairing; and D. Enhancing resident time/slowing down mucociliary clearance (Figure 3).

In the following sections, absorption enhancers utilized to overcome these barriers in nasal and pulmonary routes of administration are discussed.

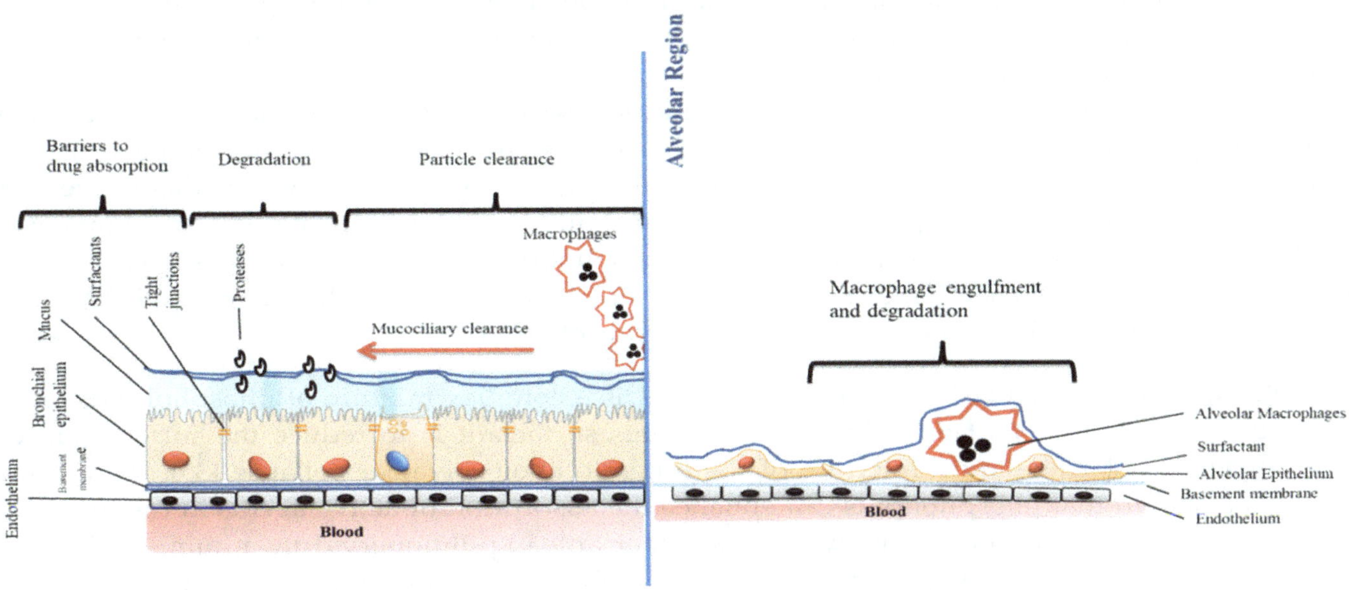

Figure 3. Hurdles for the absorption of drugs via inhalation.

3. Absorption Enhancers Investigated for Nasal and Pulmonary Drug Administration

The most common permeation enhancers investigated for nasal and pulmonary drug administration and their classification are listed in Table 1. Most of these agents have been divided into one of the following major classifications: (I) surfactants, (II) cyclodextrins, (III) protease inhibitors, (IV) cationic polymers, and (V) tight junction modulators. Each of these classifications are discussed in greater detail below.

Table 1. Common absorption permeation enhancers- application for nasal and pulmonary administration.

Class	Enhancers	Examples	References
Surfactants	Bile salts	Sodium taurocholate	[14,15]
		Sodium deoxycholate sodium	[16]
		Glycodeoxycholat	[17,18]
Surfactants	Fatty acids and derivatives	Palmitic acid	[19]
		Palmitoleic acid	
		Stearic acid	
		Oleyl alcohol	
		Oleic acid	
		Capric acid	[20,21]
		DHA, EPA	[20]
Surfactants	Phospholipids	Dipalmitoyl phophatidyl choline, soybean lecithin, phosphatidylcholine	[22,23]
Cationic polymers	Polymers	Chitosan and their derivatives	[24–26]
Enzyme inhibitors		Human neutrophil elastase inhibitor (ER143)	
Cyclodextrins		Beta-Cyclodextrin	[27]
Tight junction modulators	Claudine modulator	Clostridium perfringens enterotoxin	[28]
	ZO modulator	Zonula occludens toxin (ZOT)	[29]

3.1. *Surfactants*

Surface active agents, or surfactants, are amphiphilic molecules possessing both lipophilic and hydrophilic residues. Surfactants have various applications in pulmonary drug administration, due to their high interfacial activity; one of which is as an absorption enhancer [30]. Surfactants can enhance absorption with more than one mechanism; these include perturbing the cell membrane by leaching of membrane proteins, opening of tight junctions, or preventing enzymatic degradation of the drugs [31]. These surfactants are mainly used and studied in oral drug administration; however, there have been a few studies looking at their application in nasal and pulmonary drug delivery. Surfactants used as absorption enhancers can be classified as; (A) phospholipids [32], (B) bile salts, (such as sodium taurocholate etc.) [33], (C) non-ionic surfactants [31], (D) salt of fatty acids [20], and (E) alkyl glycosides (e.g., tetradecylmaltoside, *N*-lauryl-*b*-*d*-maltopyranoside etc.) [34].

(a) **Phospholipids**: Natural pulmonary surfactant is a complex mixture of phospholipids (90%) and proteins (10%). The main function of this surfactant is to reduce the surface tension at the alveolar air–liquid interface of the lungs to avoid alveolar collapse [35]. It has also been shown that phospholipids can enhance the absorption of active agents in the lung [36]. A review by Wauthoz extensively discussed their role in pulmonary drug administration [36]. For example, Dipalmitoylphosphatidylcholine (DPPC) is a main component of lung surfactant, representing 40% by weight [37]. DPPC has been used as a lung absorption enhancer in several studies [23,38,39]; for instance, it was used to optimize the absorption of parathyroid hormone 1-34 (PTH) from the lungs into the bloodstream [38]. Other lung surfactants, including phosphatidyl cholines (35%), phosphatidylglycerol (10%), phosphatidylinositol (2%), phosphatidylethanolamine (3%), sphingomyelin (2.5%), and neutral lipid (3%) have also been used as absorption enhancers. These natural pulmonary surfactants (PS) and their artificial substitute phospholipid hexadecanol tyloxapol (PHT) have been tested as absorption enhancers for promoting recombinant human insulin (Rh-ins) absorption in vivo from the lung in a diabetic rat model [40]. In another study, the same phospholipids were tested in vitro on Calu-3 ALI (air-liquid culture) model [41] to further investigate their absorption potential. This in vitro study demonstrated an enhanced permeation of Rh-ins and fluorescein isothiocyanate-labelled dextran (FD-4) (4000 Dalton molecular weight) through the cell layer. Hence, PS demonstrated a greater absorption enhancing effect than that of PHT. However, they could not identify the underlying mechanism of enhanced absorption. It was suggested that PS and PHT may interact directly with the tight junctions and increase the absorption via the paracellular pathway.

(b) **Bile salts**; one of the primary roles of bile salts and their derivatives in drug delivery is their ability to enhance absorption [42]. For pulmonary drug delivery applications, salts of cholate, deoxycholate, glycocholate, glycodeoxycholate, taurocholate, and taurodeoxycholate [43] have been tested as absorption enhancers. Sodium taurocholate is one of the most-used bile salts to increase bioavailability of proteins, especially insulin [33] via the pulmonary route. The ranking of enhancement by bile salts for insulin has been reported to be sodium deoxycholate > sodium cholate > sodium glycocholate > sodium glycodeoxycholate (GDCA) > sodium taurodeoxycholate [33]. Even though bile salts and derivatives have shown potential as absorption enhancers, their toxicity on the epithelial surface is a main challenge in clinical applications. In a recent study the effect of inhaled bile salts on lung surfactant function as absorption enhancers was investigated in two in vitro models and then correlated to in vivo lung effects [44]. This study demonstrated that bile salts in vitro disrupted surfactant function and in vivo induced pulmonary irritation. Therefore, even though the bile salts did not affect the barrier integrity or viability of human airway epithelial cells at the tested doses, they have shown toxicity to some extent.

(c) **Fatty acids**; Fatty acids, polyunsaturated fatty acids (PUFA), and their salts have also been investigated as absorption enhancers via the nasal and pulmonary route [21]. They have shown a tight junction modulatory effect to some extent, and enhanced permeation of drugs through the epithelial cell barrier. Although the exact mechanism is still unknown, previous studies have suggested that they may alter the membrane's permeability, increasing fluidity of the membrane or through Ca^{2+} dependent tight junction mechanisms [45]. Their potential as an absorption enhancer has been demonstrated in both in vitro [20] and in vivo studies [16]. For example, the effects of arachidonic acid as an absorption enhancer combined with amino acid Taurine enhanced absorption of fluorescein isothiocyanate 4000 (FD-4) via the pulmonary route [46]. Among the fatty acids, medium chain fatty acids such as capric acid and lauric acid have been studied extensively as absorption enhancers due to their safety and effectiveness [45,47]. The suggested mechanism for capric acid (sodium caprate) is most likely by activation of phospholipase-C and increase of intracellular calcium levels, resulting in contraction of actin microfilaments and dilation of the tight junctions [45].

(d) **Non-ionic surfactants**—Non-ionic surfactants, consisting of a hydrophilic head group and a hydrophobic tail, carry no charge and are relatively non-toxic [48]. Poloxamer 188, a non-ionic surfactant, has been widely studied as intranasal drug delivery system [49]. in vitro and in vivo studies demonstrated that poloxamer 188 played a key role in promoting intranasal absorption of both isosorbide dinitrate [49] and sumatriptan succinate [50] in rats. Incorporation of poloxamer 188 was reported to be able to influence the elasticity of nano-cubic vehicles for intranasal delivery [51]. Other non-ionic surfactants such as cremophor EL, laurate sucrose ester (SE), and sucrose cocoate have also shown absorption enhancement properties via nasal administration. SE has shown an efficient absorption-enhancing effect of poorly permeable drugs [31], furthermore, intranasal administration of an insulin formulation containing 0.5% sucrose cocoate showed a rapid and significant increase in plasma insulin level, with a concomitant decrease in blood glucose level [52]. Alkylglycosides (AGs) are a type of non-ionic surfactant class with groups such as maltose, sucrose or monosaccharides (e.g., glucose) attached to alkyl chains of variable length. Tetradecylmaltoside and *N*-lauryl-*b*-*d*-maltopyranoside are the most commonly used AGs. They have shown effective nasal absorption enhancement properties at extremely low concentrations. Pillion and his colleagues showed that AGs could be used effectively to enhance nasal absorption of insulin, calcitonin, and glucagon [53]. They synthesized a series of new glycosides with extended alkyl side-chains (C13–16) linked to maltose or sucrose and tested their efficacy as a penetration enhancer for delivery of nasal insulin in anesthetized rats [54]. Of the AGs tested, tetradecyl maltoside (TDM), a 14-carbon alkyl chain attached to a maltose ring, has been shown to be the most efficacious in enhancing nasal insulin absorption. The effects of TDM on the respiratory epithelium were shown to be reversible, with the epithelium reversing to its normal physiological barrier function 120 min after exposure to these agents. The molecular mechanism involved in these absorption-enhancing effects in vivo is unclear. It has been suggested that AGs have a direct effect on the epithelium layer, probably via the para cellular pathway [55]. Although AGs have shown absorption enhancing effect, they exhibit significant toxicity towards airway epithelial cells (Calu-3 cells), probably from a membrane-damaging effect [56].

(e) **Bio-surfactants**—Biosurfactants are surface-active substances synthesised by living cells such as bacteria, fungi, and yeast. Bio-surfactants are generally non-toxic, environmentally benign, and biodegradable. Biosurfactants have been investigated as drug absorption enhancers previously [57]. One of the most well characterized classes of biosurfactants are rhamnolipids. The effect of rhamnolipids on the epithelial permeability of FD-4 and FD-10 across Caco-2 and Calu-3 monolayers has been reported [58]. It was shown that rhamnolipids increased permeation of FD-4 and FD-10 across both cell lines at a safe concentration with a dose-dependent effect.

(f) **Animal derived surfactants**—The animal-derived surfactant poractant alfa (Curosurf®) was used to deliver polymyxin E and gentamicin to the lung in a neonatal rabbit model [59]. In this study, polymyxin E was mixed with poractant alfa and administered to a near-term rabbit. This mixture increased bactericidal effect of the antibiotics against Pseudomonas aeruginosa in vivo. This may be due to more efficient spreading mediated by interactions between drugs and surfactant.

3.2. *Enzyme Inhibitors*

Airway surface liquid and mucus contains a high number of enzymes including proteases, and nucleases that may degrade active agents before they are absorbed [60]. Among these enzymes, serine proteases and aminopeptidases constitute the majority of degrading enzymes present in the lung. Given the high number of enzymes in the lung, these may metabolize respiratory drugs before they reach the absorbing membrane. Peptide, proteins, and nucleic acid-based drugs are especially vulnerable to metabolism. Therefore, a strategy to protect drugs against enzymatic degradation within the lung and nasal cavity may be necessary in some cases. Some of the protease inhibitors studied over the last decade in pulmonary/nasal drug administration as absorption enhancers are: nafamostat mesilate [61], aprotinin [62], bacitracin [63], soybean trypsin inhibitor [63], phosphoramidon [15], leupeptin [64], and bestatin [65]. In one study, aprotinin, bacitracin, and soybean trypsin were used as protease inhibitors in combination with other absorption enhancers (sodium glycocholate, linoleic acid-surfactant mixed micelles, and *N*-lauryl-β-d-maltopyranoside) and tested on rat lung for the absorption of insulin and Asu (1,7)) eel-calcitonin (ECT) [62,63]. During the aforementioned study, rats received insulin with protease inhibitor via intra tracheal administration. The absorption of insulin from the lung was evaluated by their hypoglycemic and hypocalcemic response when used with these additives [62,63]. In the presence of protease inhibitors, the plasma concentration of glucose reached a minimum of 24.0–66.7% of baseline within 90 min of solution administration. It was also found that bacitracin (20 mM) was more effective at enhancing the pulmonary absorption of insulin than aprotinin and soybean trypsin inhibitor. In the same study, the effects of these protease inhibitors on the stability of insulin in rat lung homogenate were investigated, to elucidate the enhancing mechanisms of these protease inhibitors. All protease inhibitors were effective in reducing insulin degradation and these findings suggest that combination of absorption enhancers and protease inhibitors would be a useful approach for improving the pulmonary absorption of biologically active drugs. Studies have shown that when nafamostat mesilate, which strongly inhibits a variety of proteases, such as trypsin, plasmin, and kallikaren, was co-administered with insulin in the lung, the relative bioavailability of insulin was approximately twice that obtained when the peptide was administered alone [66].

During chronic lung inflammation and infection proteases such as neutrophil elastase (NE), a neutrophil-specific serine protease against P. aeruginosa, will be released into the lung lumen to fight pathogens involved in lung infections [67]. Excessive accumulation of NE in pulmonary fluids and tissues of patients with chronic lung infection is thought to reduce the absorption of inhaled drugs. Therefore, neutrophil elastase inhibitors (NEIs) have shown potential as absorption enhancers by protecting drug moieties from degradation by neutrophil elastase [68]. The potential use of NEIs, such as peptide chloromethyl ketones or reversible peptide aldehydes, tripeptide ketones, modified NE-specific β-lactams, or peptide boronic acids have been largely replaced by the development of EPI-HNE-4, a rapid acting and potent NE inhibitor [69] which can potentially be nebulized to CF patients [70]. However, clear clinical efficacy of this NE inhibitor remains to be demonstrated.

3.3. Cationic Polymers as Absorption Enhancers

Polymeric systems with positive charges or modified with cationic entities, incorporated on their backbone and/or side chains, are considered cationic polymers [71]. Cationic polymers have the potential to enhance absorption of macromolecules [72]. Cationated gelatins [72], cationated pullulans, poly-L-arginine, polyethylenamine (PEI), chitosan, and its derivatives are types of cationic polymers. Cationic polymers interact with the mucosal barriers and enhance the absorption of water-soluble macromolecules via tight junctions modification. For example, in the case of insulin with negative charges in neutral solutions, interaction between the cationic polymers and insulin is important to promote effective insulin absorption. An appropriate interaction can help insulin to access the cell surface; however, strong interaction can inhibit insulin absorption. PEI is a cationic and highly water-soluble polymer that has shown potential as a carrier for nasal drug administration. It was also demonstrated that the degree of positive charge was linearly correlated with absorption enhancing effect of PEI, suggesting that positive charge of PEI might be related to its absorption mechanisms for enhancing pulmonary absorption of insulin in rats [73]. Spermined dextran (SD), a cationic polymer, has been studied as absorption enhancer for pulmonary application of peptide drugs [74]. Its enhancing effects on the absorption of insulin and permeation of FD-4 through Calu-3 cells increased with an increase in the molecular weight of SD, over the range 10–70 kDa. The mechanism of action of SD is not fully understood yet, but it is hypothesized that the molecule may interact directly with the luminal surface of the mucus barriers via an ion-ion interaction, inducing the opening of tight junctions, resulting in intercellular permeation of water soluble drugs [74]. Chitosan and its derivatives are excellent examples of cationic polyelectrolytes. They have been extensively used to develop mucoadhesive polymers [25,75] and have favorable characteristics such as biocompatibility, biodegradation, and low toxicity. These aforementioned characteristics make them suitable as a pharmaceutical excipient [76]. Chitosan interacts electrostatically with the negatively charged mucin chains thereby demonstrating mucoadhesive properties. This mucoadhesion prolongs the residence time of the drug and thus enhances API absorption [77]. However, Chitosan derivatives are poorly soluble in water at physiological pH, limiting their application. Chitosan exhibits excellent mucoadhesive properties when dissolved in neutral or alkaline medium so to overcome solubility issues, different derivatives have been synthesized [78]. Chitosan oligomers [79], for example, have relatively high solubility in water compared to conventional chitosan and have been tested for their absorption enhancing potential via lung [25]. For example, the pulmonary absorption of interferon-α has been shown to be effective when using chitosan oligomers [25]. Of these chitosan oligomers, 0.5% w/v chitosan hexamer appeared to be more effective in enhancing the pulmonary absorption of IFN than other oligomers at the same concentration, and the AUC value of IFN with chitosan hexamer increased 2.6-fold when compared to control. In a recent study, O-palmitoyl chitosan, synthesized from chitosan and palmitoyl chloride, demonstrated improved mucoadhesive and absorption enhancing properties [80]. In addition, bioadhesive properties of chitosan may be useful in enhancing drug absorption following inhalation [81].

Sperminated pullulans (SP) have been shown to enhance pulmonary absorption of insulin in rats, with their enhancing effects correlated to the amino group content and their molecular weight [82]. SP acted as an enhancer for insulin absorption when a 0.1% w/v solution was applied with insulin simultaneously in vivo. Ikada et al. studied the use of negatively and positively charged gelatin microspheres for pulmonary administration of salmon calcitonin in rats [83]. The pharmacological effect after administration of salmon calcitonin in positively charged gelatin microspheres was significantly higher than that in negatively charged gelatin microspheres. Additionally, administration of salmon calcitonin in positively charged gelatin microspheres with smaller particle sizes led to a higher pharmacological effect. The pharmacological effect after pulmonary administration of salmon calcitonin in positively charged gelatin microspheres with particle sizes of 3.4 and 11.2 μm was approximately 50% [83].

Polyamines have also been tested for their absorption enhancing properties [84]. The polyamines spermidine and spermine are commonly found in all mammalian cells [84]. They are essential for the maintenance of cell growth in many tissues. Specifically, for the lungs, He et al. showed that polyamines, particularly spermine and spermidine, can effectively improve the pulmonary absorption of insulin and other water soluble macromolecules without any membrane damage of the lung tissues in rats [84]. It was suggested that the absorption-enhancing mechanism of spermine partly includes opening of the epithelial tight junctions. Sperminated dextrans have also been studied as absorption enhancers with different average molecular weights (MWs; 10, 40, and 70 kDa) and numbers of amino groups, prepared as cationized polymers [74]. Sperminated dextrans increased pulmonary absorption of insulin in rats and also permeation of FD-4 through Calu-3 cell monolayers in vitro [74].

3.4. *Tight Junction Modulators*

The intercellular spaces between adjacent epithelial cells are sealed by tight junctions (TJs). Modulation of TJs is an effective strategy for drug absorption via the paracellular pathway. The paracellular transport is not suitable for the transport of large macromolecules and is generally restricted to the compounds of molecular radii less than 11 Å. Hydrophilic drugs with low molecular weight, peptides, and proteins often have poor bioavailability. However, it has been shown that some peptide drugs, such as octreotide, desmopressin, and thyrotropin-releasing hormone are absorbed by this route in which tight junctions play a fundamental role [85]. Tight junction modulators effective on TJ proteins such as Claudin and ZO are extremely potent in opening these tight junctions, 400 fold stronger than other agents [86]. Until now they have mainly been tested on intestinal and dermal [87] tight junction barriers [88,89] and on the blood–brain barrier [90]. Of these modulators, two have been tested for pulmonary drug administration.

(A) Clostridium perfringens enterotoxin (CPE)—The C-terminal fragment of CPE (C-CPE) is known to modulate the barrier function of claudin [28]. Claudin is one of the key structural and functional components of the TJ-seal (70). Therefore, it has been suggested that claudin may be a potential target for paracellular API delivery. C-CPE is a potent absorption-enhancer and this enhancing activity is greater than clinically used enhancers. The main problem with tight junction modulators is their toxicity [91]; therefore, many variants of CPE have been synthesized to decrease toxicity [86]. In a study on nasal and pulmonary absorption of human parathyroid hormone hPTH in rats, C-CPE was used as an absorption enhancer. It was instilled into each nostril and after 4 h hPTH was delivered intranasally. A Micro-sprayer was used to spray C-CPE into rats' lungs, then after 4 h, hPTH was administered. This study showed C-CPE, and enhanced nasal but not pulmonary absorption of hPTH [89].

(B) Zonula occludens toxin (ZOT) are another tight junction modulator. Zot is a protein of Vibrio cholera, and zonulin is the Zot analogue that governs the permeability of intercellular TJs [92]. Zot and Zot derivatives are reversible TJ openers that enhance the delivery of drugs through the paracellular route. The active domain of zonula occludens toxin (ZOT) is called AT-1002 [93]. AT-1002, a hexamer peptide, induced tight junction disassembly in the epithelial layer in the trachea [29]. In this study, in vivo intratracheal administration of salmon calcitonin in rats with 1 mg of AT-1002 resulted in a 5.2-fold increase in absorption of calcitonin over the control group [29].

4. Other Strategies to Enhance Absorption

4.1. Nanoparticles (NPs)

Nanoparticles (NPs) have been used as drug carriers for overcoming mucociliary clearance and to avoid phagocytosis by alveolar macrophages, hence increasing the absorption of drugs in respiratory system [94]. It was shown that alveolar macrophages are less efficient to phagocytose ultrafine particles compared to larger particles [95] and NPs overcome the mucus barrier and achieve longer retention time at the cell surface, effectively penetrating the mucus layer and accumulating on the epithelial surface. In order to penetrate mucus, nanoparticles must avoid adhesion to mucin fibres and be small enough to avoid significant steric inhibition by the dense fibre mesh [96]. In a study by Schneider, variously sized, polystyrene-based muco-penetrating particles (MPP) were synthesized and their absorption in the lungs following inhalation investigated. They demonstrated that MPP as large as 300 nm exhibited uniform distribution and markedly enhanced retention in the lung [96]. NPs can also improve nose-to-brain drug delivery, since they are able to protect encapsulated drug from biological and/or chemical degradation, and from extracellular transport by P-gp efflux proteins [97]. Retention of bioadhesive NPs on the mucosal surface of the nasal cavity, as well as their ability of transiently opening of the tight junctions of the mucosal epithelium, should contribute to enhanced nasal absorption [98].

4.2. Liposomes

An approach to enhance mucosal penetration is to encapsulate drugs within liposomes. Liposomes consist of one or more phospholipid bilayers and can incorporate hydrophilic substances within their inner cavity and hydrophobic substances within the lipid bilayer. Liposomes and phospholipids have been investigated for the systemic absorption of proteins after intra tracheal administration [99]. It is suggested that the mechanism of absorption is driven by phospholipids in the liposomes being infused with the rapidly recycling lung surfactant that leads to enhanced uptake of the protein molecule into the systemic circulation [99]. Liposomes are also known to promote an increase in drug retention time and reduce the toxicity of drugs after administration [23]. Several factors influence drug release and absorption of drugs loaded into liposomes such as the composition of lipids and the size of the liposomes used [100]. The presence of cholesterol and phospholipids with saturated hydrocarbon chains have also been shown to increase drug residence time within the lung [23]. A number of nebulizable liposome formulations have reached clinical trial phase. For example, Arikace® (liposomal amikacin) and Pulmaquin® (liposomal ciprofloxacin) are antibacterial formulations currently in advanced stages of development.

Glycerosomes are vesicles composed of phospholipids, glycerol, and water, and have been used as novel vesicular carriers for trans-mucosal drug delivery. Glycerosomes are made from a diverse range of phospholipids and a high percent of glycerol (20–40%, v/v). They are flexible vesicular carriers, where the glycerol component alters the vesicle membrane fluidity, and are constituted by different substances such as cholesterol that enhance the lipidic bilayer stability. They also may contain basic or acidic lipid molecules which adjust the electrical charge of vesicular surfaces and decrease liposome aggregation. Glycerosomes can be prepared by the same common techniques that are used for the preparation of conventional liposomes.

As an example, curcumin was incorporated in glycerosomes for delivery into the lungs. In this study, curcumin was loaded into glycerosomes which were then combined with two polymers, sodium hyaluronate and trimethyl chitosan, to form polymer-glycerosomes [101]. The study showed that nebulized curcumin vesicles were able to protect in vitro A549 cells stressed with hydrogen peroxide, restoring healthy conditions, not only by directly scavenging free radicals but also by indirectly inhibiting the production of cytokine IL6 and IL8. Also, in vivo results in rats showed the high capacity of these glycerosomes to favor the curcumin accumulation in the lungs, confirming their potential use as a pulmonary drug delivery system. In another study, Rifampicin loaded glycerosomes, vesicles composed of phospholipids, glycerol, and water, were combined with trimethyl chitosan chloride (TMC) to prepare TMC-glycerosomes or with sodium hyaluronate (HY) to obtain HY-glycerosomes [102]. These new hybrid nanovesicles were tested as carriers for pulmonary delivery of rifampicin. Rifampicin nanoincorporation in vesicles reduced the in vitro drug toxicity on A549 cells, as well as increasing its efficacy against Staphylococcus aureus. Finally, the in vivo biodistribution and accumulation, evaluated after intra-tracheal administration to rats, confirmed the improvement of rifampicin accumulation in lung.

4.3. Dendrimers

Dendrimers possess high water solubility, and as highly efficient absorption promoters, they can easily penetrate through barriers. In addition, they can be used as carriers for different routes of drug administration [103,104]. Dendrimers have been studied intensively as a drug carrier in delivery systems [103,104]. As a novel class of artificial macromolecules, polyamidoamine (PAMAM) dendrimers have shown excellent performance in drug delivery systems due to their unique physical and chemical properties [105]. PAMAM dendrimers with generation 0 to generation 3 (G0–G3) and concentrations (0.1–1.0%) were tested in terms of their capacity to enhance pulmonary absorption of macromolecules [105]. The results showed that treatment with a 0.1% G3 PAMAM dendrimer could increase the secretion of organic cation transporters (OCTs), OCT1, OCT2, and OCT3, which might be related to the absorption-enhancing mechanisms of the pulmonary absorption of the macromolecule.

4.4. Exosomes

Exosomes are a subgroup of 30–100 nm size extracellular vesicles (EVs) secreted by cells into the extracellular environment. EVs have the distinct advantage that their membranes are structurally similar to the cell membrane. This means that EVs lipid composition, fluidity, protein membranes, and other fusogenic proteins are similar to what is found in cell membranes. Because of this unique property, cellular uptake of EVs surpasses that of more traditional carriers, such as liposomes or nanoparticles. Exosomes can be used as a biological nano-platform for enhanced drug delivery [106]. Their advantages include their small size for penetration into deep tissues, slightly negative zeta potential for long circulation, and deformable cytoskeleton, as well as their similarity to cell membranes [107]. In addition, some exosomes also exhibit an increased capacity to escape degradation or clearance by the immune system [108]. Exosomes have been developed as drug delivery vehicles for a variety of drugs [109,110]. Tumor-derived exosomes are of great significance for guiding the targeted therapy of lung cancer, and exosomes themselves can be a target for treatment. For example, GW4869, a neutral sphingomyelase inhibitor (regulates ceramide biosynthesis, promotes exosomes inward budding), tested in mice, demonstrated inhibition of exosomes production with reduced metastasis in lung cancer [111]. In another study, exosomes derived from curcumin-treated cells alleviated oxidative stress, tight junctions (ZO-1, claudin, occludin), adherent junction (VE-cadherin) proteins, and endothelial cell layer permeability [112]. A nano-formulation consisting of exosomes loaded with paclitaxel (PTX), a commonly used chemotherapeutic agent, developed by Batrakova et al. [113], showed efficacy in the treatment of multi-drug resistant cancer cells. Incorporation of PTX into exosomes increased cytotoxicity more than 50 times in drug resistant MDCKMDR1 (Pgp+) cells and showed a potent anticancer effect in the murine Lewis lung carcinoma pulmonary metastases model. It was shown that exosomes loaded with PTX may alter drug intracellular trafficking and bypass the drug efflux system. The potential of intranasally administered exosomes as delivery vehicles for the treatment of neuro inflammatory diseases has also been investigated. After intranasal administration of exosomes loaded with potent antioxidant, considerable amounts of catalase were detected in a Parkinson's disease (PD) mouse brain model. It provided significant neuroprotective effects in in vitro and in vivo models of PD [114]. Low molecular antioxidant [115], anticancer agents, doxorubicin (Dox) [116], and a model drug rhodamine [117], have also been loaded into exosomes or exosome-like vesicles for nasal drug delivery to enhance absorption and efficacy.

4.5. Cell Penetrating Peptides (CPPs)

Improving the translocation of drugs across the plasma membrane will significantly enhance their absorption. Therefore, using cell penetrating peptides (CPPs) to enhance drug penetration has the potential to significantly reduce the quantity of drug to be administered, thus reducing possible side effects. Cell-penetrating peptides are short peptides that enable cellular intake/uptake of various molecular moieties with poor permeability across epithelial and endothelial barriers [118]. Several types of cargoes, for example, proteins, nucleic acid based macromolecules such as siRNA, plasmid DNA, and small drug molecules, can be transported by CPPs to overcome the natural cellular biological barriers [119]. The mechanism of action of CPPs is still a matter of some debate. Some research suggests CPPs could pass through the plasma membrane via an energy-independent pathway, with others claiming the formation of micro-micelles at the membrane [120], or direct translocation through the lipid bilayer [121]. Multiple studies have consolidated the high efficiency of CPP-mediated drug delivery in vitro. For instance, CPPs have been used successfully to deliver macromolecules [122], oligonucleotides [119,123], and peptides [124] across different cellular barriers. Specifically, CPPs have been recently investigated in nasal and pulmonary drug administration [125–127], where they have been used as a conjugate to liposomes and nanoparticles to enhance absorption of model DNA [128]. Co-administration of CPPs could improve nose-to-brain drug transport. In Kamei's study, it was demonstrated that, insulin was transported into the brain when co-administered with amphipathic CPP, and eventually insulin reached the deeper regions of the brain such as the hippocampus in both mice and rat [126]. The immunohistological examination of the hippocampus demonstrated enhanced nose-to-brain delivery of insulin had a partial neuroprotective effect but unexpectedly increased amyloid β plaque deposition. Therefore, CPPs seem to hold great promise as delivery agents for biomacromolecules. However, CPP-mediated delivery is apparently not tissue- or cell-type specific, so for specific targeting purposes additional agents need to be included in the drug delivery system.

4.6. Surface Modification

To enhance the absorption of poorly permeable drugs, another strategy is to modify the inhaled particle surface with agents that enhance their absorption. For example, by coating particles with lipids, the disturbance of the particles on the cellular layer can be reduced [129]. Moreover, the lipid-coated particles can be readily enfolded by the surfactant layer to form vesicular structures that can fuse with the cell membrane. Polymer coating of nanoparticles and liposomes is another strategy to enhance the mucosal penetration of particles via nasal/pulmonary administration [130]. For example, spray dried polymer coated liposomes composed of soy phosphatidylcholine and phospholipid dimyristoyl phosphatidylglycerol coated with alginate, chitosan, or trimethyl chitosan, increased penetration of liposomes through the nasal mucosa over uncoated liposomes when delivered as a dry powder [130]. Surface-modified liposomes for pulmonary administration of peptides were also investigated. For example, chitosan oligosaccharide (oligoCS) and polyvinyl alcohol (PVA-R) with a hydrophobic anchor were used as surface modifiers [131]. The effect of surface modified liposomes on potential toxicity via inhalation was evaluated in vitro and in vivo. In vitro studies on alveolar epithelial cells (A549 cells) demonstrated that PVA-R modification reduced interaction with this cell line, whereas oligoCS modification electrostatically enhanced cellular interaction. The therapeutic efficacy of a peptide (elcatonin) after pulmonary administration to rats was significantly enhanced and prolonged for 48 h after separate administration with oligoCS- or PVA-R-modified liposomes. Furthermore, oligoCS-modified liposomes increased residency of liposomes in the lung and had a tight junction opening effect. On the other hand, PVA-R-modified liposomes induced long-term retention of elcatonin in the lung fluid, leading to sustained absorption. Lactoferrin, a natural iron binding protein whose receptor is highly expressed in both respiratory epithelial cells and neurons, was utilized to facilitate the nasal delivery of nucleic based therapeutic agents. For example, a Lactoferrin-modified PEG-*co*-PCL NPs was recently developed to enhance brain delivery of a neuroprotective peptide—NAPVSIPQ following intranasal administration [132]. In another study, rotigotine, dopamine agonist for the treatment of PD, was loaded in lactoferrin (Lf) modified poly(ethylene glycol)–poly(lactic-*co*-glycolic acid) (PEG-PLGA) nanoparticles. Following intranasal administration, brain delivery of rotigotine was more effective with Lf-NPs than with NPs alone. The brain distribution of rotigotine was heterogeneous, with a higher concentration in the striatum, the primary region affected in PD. This strongly suggested that Lf-NPs enable the targeted delivery of rotigotine for the treatment of PD.

4.7. Cyclodextrins (CDs)

Cyclodextrins (CDs) are a distinct family of chemical reagents that contain six, seven, or eight monosaccharide units in a cyclized ring with a central cavity that can accommodate other agents [133]. Hydrophobic drug molecules or hydrophobic parts of drugs are introduced into the CD apolar cavities, thereby presenting the potential to modify the properties of the inhaled drug. For example, Shimpi et al. showed that CDs have an effect on absorption of hydrophilic macromolecules through the pulmonary and nasal routes [27]. They have demonstrated many benefits in pulmonary drug administration, such as improvements in aqueous solubility, systemic absorption and bioavailability of drugs. It has also been shown that modified CDs, such as methylated β-cyclodextrin (M-β-CD), dimethyl-β-cyclodextrin (DM-β-CD), and hydroxypropyl-beta-cyclodextrin (HP-β-CD) as its derivatives notably enhance intranasal absorption of drugs [134]. β-cyclodextrins (β-CD) have been broadly studied as an intranasal absorption enhancer [49]. The effect of CDs on the respiratory cell layer permeability was investigated in vitro and shown to be concentration-dependent and variable according to the type of CDs, type of chemical modification, and degree of substitution [135]. It has been shown that CDs, in general, do not cause a decrease in cell viability at concentrations $\leq$1 mM, whereas differences between various CDs were observed at concentrations $\geq$2 mM [136,137]. HP-β-CD and natural-CDs are safest in terms of cytotoxicity, while M-β-CD were the least safe for pulmonary administration [138]. Particularly, it has been shown that CDs are more effective in animal studies compared to in vitro studies as absorption enhancers [134].

The mechanism of absorption enhancement with CDs is still unclear; however, there are reports that M-β-CD increase transcellular, as well as paracellular, movement of peptide drugs [135]. CDs may also have a direct disruptive effect on the alveolar epithelial membrane as evidenced by the extraction of membrane lipids and proteins [139]. CDs derivatives can also stimulate transmucosal absorption of peptide drugs. Importantly, M-β-CD, such as DM-β-CD, strongly enhance transmucosal insulin absorption, whereas unmodified-cyclodextrin has little effect on insulin absorption [139]. It is suggested that both DM-β-CD and tetradecyl-beta-maltoside cyclodextrin (TDM-CD) enhance absorption of insulin by different mechanisms. It has been demonstrated that CDs enhance transmucosal absorption of insulin by formation of an inclusion complex, with insulin or by direct action on the membrane [139]. The latter may involve removal of membrane proteins, complexation with different membrane components, or inhibition of proteolytic enzyme activity. However, it has been claimed that TDM-CD may act by opening cell–cell tight junctions. There is a commercial product of CDs available in the market called Kleptose® HPB (hydroxypropylβ-cyclodextrin) which has been suggested as an attractive excipient for nasal and pulmonary drug administration due to its potential in solubilizing drugs, enhancing absorption of drugs, and low toxicity profile.

5. Products in Development

Currently, there are few products in development that employ an absorption-enhancing technology for nasal and pulmonary formulations, as seen in Table 2.

Table 2. Nasal and Inhalation products in development that employ penetration enhancers.

Technology	Development Stage	Biological Products	Company	Absorption Enhancer Used in the Technology
Cyclopenta Decalactone	Marketed Phase 2	Testosterone (Testim) Nocturia	CPEX Pharmaceuticals Serenity	Surfactant
ChiSys™ PecSys™	Phase 2 Phase 2 Phase 3	Intranasal Apomorphine Intranasal Diazepam Intranasal fentanyl citrate (NasalFent)	Archimedes Pharma Ltd.	Chitosan based delivery
Intravail™	Phase 1 Phase 2 Phase 1	Proteins (IFN-β, EPO) and peptides (PTH, GLP-1), Sumatriptan Naltrexone, Nalmefene	Neurelis, Inc. (Aegis Therapeutics Inc.) Opiant Pharmaceuticals	Cationic polymers-Alkyl saccharide
GelSite® GelVac™ nasal dry powder	Phase 1	Vaccines	Carrington Labs (Delsite Biotech)	Cationic polymers-Poly saccharide
μco™	Phase II Phase 1	Granisetron-zolmitriptan Peptides: (insulin, PTH, FSH, GHRP) Nasal epinephrine formulation	SNBL, Ltd. G2B Pharma Inc.	Polymer-Micro crystalline cellulose (Powder)

6. Conclusions

Several technologies for enhancing the absorption of poorly permeable therapeutic biomolecules have progressed from early studies. They have demonstrated permeation enhancement in isolated barrier model, and a number of absorption-enhancing technologies, especially for nasal applications, are now in clinical trials. These absorption enhancers increase systemic absorption of biomolecules as indicated by improved bioavailability or bioactivity, and appear to represent possible alternatives to existing products, which have sub-optimal bioavailability. Still, one of the challenges towards clinical application of these agents is their lack of safety. Understanding the mechanism of absorption enhancement may be very useful toward reducing their side effects and improving their efficacy before these could be considered as future platforms for inhalation formulation of drugs with poor permeability.

References

1. Helmstadter, A. Endermatic, epidermatic, enepidermatic-the early history of penetration enhancers. *Int. J. Pharm.* **2011**, *416*, 12–15. [CrossRef] [PubMed]
2. Thwala, L.N.; Preat, V.; Csaba, N.S. Emerging delivery platforms for mucosal administration of biopharmaceuticals: A critical update on nasal, pulmonary and oral routes. *Expert Opin. Drug Deliv.* **2017**, *14*, 23–36. [CrossRef] [PubMed]

3. Turker, S.; Onur, E.; Ozer, Y. Nasal route and drug delivery systems. *Pharm. World Sci.* **2004**, *26*, 137–142. [CrossRef] [PubMed]
4. Agu, R.U.; Ugwoke, M.I.; Armand, M.; Kinget, R.; Verbeke, N. The lung as a route for systemic delivery of therapeutic proteins and peptides. *Respir. Res.* **2001**, *2*, 198–209. [PubMed]
5. Fan, Y.; Chen, M.; Zhang, J.Q.; Maincent, P.; Xia, X.F.; Wu, W. Updated progress of nanocarrier-based intranasal drug delivery systems for treatment of brain diseases. *Crit. Rev. Ther. Drug* **2018**, *35*, 433–467. [CrossRef] [PubMed]
6. Zhu, Z.T.; Pan, J.H.; Wu, X.H.; Jiang, Z.T. [screen absorption enhancer for intranasal administration preparations of paeoniflorin based on nasal perfusion method in rats]. *Zhongguo Zhong yao za zhi = Zhongguo zhongyao zazhi = China J. Chin. Mater. Med.* **2017**, *42*, 493–497.
7. Sleigh, M.A.; Blake, J.R.; Liron, N. The propulsion of mucus by cilia. *Am. Rev. Respir. Dis.* **1988**, *137*, 726–741. [CrossRef] [PubMed]
8. Clunes, M.T.; Boucher, R.C. Cystic fibrosis: The mechanisms of pathogenesis of an inherited lung disorder. *Drug Discov. Today Dis. Mech.* **2007**, *4*, 63–72. [CrossRef] [PubMed]
9. Verkman, A.S.; Song, Y.; Thiagarajah, J.R. Role of airway surface liquid and submucosal glands in cystic fibrosis lung disease. *Am. J. Physiol. Cell Physiol.* **2003**, *284*, C2–C15. [CrossRef] [PubMed]
10. Rosen, H.; Abribat, T. The rise and rise of drug delivery. *Nat. Rev. Drug Discov.* **2005**, *4*, 381–385. [CrossRef] [PubMed]
11. Ali, M.S.; Pearson, J.P. Upper airway mucin gene expression: A review. *Laryngoscope* **2007**, *117*, 932–938. [CrossRef] [PubMed]
12. Mainardes, R.M.; Urban, M.C.; Cinto, P.O.; Chaud, M.V.; Evangelista, R.C.; Gremiao, M.P. Liposomes and micro/nanoparticles as colloidal carriers for nasal drug delivery. *Curr. Drug Deliv.* **2006**, *3*, 275–285. [CrossRef] [PubMed]
13. Inoue, D.; Tanaka, A.; Kimura, S.; Kiriyama, A.; Katsumi, H.; Yamamoto, A.; Ogawara, K.I.; Kimura, T.; Higaki, K.; Yutani, R.; et al. The relationship between in vivo nasal drug clearance and in vitro nasal mucociliary clearance: Application to the prediction of nasal drug absorption. *Eur. J. Pharm. Sci.* **2018**, *117*, 21–26. [CrossRef] [PubMed]
14. Karasulu, E.; Yavasoglu, A.; Evrensanal, Z.; Uvanikgil, Y.; Karasulu, H.Y. Permeation studies and histological examination of sheep nasal mucosa following administration of different nasal formulations with or without absorption enhancers. *Drug Deliv.* **2008**, *15*, 219–225. [CrossRef] [PubMed]
15. Kobayashi, S.; Kondo, S.; Juni, K. Study on pulmonary delivery of salmon-calcitonin in rats—Effects of protease inhibitors and absorption enhancers. *Pharm. Res.-Dordr.* **1994**, *11*, 1239–1243. [CrossRef]
16. Chavanpatil, M.D.; Vavia, P.R. The influence of absorption enhancers on nasal absorption of acyclovir. *Eur. J. Pharm. Biopharm.* **2004**, *57*, 483–487. [CrossRef] [PubMed]
17. Kim, I.W.; Yoo, H.; Song, I.S.; Chung, Y.B.; Moon, D.C.; Chung, S.J.; Shim, C.K. Effect of excipients on the stability and transport of recombinant human epidermal growth factor (rhegf) across caco-2 cell monolayers. *Arch. Pharm. Res.* **2003**, *26*, 330–337. [CrossRef] [PubMed]
18. Ikeda, K.; Murata, K.; Kobayashi, M.; Noda, K. Enhancement of bioavailability of dopamine via nasal route in beagle dogs. *Chem. Pharm. Bull.* **1992**, *40*, 2155–2158. [CrossRef] [PubMed]
19. Amancha, K.P.; Hussain, A. Effect of protease inhibitors on pulmonary bioavailability of therapeutic proteins and peptides in the rat. *Eur. J. Pharm. Sci.* **2015**, *68*, 1–10. [CrossRef] [PubMed]
20. Ghadiri, M.; Canney, F.; Pacciana, C.; Colombo, G.; Young, P.M.; Traini, D. The use of fatty acids as absorption enhancer for pulmonary drug delivery. *Int. J. Pharm.* **2018**, *541*, 93–100. [CrossRef]
21. Ghadiri, M.; Mamlouk, M.; Spicer, P.; Jarolimek, W.; Grau, G.E.R.; Young, P.M.; Traini, D. Effect of polyunsaturated fatty acids (pufas) on airway epithelial cells' tight junction. *Pulm. Pharmacol. Ther.* **2016**, *40*, 30–38. [CrossRef] [PubMed]
22. Li, F.; Yang, X.L.; Yang, Y.A.; Li, P.; Yang, Z.L.; Zhang, C.F. Phospholipid complex as an approach for bioavailability enhancement of echinacoside. *Drug Dev. Ind. Pharm.* **2015**, *41*, 1777–1784. [CrossRef] [PubMed]
23. Chono, S.; Fukuchi, R.; Seki, T.; Morimoto, K. Aerosolized liposomes with dipalmitoyl phosphatidylcholine enhance pulmonary insulin delivery. *J. Control. Release* **2009**, *137*, 104–109. [CrossRef] [PubMed]

24. Benediktsdottir, B.E.; Gudjonsson, T.; Baldursson, O.; Masson, M. N-alkylation of highly quaternized chitosan derivatives affects the paracellular permeation enhancement in bronchial epithelia in vitro. *Eur. J. Pharm. Biopharm.* **2014**, *86*, 55–63. [CrossRef] [PubMed]
25. Yamada, K.; Odomi, M.; Okada, N.; Fujita, T.; Yamamoto, A. Chitosan oligomers as potential and safe absorption enhancers for improving the pulmonary absorption of interferon-alpha in rats. *J. Pharm. Sci.-US* **2005**, *94*, 2432–2440. [CrossRef] [PubMed]
26. Yamamoto, A.; Yamada, K.; Muramatsu, H.; Nishinaka, A.; Okumura, S.; Okada, N.; Fujita, T.; Muranishi, S. Control of pulmonary absorption of water-soluble compounds by various viscous vehicles. *Int. J. Pharm.* **2004**, *282*, 141–149. [CrossRef] [PubMed]
27. Shimpi, S.; Chauhan, B.; Shimpi, P. Cyclodextrins: Application in Different Routes of Drug Administration. *Acta Pharm.* **2005**, *55*, 139–156. [PubMed]
28. Suzuki, H.; Kondoh, M.; Li, X.; Takahashi, A.; Matsuhisa, K.; Matsushita, K.; Kakamu, Y.; Yamane, S.; Kodaka, M.; Isoda, K.; et al. A toxicological evaluation of a claudin modulator, the c-terminal fragment of clostridium perfringens enterotoxin, in mice. *Pharmazie* **2011**, *66*, 543–546. [PubMed]
29. Gopalakrishnan, S.; Pandey, N.; Tamiz, A.P.; Vere, J.; Carrasco, R.; Somerville, R.; Tripathi, A.; Ginski, M.; Paterson, B.M.; Alkan, S.S. Mechanism of action of zot-derived peptide at-1002, a tight junction regulator and absorption enhancer. *Int. J. Pharm.* **2009**, *365*, 121–130. [CrossRef] [PubMed]
30. Shubber, S.; Vllasaliu, D.; Rauch, C.; Jordan, F.; Illum, L.; Stolnik, S. Mechanism of mucosal permeability enhancement of criticalsorb (r) (solutol (r) hs15) investigated in vitro in cell cultures. *Pharm. Res.-Dordr* **2015**, *32*, 516–527. [CrossRef] [PubMed]
31. Li, Y.; Li, J.; Zhang, X.; Ding, J.; Mao, S. Non-ionic surfactants as novel intranasal absorption enhancers: In vitro and in vivo characterization. *Drug Deliv.* **2016**, *23*, 2272–2279. [PubMed]
32. Brockman, J.M.; Wang, Z.D.; Notter, R.H.; Dluhy, R.A. Effect of hydrophobic surfactant proteins sp-b and sp-c on binary phospholipid monolayers ii. Infrared external reflectance-absorption spectroscopy. *Biophys. J.* **2003**, *84*, 326–340. [CrossRef]
33. Johansson, F.; Hjertberg, E.; Eirefelt, S.; Tronde, A.; Bengtsson, U.H. Mechanisms for absorption enhancement of inhaled insulin by sodium taurocholate. *Eur. J. Pharm. Sci.* **2002**, *17*, 63–71. [CrossRef]
34. Chen-Quay, S.C.; Eiting, K.T.; Li, A.W.A.; Lamharzi, N.; Quay, S.C. Identification of tight junction modulating lipids. *J. Pharm. Sci.-US* **2009**, *98*, 606–619. [CrossRef] [PubMed]
35. Griese, M. Pulmonary surfactant in health and human lung diseases: State of the art. *Eur. Respir. J.* **1999**, *13*, 1455–1476. [CrossRef] [PubMed]
36. Wauthoz, N.; Amighi, K. Phospholipids in pulmonary drug delivery. *Eur. J. Lipid Sci. Technol.* **2014**, *116*, 1114–1128. [CrossRef]
37. Veldhuizen, R.; Nag, K.; Orgeig, S.; Possmayer, F. The role of lipids in pulmonary surfactant. *BBA-Mol. Basis Dis.* **1998**, *1408*, 90–108. [CrossRef]
38. Hoyer, H.; Perera, G.; Bernkop-Schnurch, A. Noninvasive delivery systems for peptides and proteins in osteoporosis therapy: A retroperspective. *Drug Dev. Ind. Pharm.* **2010**, *36*, 31–44. [CrossRef] [PubMed]
39. Ventura, C.A.; Fresta, M.; Paolino, D.; Pedotti, S.; Corsaro, A.; Puglisi, G. Biomembrane model interaction and percutaneous absorption of papaverine through rat skin: Effects of cyclodextrins as penetration enhancers. *J. Drug Target* **2001**, *9*, 379–393. [CrossRef] [PubMed]
40. Zheng, J.H.; Zhang, G.; Lu, Y.; Fang, F.; He, J.K.; Li, N.; Talbi, A.; Zhang, Y.; Tang, Y.; Zhu, J.B.; et al. Effect of pulmonary surfactant and phospholipid hexadecanol tyloxapol on recombinant human-insulin absorption from intratracheally administered dry powders in diabetic rats. *Chem. Pharm. Bull.* **2010**, *58*, 1612–1616. [CrossRef] [PubMed]
41. Zheng, J.H.; Zheng, Y.; Chen, J.Y.; Fang, F.; He, J.K.; Li, N.; Tang, Y.; Zhu, J.B.; Chen, X.J. Enhanced pulmonary absorption of recombinant human insulin by pulmonary surfactant and phospholipid hexadecanol tyloxapol through calu-3 monolayers. *Pharmazie* **2012**, *67*, 448–451. [PubMed]
42. Stojancevic, M.; Pavlovic, N.; Golocorbin-Kon, S.; Mikov, M. Application of bile acids in drug formulation and delivery. *Front. Life Sci.* **2013**, *7*, 112–122. [CrossRef]
43. Moghimipour, E.; Ameri, A.; Handali, S. Absorption-enhancing effects of bile salts. *Molecules* **2015**, *20*, 14451–14473. [CrossRef] [PubMed]

44. Sørli, J.B.; Balogh Sivars, K.; Da Silva, E.; Hougaard, K.S.; Koponen, I.K.; Zuo, Y.Y.; Weydahl, I.E.K.; Åberg, P.M.; Fransson, R. Bile salt enhancers for inhalation: Correlation between in vitro and in vivo lung effects. *Int. J. Pharm.* **2018**, *550*, 114–122. [CrossRef] [PubMed]
45. Del Vecchio, G.; Tscheik, C.; Tenz, K.; Helms, H.C.; Winkler, L.; Blasig, R.; Blasig, I.E. Sodium caprate transiently opens claudin-5-containing barriers at tight junctions of epithelial and endothelial cells. *Mol. Pharm.* **2012**, *9*, 2523–2533. [CrossRef] [PubMed]
46. Miyake, M.; Minami, T.; Yamazaki, H.; Emoto, C.; Mukai, T.; Toguchi, H. Arachidonic acid with taurine enhances pulmonary absorption of macromolecules without any serious histopathological damages. *Eur. J. Pharm. Biopharm.* **2017**, *114*, 22–28. [CrossRef] [PubMed]
47. Coyne, C.B.; Ribeiro, C.M.P.; Boucher, R.C.; Johnson, L.G. Acute mechanism of medium chain fatty acid-induced enhancement of airway epithelial permeability. *J. Pharmacol. Exp. Ther.* **2003**, *305*, 440–450. [CrossRef] [PubMed]
48. Ujhelyi, Z.; Fenyvesi, F.; Varadi, J.; Feher, P.; Kiss, T.; Veszelka, S.; Deli, M.; Vecsernyes, M.; Bacskay, I. Evaluation of cytotoxicity of surfactants used in self-micro emulsifying drug delivery systems and their effects on paracellular transport in caco-2 cell monolayer. *Eur. J. Pharm. Sci.* **2012**, *47*, 564–573. [CrossRef] [PubMed]
49. Na, L.; Mao, S.; Wang, J.; Sun, W. Comparison of different absorption enhancers on the intranasal absorption of isosorbide dinitrate in rats. *Int. J. Pharm.* **2010**, *397*, 59–66. [CrossRef] [PubMed]
50. Kreuter, J. Mechanism of polymeric nanoparticle-based drug transport across the blood-brain barrier (bbb). *J. Microencapsul.* **2013**, *30*, 49–54. [CrossRef] [PubMed]
51. Salama, H.A.; Mahmoud, A.A.; Kamel, A.O.; Abdel Hady, M.; Awad, G.A.S. Phospholipid based colloidal poloxamer–nanocubic vesicles for brain targeting via the nasal route. *Colloids Surf. B Biointerfaces* **2012**, *100*, 146–154. [CrossRef] [PubMed]
52. Ahsan, F.; Arnold, J.J.; Meezan, E.; Pillion, D.J. Sucrose cocoate, a component of cosmetic preparations, enhances nasal and ocular peptide absorption. *Int. J. Pharm.* **2003**, *251*, 195–203. [CrossRef]
53. Maggio, E.T.; Pillion, D.J. High efficiency intranasal drug delivery using intravail (r) alkylsaccharide absorption enhancers. *Drug Deliv. Transl. Res.* **2013**, *3*, 16–25. [CrossRef] [PubMed]
54. Pillion, D.J.; Ahsan, F.; Arnold, J.J.; Balusubramanian, B.M.; Piraner, O.; Meezan, E. Synthetic long-chain alkyl maltosides and alkyl sucrose esters as enhancers of nasal insulin absorption. *J. Pharm. Sci.-US* **2002**, *91*, 1456–1462. [CrossRef] [PubMed]
55. Ahsan, F.; Arnold, J.; Meezan, E.; Pillion, D.J. Enhanced bioavailability of calcitonin formulated with alkylglycosides following nasal and ocular administration in rats. *Pharm. Res.-Dordr.* **2001**, *18*, 1742–1746. [CrossRef]
56. Vllasaliu, D.; Shubber, S.; Fowler, R.; Garnett, M.; Alexander, C.; Stolnik, S. Epithelial toxicity of alkylglycoside surfactants. *J. Pharm. Sci.-US* **2013**, *102*, 114–125. [CrossRef] [PubMed]
57. Wallace, C.J.; Medina, S.H.; ElSayed, M.E.H. Effect of rhamnolipids on permeability across caco-2 cell monolayers. *Pharm. Res.-Dordr.* **2014**, *31*, 887–894. [CrossRef] [PubMed]
58. Perinelli, D.R.; Vllasaliu, D.; Bonacucina, G.; Come, B.; Pucciarelli, S.; Ricciutelli, M.; Cespi, M.; Itri, R.; Spinozzi, F.; Palmieri, G.F.; et al. Rhamnolipids as epithelial permeability enhancers for macromolecular therapeutics. *Eur. J. Pharm. Biopharm.* **2017**, *119*, 419–425. [CrossRef] [PubMed]
59. Basabe-Burgos, O.; Zebialowicz, J.; Stichtenoth, G.; Curstedt, T.; Bergman, P.; Johansson, J.; Rising, A. Natural derived surfactant preparation as a carrier of polymyxin e for treatment of *pseudomonas aeruginosa* pneumonia in a near-term rabbit model. *J. Aerosol. Med. Pulm. Drug Deliv.* **2018**. [CrossRef] [PubMed]
60. Candiano, G.; Bruschi, M.; Pedemonte, N.; Musante, L.; Ravazzolo, R.; Liberatori, S.; Bini, L.; Galietta, L.J.; Zegarra-Moran, O. Proteomic analysis of the airway surface liquid: Modulation by proinflammatory cytokines. *Am. J. Physiol. Lung Cell. Mol. Physiol.* **2007**, *292*, L185–L198. [CrossRef] [PubMed]
61. Morita, T.; Yamamoto, A.; Takakura, Y.; Hashida, M.; Sezaki, H. Improvement of the pulmonary absorption of (asu(1,7))-eel calcitonin by various protease inhibitors in rats. *Pharm. Res.-Dordr.* **1994**, *11*, 909–913. [CrossRef]
62. Yamamoto, A.; Umemori, S.; Muranishi, S. Absorption enhancement of intrapulmonary administered insulin by various absorption enhancers and protease inhibitors in rats. *J. Pharm. Pharmacol.* **1994**, *46*, 14–18. [CrossRef] [PubMed]

63. Yamamoto, A.; Fujita, T.; Muranishi, S. Pulmonary absorption enhancement of peptides by absorption enhancers and protease inhibitors. *J. Control. Release* **1996**, *41*, 57–67. [CrossRef]
64. Yamahara, H.; Morimoto, K.; Lee, V.H.L.; Kim, K.J. Effects of protease inhibitors on vasopressin transport across rat alveolar epithelial-cell monolayers. *Pharm. Res.-Dordr.* **1994**, *11*, 1617–1622. [CrossRef]
65. Machida, M.; Hayashi, M.; Awazu, S. The effects of absorption enhancers on the pulmonary absorption of recombinant human granulocyte colony-stimulating factor (rhg-csf) in rats. *Biol. Pharm. Bull.* **2000**, *23*, 84–86. [CrossRef] [PubMed]
66. Okumura, K.; Iwakawa, S.; Yoshida, T.; Seki, T.; Komada, F. Intratracheal delivery of insulin absorption from solution and aerosol by rat lung. *Int. J. Pharm.* **1992**, *88*, 63–73. [CrossRef]
67. Hirche, T.O.; Benabid, R.; Deslee, G.; Gangloff, S.; Achilefu, S.; Guenounou, M.; Lebargy, F.; Hancock, R.E.; Belaaouaj, A. Neutrophil elastase mediates innate host protection against pseudomonas aeruginosa. *J. Immunol.* **2008**, *181*, 4945–4954. [CrossRef] [PubMed]
68. Gibbons, A.; McElvaney, N.G.; Cryan, S.A. A dry powder formulation of liposome-encapsulated recombinant secretory leukocyte protease inhibitor (rslpi) for inhalation: Preparation and characterisation. *AAPS PharmSciTech* **2010**, *11*, 1411–1421. [CrossRef] [PubMed]
69. Delacourt, C.; Herigault, S.; Delclaux, C.; Poncin, A.; Levame, M.; Harf, A.; Saudubray, F.; Lafuma, C. Protection against acute lung injury by intravenous or intratracheal pretreatment with epi-hne-4, a new potent neutrophil elastase inhibitor. *Am. J. Respir Cell Mol. Biol.* **2002**, *26*, 290–297. [CrossRef] [PubMed]
70. Grimbert, D.; Vecellio, L.; Delepine, P.; Attucci, S.; Boissinot, E.; Poncin, A.; Gauthier, F.; Valat, C.; Saudubray, F.; Antonioz, P.; et al. Characteristics of epi-hne4 aerosol: A new elastase inhibitor for treatment of cystic fibrosis. *J. Aerosol. Med.* **2003**, *16*, 121–129. [CrossRef] [PubMed]
71. Schulz, J.D.; Gauthier, M.A.; Leroux, J.C. Improving oral drug bioavailability with polycations? *Eur. J. Pharm. Biopharm.* **2015**, *97*, 427–437. [CrossRef] [PubMed]
72. Seki, T. Enhancement of insulin absorption through mucosal membranes using cationic polymers. *Yakugaku Zasshi* **2010**, *130*, 1115–1121. [CrossRef] [PubMed]
73. Zhang, H.; Huang, X.; Sun, Y.; Lu, G.; Wang, K.; Wang, Z.; Xing, J.; Gao, Y. Improvement of pulmonary absorption of poorly absorbable macromolecules by hydroxypropyl-β-cyclodextrin grafted polyethylenimine (hp-β-cd-pei) in rats. *Int. J. Pharm.* **2015**, *489*, 294–303. [CrossRef] [PubMed]
74. Morimoto, K.; Fukushi, N.; Chono, S.; Seki, T.; Tabata, Y. Spermined dextran, a cationized polymer, as absorption enhancer for pulmonary application of peptide drugs. *Pharmazie* **2008**, *63*, 180–184. [PubMed]
75. Zhang, J.; Zhu, X.; Jin, Y.; Shan, W.; Huang, Y. Mechanism study of cellular uptake and tight junction opening mediated by goblet cell-specific trimethyl chitosan nanoparticles. *Mol. Pharm.* **2014**, *11*, 1520–1532. [CrossRef] [PubMed]
76. Yamada, K. Control of pulmonary absorption of drugs by various pharmaceutical excipients. *Yakugaku Zasshi* **2007**, *127*, 631–641. [CrossRef] [PubMed]
77. Roy, S.; Pal, K.; Anis, A.; Pramanik, K.; Prabhakar, B. Polymers in mucoadhesive drug-delivery systems: A brief note. *Des. Monomers Polym.* **2009**, *12*, 483–495. [CrossRef]
78. Botelho da Silva, S.; Krolicka, M.; van den Broek, L.A.M.; Frissen, A.E.; Boeriu, C.G. Water-soluble chitosan derivatives and ph-responsive hydrogels by selective c-6 oxidation mediated by tempo-laccase redox system. *Carbohydr. Polym.* **2018**, *186*, 299–309. [CrossRef] [PubMed]
79. Jeon, Y.J.; Shahidi, F.; Kim, S.K. Preparation of chitin and chitosan oligomers amd their applications in physiological functional foods. *Food Rev. Int.* **2000**, *16*, 159–176. [CrossRef]
80. Zariwala, M.G.; Bendre, H.; Markiv, A.; Farnaud, S.; Renshaw, D.; Taylor, K.M.; Somavarapu, S. Hydrophobically modified chitosan nanoliposomes for intestinal drug delivery. *Int. J. Nanomed.* **2018**, *13*, 5837–5848. [CrossRef] [PubMed]
81. Sonia, T.A.; Rekha, M.R.; Sharma, C.P. Bioadhesive hydrophobic chitosan microparticles for oral delivery of insulin: In vitro characterization and in vivo uptake studies. *J. Appl. Polym. Sci.* **2011**, *119*, 2902–2910. [CrossRef]
82. Seki, T.; Fukushi, N.; Maru, H.; Kimura, S.; Chono, S.; Egawa, Y.; Morimoto, K.; Ueda, H.; Morimoto, Y. Effects of sperminated pullulans on the pulmonary absorption of insulin. *Yakugaku Zasshi* **2011**, *131*, 307–314. [CrossRef] [PubMed]

83. Morimoto, K.; Katsumata, H.; Yabuta, T.; Iwanaga, K.; Kakemi, M.; Tabata, Y.; Ikada, Y. Gelatin microspheres as a pulmonary delivery system: Evaluation of salmon calcitonin absorption. *J. Pharm. Pharmacol.* **2000**, *52*, 611–617. [CrossRef] [PubMed]
84. He, L.; Gao, Y.; Lin, Y.; Katsumi, H. Improvement of pulmonary absorption of insulin and other water-soluble compounds by polyamines in rats. *J. Control. Release* **2007**, *122*, 94–101. [CrossRef] [PubMed]
85. Pauletti, G.M.; Okumu, F.W.; Borchardt, R.T. Effect of size and charge on the passive diffusion of peptides across caco-2 cell monolayers via the paracellular pathway. *Pharm. Res.-Dordr.* **1997**, *14*, 164–168. [CrossRef]
86. Smedley, J.G.; Saputo, J.; Parker, J.C.; Fernandez-Miyakawa, M.E.; Robertson, S.L.; McClane, B.A.; Uzal, F.A. Noncytotoxic *clostridium perfringens* enterotoxin (cpe) variants localize cpe intestinal binding and demonstrate a relationship between cpe-induced cytotoxicity and enterotoxicity. *Infect. Immun.* **2008**, *76*, 3793–3800. [CrossRef] [PubMed]
87. Nakajima, M.; Nagase, S.; Iida, M.; Takeda, S.; Yamashita, M.; Watari, A.; Shirasago, Y.; Fukasawa, M.; Takeda, H.; Sawasaki, T.; et al. Claudin-1 binder enhances epidermal permeability in a human keratinocyte model. *J. Pharmacol. Exp. Ther.* **2015**, *354*, 440–447. [CrossRef] [PubMed]
88. Saaber, D.; Wollenhaupt, S.; Baumann, K.; Reichl, S. Recent progress in tight junction modulation for improving bioavailability. *Expert Opin. Drug Dis.* **2014**, *9*, 367–381. [CrossRef] [PubMed]
89. Uchida, H.; Kondoh, M.; Hanada, T.; Takahashi, A.; Hamakubo, T.; Yagi, K. A claudin-4 modulator enhances the mucosal absorption of a biologically active peptide. *Biochem. Pharmacol.* **2010**, *79*, 1437–1444. [CrossRef] [PubMed]
90. Helms, H.C.; Waagepetersen, H.S.; Nielsen, C.U.; Brodin, B. Paracellular tightness and claudin-5 expression is increased in the bcec/astrocyte blood-brain barrier model by increasing media buffer capacity during growth. *AAPS J.* **2010**, *12*, 759–770. [CrossRef] [PubMed]
91. Deli, M.A. Potential use of tight junction modulators to reversibly open membranous barriers and improve drug delivery. *BBA-Biomembranes* **2009**, *1788*, 892–910. [CrossRef] [PubMed]
92. Fasano, A.; Not, T.; Wang, W.L.; Uzzau, S.; Berti, I.; Tommasini, A.; Goldblum, S.E. Zonulin, a newly discovered modulator of intestinal permeability, and its expression in coeliac disease. *Lancet* **2000**, *355*, 1518–1519. [CrossRef]
93. Li, M.; Oliver, E.; Kitchens, K.M.; Vere, J.; Alkan, S.S.; Tamiz, A.P. Structure-activity relationship studies of permeability modulating peptide at-1002. *Bioorg. Med. Chem. Lett.* **2008**, *18*, 4584–4586. [CrossRef] [PubMed]
94. Porter, A.E.; Muller, K.; Skepper, J.; Midgley, P.; Welland, M. Uptake of c60 by human monocyte macrophages, its localization and implications for toxicity: Studied by high resolution electron microscopy and electron tomography. *Acta Biomater.* **2006**, *2*, 409–419. [CrossRef] [PubMed]
95. Kreyling, W.G.; Semmler-Behnke, M.; Moller, W. Ultrafine particle-lung interactions: Does size matter? *J. Aerosol. Med.* **2006**, *19*, 74–83. [CrossRef] [PubMed]
96. Schneider, C.S.; Xu, Q.; Boylan, N.J.; Chisholm, J.; Tang, B.C.; Schuster, B.S.; Henning, A.; Ensign, L.M.; Lee, E.; Adstamongkonkul, P.; et al. Nanoparticles that do not adhere to mucus provide uniform and long-lasting drug delivery to airways following inhalation. *Sci. Adv.* **2017**, *3*, e1601556. [CrossRef] [PubMed]
97. Mistry, A.; Stolnik, S.; Illum, L. Nanoparticles for direct nose-to-brain delivery of drugs. *Int. J. Pharm.* **2009**, *379*, 146–157. [CrossRef] [PubMed]
98. Kulkarni, A.D.; Vanjari, Y.H.; Sancheti, K.H.; Belgamwar, V.S.; Surana, S.J.; Pardeshi, C.V. Nanotechnology-mediated nose to brain drug delivery for parkinson's disease: A mini review. *J. Drug Target* **2015**, *23*, 775–788. [CrossRef] [PubMed]
99. Hussain, A.; Arnold, J.J.; Khan, M.A.; Ahsan, F. Absorption enhancers in pulmonary protein delivery. *J. Control. Release* **2004**, *94*, 15–24. [CrossRef] [PubMed]
100. Cupri, S.; Graziano, A.C.E.; Cardile, V.; Skwarczynski, M.; Toth, I.; Pignatello, R. A study on the encapsulation of an occludin lipophilic derivative in liposomal carriers. *J. Liposome Res.* **2015**, *25*, 287–293. [CrossRef] [PubMed]
101. Manca, M.L.; Peris, J.E.; Melis, V.; Valenti, D.; Cardia, M.C.; Lattuada, D.; Escribano-Ferrer, E.; Fadda, A.M.; Manconi, M. Nanoincorporation of curcumin in polymer-glycerosomes and evaluation of their in vitro–in vivo suitability as pulmonary delivery systems. *Rsc. Adv.* **2015**, *5*, 105149–105159. [CrossRef]
102. Melis, V.; Manca, M.L.; Bullita, E.; Tamburini, E.; Castangia, I.; Cardia, M.C.; Valenti, D.; Fadda, A.M.; Peris, J.E.; Manconi, M. Inhalable polymer-glycerosomes as safe and effective carriers for rifampicin delivery to the lungs. *Colloid Surf. B* **2016**, *143*, 301–308. [CrossRef] [PubMed]

103. Bai, S.; Thomas, C.; Ahsan, F. Dendrimers as a carrier for pulmonary delivery of enoxaparin, a low-molecular weight heparin. *J. Pharm. Sci.-US* **2007**, *96*, 2090–2106. [CrossRef] [PubMed]
104. Inapagolla, R.; Guru, B.R.; Kurtoglu, Y.E.; Gao, X.; Lieh-Lai, M.; Bassett, D.J.P.; Kannan, R.M. In vivo efficacy of dendrimer–methylprednisolone conjugate formulation for the treatment of lung inflammation. *Int. J. Pharm.* **2010**, *399*, 140–147. [CrossRef] [PubMed]
105. Lu, J.; Li, N.; Gao, Y.; Guo, Y.; Liu, H.; Chen, X.; Zhu, C.; Dong, Z.; Yamamoto, A. The Effect of Absorption-Enhancement and the Mechanism of the PAMAM Dendrimer on Poorly Absorbable Drugs. *Molecules* **2018**, *23*, 2001. [CrossRef] [PubMed]
106. Luan, X.; Sansanaphongpricha, K.; Myers, I.; Chen, H.; Yuan, H.; Sun, D. Engineering exosomes as refined biological nanoplatforms for drug delivery. *Acta Pharmacol. Sin.* **2017**, *38*, 754. [CrossRef] [PubMed]
107. Vader, P.; Mol, E.A.; Pasterkamp, G.; Schiffelers, R.M. Extracellular vesicles for drug delivery. *Adv. Drug Deliv. Rev.* **2016**, *106*, 148–156. [CrossRef] [PubMed]
108. Hood, J.L. Post isolation modification of exosomes for nanomedicine applications. *Nanomedicine (London, England)* **2016**, *11*, 1745–1756. [CrossRef] [PubMed]
109. Batrakova, E.V.; Kim, M.S. Using exosomes, naturally-equipped nanocarriers, for drug delivery. *J. Control. Release* **2015**, *219*, 396–405. [CrossRef] [PubMed]
110. Harding, C.V.; Heuser, J.E.; Stahl, P.D. Exosomes: Looking back three decades and into the future. *J. Cell Biol.* **2013**, *200*, 367–371. [CrossRef] [PubMed]
111. Fabbri, M.; Paone, A.; Calore, F.; Galli, R.; Gaudio, E.; Santhanam, R.; Lovat, F.; Fadda, P.; Mao, C.; Nuovo, G.J.; et al. Micrornas bind to toll-like receptors to induce prometastatic inflammatory response. *Proc. Natl. Acad. Sci. USA* **2012**, *109*, E2110–E2116. [CrossRef] [PubMed]
112. Kalani, A.; Kamat, P.K.; Chaturvedi, P.; Tyagi, S.C.; Tyagi, N. Curcumin-primed exosomes mitigate endothelial cell dysfunction during hyperhomocysteinemia. *Life Sci.* **2014**, *107*, 1–7. [CrossRef] [PubMed]
113. Batrakova, E.V.; Kim, M.S.; Haney, M.J.; Zhao, Y.; Deygen, I.; Klyachko, N.L.; Kabanov, A.V. Development of exosome-encapsulated paclitaxel to treat cancer metastases. *In Vitro Cell Dev.* **2017**, *53*, S9.
114. Haney, M.J.; Klyachko, N.L.; Zhao, Y.; Gupta, R.; Plotnikova, E.G.; He, Z.; Patel, T.; Piroyan, A.; Sokolsky, M.; Kabanov, A.V.; et al. Exosomes as drug delivery vehicles for parkinson's disease therapy. *J. Control. Release* **2015**, *207*, 18–30. [CrossRef] [PubMed]
115. Zhuang, X.; Xiang, X.; Grizzle, W.; Sun, D.; Zhang, S.; Axtell, R.C.; Ju, S.; Mu, J.; Zhang, L.; Steinman, L.; et al. Treatment of brain inflammatory diseases by delivering exosome encapsulated anti-inflammatory drugs from the nasal region to the brain. *Mol. Ther.* **2011**, *19*, 1769–1779. [CrossRef] [PubMed]
116. Tian, Y.; Li, S.; Song, J.; Ji, T.; Zhu, M.; Anderson, G.J.; Wei, J.; Nie, G. A doxorubicin delivery platform using engineered natural membrane vesicle exosomes for targeted tumor therapy. *Biomaterials* **2014**, *35*, 2383–2390. [CrossRef] [PubMed]
117. Yang, T.; Martin, P.; Fogarty, B.; Brown, A.; Schurman, K.; Phipps, R.; Yin, V.P.; Lockman, P.; Bai, S. Exosome delivered anticancer drugs across the blood-brain barrier for brain cancer therapy in danio rerio. *Pharm. Res.* **2015**, *32*, 2003–2014. [CrossRef] [PubMed]
118. Foged, C.; Nielsen, H.M. Cell-penetrating peptides for drug delivery across membrane barriers. *Expert Opin. Drug Deliv.* **2008**, *5*, 105–117. [CrossRef] [PubMed]
119. McClorey, G.; Banerjee, S. Cell-penetrating peptides to enhance delivery of oligonucleotide-based therapeutics. *Biomedicines* **2018**, *6*, 51. [CrossRef] [PubMed]
120. Derossi, D.; Calvet, S.; Trembleau, A.; Brunissen, A.; Chassaing, G.; Prochiantz, A. Cell internalization of the third helix of the antennapedia homeodomain is receptor-independent. *J. Biol. Chem.* **1996**, *271*, 18188–18193. [CrossRef] [PubMed]
121. Thorén, P.E.G.; Persson, D.; Esbjörner, E.K.; Goksör, M.; Lincoln, P.; Nordén, B. Membrane binding and translocation of cell-penetrating peptides. *Biochemistry-US* **2004**, *43*, 3471–3489. [CrossRef] [PubMed]
122. Tan, J.; Cheong, H.; Park, Y.S.; Kim, H.; Zhang, M.; Moon, C.; Huang, Y.Z. Cell-penetrating peptide-mediated topical delivery of biomacromolecular drugs. *Curr. Pharm. Biotechnol.* **2014**, *15*, 231–239. [CrossRef] [PubMed]
123. Kato, T.; Yamashita, H.; Misawa, T.; Nishida, K.; Kurihara, M.; Tanaka, M.; Demizu, Y.; Oba, M. Plasmid DNA delivery by arginine-rich cell-penetrating peptides containing unnatural amino acids. *Bioorg. Med. Chem.* **2016**, *24*, 2681–2687. [CrossRef] [PubMed]

124. Eudes, F.; Shim, Y.S. Cell-penetrating peptides trojan horse for DNA and protein delivery in plant. *In Vitro Cell Dev.* **2010**, *46*, S112–S113.
125. Dos Reis, L.G.; Svolos, M.; Hartwig, B.; Windhab, N.; Young, P.M.; Traini, D. Inhaled gene delivery: A formulation and delivery approach. *Expert Opin. Drug Deliv.* **2017**, *14*, 319–330. [CrossRef] [PubMed]
126. Kamei, N. Nose-to-brain delivery of peptide drugs enhanced by coadministration of cell-penetrating peptides: Therapeutic potential for dementia. *Yakugaku Zasshi* **2017**, *137*, 1247–1253. [CrossRef] [PubMed]
127. Kamei, N.; Tanaka, M.; Choi, H.; Okada, N.; Ikeda, T.; Itokazu, R.; Takeda-Morishita, M. Effect of an enhanced nose-to-brain delivery of insulin on mild and progressive memory loss in the senescence-accelerated mouse. *Mol. Pharm.* **2017**, *14*, 916–927. [CrossRef] [PubMed]
128. Zhang, X.; Lin, C.; Lu, A.; Lin, G.; Chen, H.; Liu, Q.; Yang, Z.; Zhang, H. Liposomes equipped with cell penetrating peptide br2 enhances chemotherapeutic effects of cantharidin against hepatocellular carcinoma. *Drug Deliv.* **2017**, *24*, 986–998. [CrossRef] [PubMed]
129. Xu, Y.; Li, S.; Luo, Z.; Ren, H.; Zhang, X.; Huang, F.; Zuo, Y.Y.; Yue, T. Role of lipid coating in the transport of nanodroplets across the pulmonary surfactant layer revealed by molecular dynamics simulations. *Langmuir* **2018**, *34*, 9054–9063. [CrossRef] [PubMed]
130. Chen, K.H.; Di Sabatino, M.; Albertini, B.; Passerini, N.; Kett, V.L. The effect of polymer coatings on physicochemical properties of spray-dried liposomes for nasal delivery of bsa. *Eur. J. Pharm. Sci.* **2013**, *50*, 312–322. [CrossRef] [PubMed]
131. Murata, M.; Nakano, K.; Tahara, K.; Tozuka, Y.; Takeuchi, H. Pulmonary delivery of elcatonin using surface-modified liposomes to improve systemic absorption: Polyvinyl alcohol with a hydrophobic anchor and chitosan oligosaccharide as effective surface modifiers. *Eur. J. Pharm. Biopharm.* **2012**, *80*, 340–346. [CrossRef] [PubMed]
132. Liu, Z.Y.; Jiang, M.Y.; Kang, T.; Miao, D.Y.; Gu, G.Z.; Song, Q.X.; Yao, L.; Hu, Q.Y.; Tu, Y.F.; Pang, Z.Q.; et al. Lactoferrin-modified peg-co-pcl nanoparticles for enhanced brain delivery of nap peptide following intranasal administration. *Biomaterials* **2013**, *34*, 3870–3881. [CrossRef] [PubMed]
133. Marttin, E.; Verhoef, J.C.; Merkus, F.W.H.M. Efficacy, safety and mechanism of cyclodextrins as absorption enhancers in nasal delivery of peptide and protein drugs. *J. Drug Target* **1998**, *6*, 17–36. [CrossRef] [PubMed]
134. Schipper, N.G.M.; Verhoef, J.; Romeijn, S.G.; Merkus, F.W.H.M. Absorption enhancers in nasal insulin delivery and their influence on nasal ciliary functioning. *J. Control. Release* **1992**, *21*, 173–185. [CrossRef]
135. Salem, L.B.; Bosquillon, C.; Dailey, L.A.; Delattre, L.; Martin, G.P.; Evrard, B.; Forbes, B. Sparing methylation of beta-cyclodextrin mitigates cytotoxicity and permeability induction in respiratory epithelial cell layers in vitro. *J. Control. Release* **2009**, *136*, 110–116. [CrossRef] [PubMed]
136. Kiss, T.; Fenyvesi, F.; Bacskay, I.; Varadi, J.; Fenyvesi, E.; Ivanyi, R.; Szente, L.; Tosaki, A.; Vecsernyes, M. Evaluation of the cytotoxicity of beta-cyclodextrin derivatives: Evidence for the role of cholesterol extraction. *Eur. J. Pharm. Sci.* **2010**, *40*, 376–380. [CrossRef] [PubMed]
137. Roka, E.; Ujhelyi, Z.; Deli, M.; Bocsik, A.; Fenyvesi, E.; Szente, L.; Fenyvesi, F.; Vecsernyes, M.; Varadi, J.; Feher, P.; et al. Evaluation of the cytotoxicity of alpha-cyclodextrin derivatives on the caco-2 cell line and human erythrocytes. *Molecules* **2015**, *20*, 20269–20285. [CrossRef] [PubMed]
138. Matilainen, L.; Toropainen, T.; Vihola, H.; Hirvonen, J.; Jarvinen, T.; Jarho, P.; Jarvinen, K. In vitro toxicity and permeation of cyclodextrins in calu-3 cells. *J. Control. Release* **2008**, *126*, 10–16. [CrossRef] [PubMed]
139. Hussain, A.; Yang, T.; Zaghloul, A.-A.; Ahsan, F. Pulmonary absorption of insulin mediated by tetradecyl-β-maltoside and dimethyl-β-cyclodextrin. *Pharm. Res.* **2003**, *20*, 1551–1557. [CrossRef] [PubMed]

Fast Dissolving of Ferulic Acid via Electrospun Ternary Amorphous Composites Produced by a Coaxial Process

Weidong Huang [1,2], Yaoyao Yang [3], Biwei Zhao [3], Gangqiang Liang [3], Shiwei Liu [3], Xian-Li Liu [2,*] and Deng-Guang Yu [3,*]

1 School of Chemistry and Chemical Engineering, Hubei Polytechnic University, Huangshi 435003, China; neweydong@hbpu.edu.cn
2 Hubei Key Laboratory of Mine Environmental Pollution Control and Remediation, Hubei Polytechnic University, Huangshi 435003, China
3 School of Materials Science and Engineering, University of Shanghai for Science and Technology, Shanghai 200093, China; yyyang@usst.edu.cn (Y.Y.); 1526410303@st.usst.edu.cn (B.Z.); 1526410214@st.usst.edu.cn (G.L.); 1526410109@st.usst.edu.cn (S.L.)
* Correspondence: liuxianli@hbpu.edu.cn (X.-L.L.); ydg017@usst.edu.cn (D.-G.Y.);

Abstract: Enhancing the dissolution of insoluble active ingredients comprises one of the most important issues in the pharmaceutical and biomaterial fields. Here, a third generation solid dispersion (3rd SD) of ferulic acid was designed and fabricated by a modified coaxial electrospinning process. A traditional second generation SD (2nd SD) was also prepared by common one-fluid blending electrospinning and was used as a control. With poly(vinyl alcohol) as the fiber matrix and polyvinylpyrrolidone K10 as an additive in the 3rd SDs, the two electrospinning processes were investigated. The prepared 2nd and 3rd SDs were subjected to a series of characterizations, including X-ray diffraction (XRD), scanning electron microscope (SEM), hydrophilicity and in vitro drug dissolving experiments. The results demonstrate that both SDs were monolithic nanocomposites and that the drugs were amorphously distributed within the matrix. However, the 3rd SDs had better morphology with smaller size, narrower size distribution, and smaller water contact angles than the 2nd SDs. Dissolution tests verified that the 3rd SDs could release their loaded cargoes within 60 s, which was over three times faster than the 2nd SDs. Therefore, a combined strategy based on the modified coaxial electrospinning and the logical selections of drug carriers is demonstrated for creating advanced biomaterials.

Keywords: amorphous composite; coaxial electrospinning; fast dissolution; insoluble drug; solid dispersion

---

1. Introduction

Many drugs are insoluble or poorly water soluble, and improving their dissolution is one of the central challenges in pharmaceutics [1–4]. Among the different kinds of strategies that have been broadly investigated to resolve this problem, drug solid dispersions (SDs) are some of the most promising ways with many commercial products [5–9]. New methods for creating new kinds of high-performance SDs are always desired and are thus becoming a rapidly developing branch of pharmaceutical technologies [10–15].

Over the past half century, first generation SDs (1st SDs) have progressed to second (2nd SDs) and third generation SDs (3rd SDs) [16,17]. Figure 1 is a schematic of the differences in their characteristics. Often, 1st and 2nd SDs are binary systems with the drug distributed in carriers.

In 1st SDs, carriers are mainly crystalline pharmaceutical excipients; in 2nd SDs, amorphous polymers are frequently used as host polymers. The concept of 3rd SDs has gained the interest of researchers in related fields [18]. This new type of SD is typically a ternary or quaternary system with one or two additives (such as surfactants and other polymeric excipients) that, together with the drug and host polymer, are combined to exert a synergistic effect on drug-dissolution improvement [17,18]. The polymer-based SDs are amorphous composites. When an amorphous polymer is exploited not only for drug dissolution but also for controlling drug release, the SD is often termed a 4th generation SD [19,20].

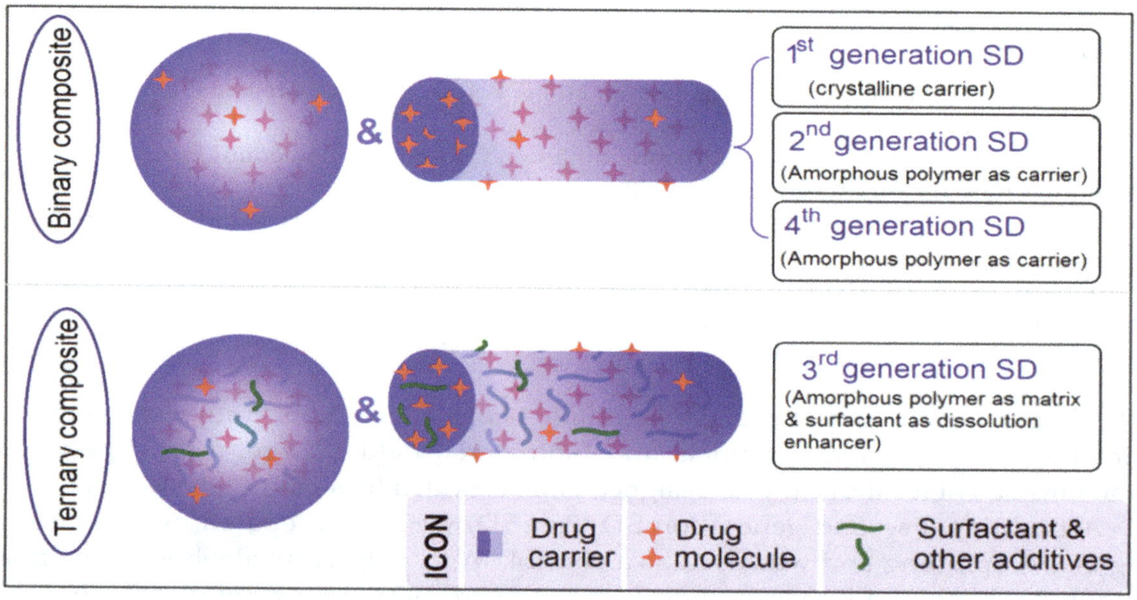

Figure 1. A diagram showing the development of solid dispersions (SDs) from the initial first generation to the third and fourth generations.

Considering the present nano-era, SDs are inevitably advancing to nanoproduction because a fine size always means large surface area for functional performance. Among different pharmaceutical nanotechnologies, electrospinning is distinct from others because of its high effectiveness, easy implementation, and low cost for creating polymer nanofibers [21–28]. Electrospinning and also electrospraying are simple, one-step, "top-down" electrohydrodynamic atomization (EHDA) processes that have quickly developed from the traditional one-fluid blending process to two-fluid (side-by-side and coaxial) processes, and also to tri-axial processes [29–33]. Some studies have demonstrated that single-fluid EHDA and traditional coaxial EHDA are powerful tools for creating SDs [34,35].

For SDs produced from a co-dissolving solution using the one-fluid blending process, several amorphous water-soluble polymers have been investigated. These polymers include poly(ethylene oxide), polyvinylpyrrolidone (PVP), poly(vinyl alcohol) (PVA), gelatin, and some other natural products, e.g., water-soluble polysaccharides [36,37]. Among them, PVA has wide-ranging applications in the pharmaceutical, cosmetic, food, medical and packaging industries. In the field of biomaterials, PVA gels are exploited as drug carriers directly or in the form of particles added to other carriers for tablet formulation. However, these studies have focused only on drug-sustained release; cross-linking is often carried out for creating insoluble nonwoven mats [36]. For SDs, the role of the carrier in forming SDs is very important [38,39]. PVA, as a highly water soluble, highly biocompatible and nontoxic polymer, is a good candidate carrier for promoting drug dissolution [36,37].

Ferulic acid (FA), an abundant polyphenol in maize bran and vegetables, was utilized as a model of a poorly water-soluble drug. It has been explored for a wide variety of potential applications such as age-related diseases, cancer, cardiovascular diseases and diabetes [40]. However, its poor solubility has greatly limited its oral bioavailability [41]. Thus, based on our previous work on the fabrication of SD using traditional coaxial electrospinning [42], here, the usage of advanced modified coaxial electrospinning to prepare 3rd SDs was investigated for the first time.

2. Materials and Methods

2.1. Materials

PVA (M_w = 170,000 g/mol; 88% hydrolyzed) was bought from Shanghai Meimengjia Chemical Co., Ltd. (Shanghai, China). FA (purity > 99%) was purchased from Shanghai Rong-Chuang Biotechnology Co., Ltd. (Shanghai, China). PVP K10 with a molecular weight of 10,000 g/mol was obtained from Sigma-Aldrich Co., Ltd. (Shanghai, China). Anhydrous ethanol and methylene blue were bought from Shanghai Chemical Reagents Co., Ltd. (Shanghai, China).

2.2. Electrospinning

The electrospinning system had the following four parts: a power supply (ZGF60kV-2mA, Wuhan Hua-Tian Corp., Wuhan, China), two fluid drivers (KDS100 and KDS200, Cole-Parmer, Vernon Hills, IL, USA), a collector and a homemade concentric spinneret. After some optimization experiments, the preparation conditions were determined as follows: an applied voltage of 14 kV, a spinneret-collector distance of 15 cm, and a fixed core fluid flow rate of 1.0 mL/h. The environmental temperature and humidity were 21 $\pm$ 4 °C and 51 $\pm$ 5%, respectively. The properties of the working fluids, including conductivity, surface tension and viscosity were measured using a conductivity meter (DDS-11, Shanghai Rex Co-perfect Instrument Co., Ltd., Shanghai, China), a surface tension tensiometer (BZY-1, Shanghai Hengping Instrument & Meter Factory, Shanghai, China), and a rotary viscometer (NDJ 279, Machinery & Electronic Factory of Tongji University, Shanghai, China), respectively. All the experiments were repeated three times.

2.3. Morphology

The nanofibers' morphologies were studied with the aid of a Quanta FEG450 scanning electron microscope (FE-SEM; FEI Corporation, Hillsboro, OR, USA). Samples were platinum sputter-coated under a nitrogen atmosphere for 100 s prior to visualization. Fiber diameters were calculated using the ImageJ software (National Institutes of Health, Bethesda, MD, USA) to measure the fibers at 100 different points.

2.4. Physical Form and Compatibility

X-ray diffraction (XRD) patterns were collected on a D/Max-BR diffractometer (Rigaku, Tokyo, Japan) over the 2θ range 5 to 60°. The instrument was supplied with Cu Kα radiation at 40 mV and 30 mA. Differential scanning calorimetry (DSC) was carried out using an MDSC 2910 differential scanning calorimeter (TA Instruments Co., New Castle, DE, USA). Sealed samples were heated at 10 °C·min^{-1} from 21 to 250 °C. The nitrogen gas flow rate was kept at 40 mL·min^{-1}. Fourier transform infrared (FTIR) spectroscopy was carried out on a Nicolet-Nexus 670 FTIR spectrometer (Nicolet Instrument Corporation, Madison, WI, USA) at a range of 500 to 4000 cm^{-1} and a resolution of 2 cm^{-1}.

2.5. Property and Functional Performances

A DSA100 drop analysis instrument (Krüss GmbH, Hamburg, Germany) was exploited to measure the surface contact angle (WCA) of nanofiber mats. Distilled water droplets (3 μL) were placed onto the sample's surface. Six different regions of each surface were measured, and the obtained data were averaged.

FA has a maximum UV absorbance at λ_{max} = 321 nm and a shoulder at 278 nm. A calibration curve was thus constructed at 321 nm with the aid of a Lambda 750S spectrophotometer (Perkin Elmer,

Waltham, MA, USA). This took the form $C = 17.74A + 0.14$ ($R^2 = 0.9996$), where C is the concentration of FA (μg/mL) and A is the absorbance (linear range: 1–20 μg/mL).

Drug release was quantified following the Chinese Pharmacopoeia Method II (a paddle method) on RCZ-8A dissolution apparatus (Tianjin University Radio Factory, Tianjin, China) at 50 rpm and 37 °C. Then, 30 mg of each sample was placed into 600 mL of phosphate buffered saline (PBS, pH = 7.0, 0.1 M). At predetermined time points, 5 mL aliquots were withdrawn, and 5 mL of fresh preheated PBS was added to maintain a constant volume. The absorbance of the aliquots at $\lambda_{max} = 321$ nm was used to determine the amount of FA released at each time point (with suitable dilution performed where required, to ensure the absorbance lay within the calibration range). Dissolution tests for each sample were performed six times.

2.6. Statistical Method

All experiments for statistical analysis were repeated with a minimum of $n = 6$. Statistical analysis was performed using two-way analysis of variance (ANOVA). Statistically significant values were defined at $\alpha = 0.05$.

3. Results and Discussion

3.1. One System but Two Different Electrospinning Processes

Figure 2 is a schematic of the homemade electrospinning system that can be used to implement both one-fluid blending electrospinning and two-fluid coaxial processes. When the sheath fluid flow rate (*Fs*) was turned off, i.e., *Fs* = 0 mL/h, it was a typical one-fluid blending spinning process; when *Fs* > 0 mL/h, it became a two-fluid coaxial spinning process. In the literature, almost all single-fluid electrospinning processes are carried out using a metal capillary as a spinneret, and all double coaxial processes are carried out using a concentric spinneret [17,32]. In the present study, one system with a key component (concentric spinneret) was used for both processes. An image of the working system is shown in Figure 3a. The system consisted of two syringe pumps, a collector, a concentric spinneret (inset of Figure 3a), and a power supply. The power supply was connected with the spinneret through an crocodile clip (Figure 3b).

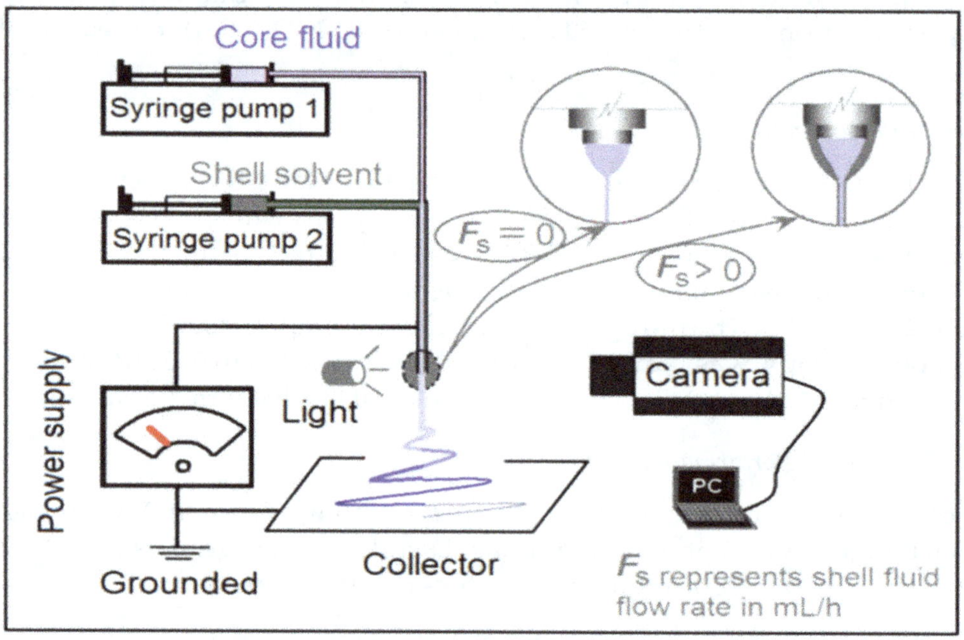

Figure 2. Schematic of the electrospinning system.

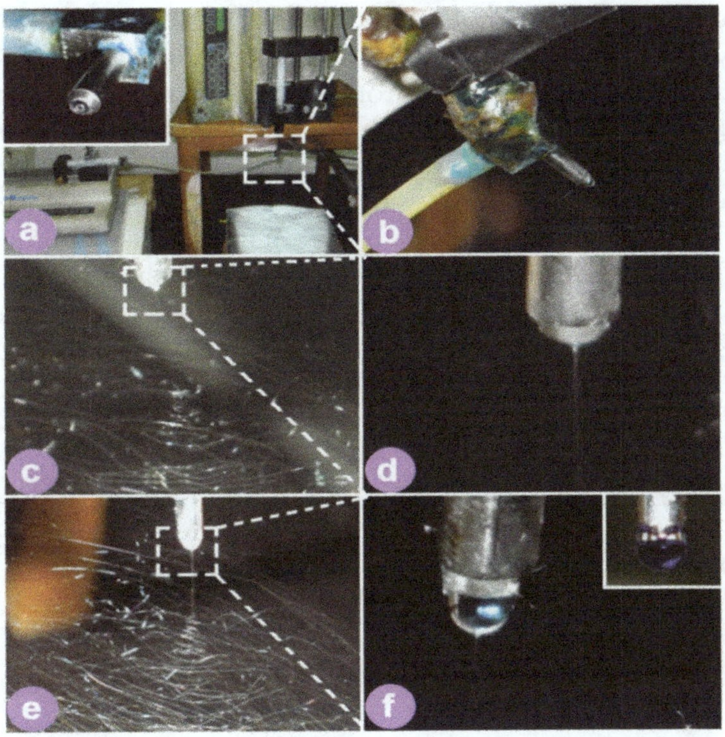

Figure 3. Two electrospinning processes. (**a**) An image of the working system; the inset is the concentric spinneret. (**b**) The connection between the spinneret and the power supply. (**c**) An image of the one-fluid electrospinning process. (**d**) An enlarged image of the Taylor cone in a single-fluid process. (**e**) An image of the coaxial process. (**f**) An enlarged image of the Taylor cone in a two-fluid coaxial process.

In the preparation of 2nd SDs, a blending solution composed of 13% (*w*/*v*) PVA and 2.0% (*w*/*v*) FA in 50% (*v*/*v*) aqueous ethanol was used as the working fluid for the one-fluid blending electrospinning. In the preparation of 3rd SDs using the modified coaxial process, 50% (*v*/*v*) aqueous ethanol was used as the sheath fluid. A co-dissolving solution composed of 13% (*w*/*v*) PVA, 2% (*w*/*v*) PVP K10, and 2% (*w*/*v*) FA in 50% (*v*/*v*) aqueous ethanol was exploited as the core working liquid. For observing the experimental processes, methylene blue (5 ng/mL in 50% (*v*/*v*) aqueous ethanol) was mixed into the core solutions. Details for the preparation are included in Table 1.

Table 1. Parameters for solid dispersion (SD) preparations.

No.	Electrospinning	Sheath Fluid	Core Fluid	Flow Rate (mL/h)	
				Sheath	Core
2nd	Blending	–	13% (*w*/*v*) PVA and 2% (*w*/*v*) FA in 50% (*v*/*v*) aqueous ethanol	–	1.0
3rd	Modified coaxial process	50% (*v*/*v*) aqueous ethanol	13% (*w*/*v*) PVA, 2% (*w*/*v*) PVP K10 and 2% (*w*/*v*) FA in 50% (*v*/*v*) aqueous ethanol	0.2	1.0

Abbreviation: PVP = polyvinylpyrrolidone, PVA = poly(vinyl alcohol), and FA = Ferulic acid.

Figure 3c shows a single-fluid electrospinning process, where a Taylor cone (Figure 3d) was adjacent to a straight fluid jet and to bending and whipping loops for drawing the fluid jets. Similarly, when coaxial electrospinning was carried out (Figure 3e), a straight fluid jet was ejected out from a compound Taylor cone (Figure 3f), which was followed by a series of enlarged loops. The inset of Figure 3f shows an initial droplet before applying a high voltage, suggesting an easy diffusion of the methylene blue dye from the core solution to the sheath solvent in the static state.

As shown in Table 2, the addition of PVP K10 into the PVA and FA co-dissolving solutions increased their viscosity and slightly elevated their surface tension and conductivity. These changes had little influence on their filament-forming property. However, when the sheath solvent mixture was exploited to surround the core spinnable fluid, it generated a significant influence on the working processes. The coaxial working process was initiated more easily, the Taylor cone was rounder, and the straight fluid jet was shorter than the cases in the single-fluid process, which is obvious from a comparison of Figure 3c,d with Figure 3e,f. In the electrical field, the electronic energy always gathered on the surface of fluid jets. The small viscosity and surface tension of the sheath solvent mixture (Table 2) played their positive roles for a stable and continuous electrospinning process, offsetting the negative influences of a small conductivity.

Table 2. The properties of the three working fluids during the electrospinning processes (n = 6).

Electrospinning Working Fluid	Viscosity (cp)	Surface Tension ($N{\cdot}m^{-1} \times 10^{-3}$)	Conductivity ($\mu S{\cdot}cm^{-1}$)
Fluid for the blending process	212.4 ± 4.5	87.6 ± 1.2	57.4 ± 0.5
Core fluid of the coaxial process	343.7 ± 6.8	93.3 ± 0.7	57.8 ± 0.5
Sheath fluid of the coaxial process	2.87 ± 0.04	27.5 ± 0.4	0.87 ± 0.02

3.2. Morphology

One-fluid and modified coaxial processes were both able to create composite nanofibers that were assessed by SEM. All of them had a linear morphology without any discernible bead or spindle. However, the differences in the two types of nanofibers were significant. As shown in Figure 4a,b, the 2nd SDs had an average diameter of 560 ± 140 nm (Figure 4c). The 3rd SDs from the modified coaxial process (Figure 4d,e) had an average diameter of 220 ± 40 nm (Figure 4f), meaning a higher quality than the 2nd SDs in terms of a smaller diameter and more concentrated size distribution. The sheath solvents in the modified coaxial process retained a stable and robust spinning process and enabled a longer time drawing on the fluid jets to further downsize the nanofibers.

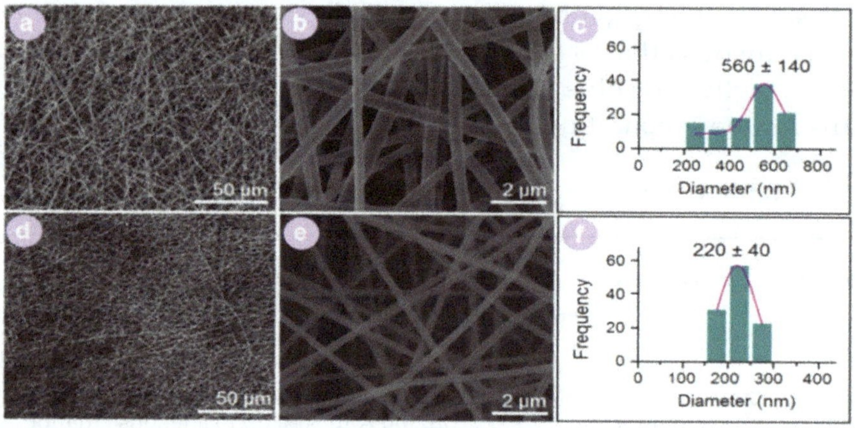

Figure 4. Scanning electron microscope (SEM) images of electrospun nanofibers and their size distributions. (**a**,**b**) Morphology of 2nd SDs with different magnifications. (**c**) Diameter distribution of 2nd SDs. (**d**,**e**) Morphology of 3rd SDs with different magnifications. (**f**) Diameter distribution of 3rd SDs.

3.3. Physical Forms

The X-ray powder diffraction (XRD) patterns of the crude materials (FA, PVA, and PVP K10), 2nd SDs, and 3rd SDs are shown in Figure 5a. The numerous sharp peaks in the patterns of FA suggest that the raw FA particles were crystalline. In sharp contrast, the two halos in the patterns of PVP

K10 suggest that the raw PVP particles were an amorphous polymer matrix. The semi-crystalline, hydrophilic nature of PVA was demonstrated by the single blunt peak. However, both binary and ternary SDs had no sharp peak of the drug and had only one clear hump. These results suggest that both of them were monolithic and amorphous regardless of the two or three components present within the nanofibers. DSC thermograms of the crude powders (FA, PVA, and PVP K10), 2nd SDs, and 3rd SDs are shown in Figure 5b. These data concur with the XRD results. FA and PVA each had a single melting point at 174 and 231 °C, respectively. PVP had a blunt dehydrated endothermic peak before 100 °C, followed by a small conversion slope from the glass state to a rubber state around 170 °C (the inset of Figure 5b). However, in the curves of 2nd SDs and 3rd SDs, no peaks of FA could be detected along with the peaks from PVP and PVA, suggesting that FA was completely converted into an amorphous state. Meanwhile, the drug FA generated some plasticization effects on PVA, moving the melting points from 231 °C to 228 °C and 227 °C for 2nd SDs and 3rd SDs, respectively.

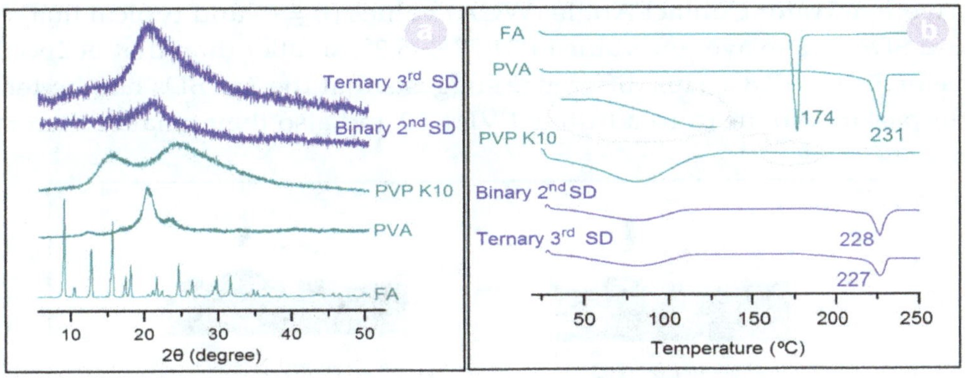

Figure 5. (**a**) XRD patterns; (**b**) DSC thermograms.

Shown in Figure 6a are the FTIR spectra of the crude powders (FA, PVA, and PVP K10) and their binary 2nd SDs and ternary 3rd SDs. Their molecular formulae are shown in Figure 6b. The FTIR spectra of FA powders have a series of sharp peaks, such as 1689 and 1663 cm^{-1} (Figure 6a). These peaks should result from the stretching vibration of C=O groups, giving a hint that they were in a different crystal lattice (Figure 6b). FA molecules have both OH and C=O groups, PVA molecules have numerous OH groups and PVP molecules have numerous C=O groups. When electrospun into binary 2nd SDs or ternary 3rd SDs, they were compatible because of the favorable secondary interactions between the drug and the polymers.

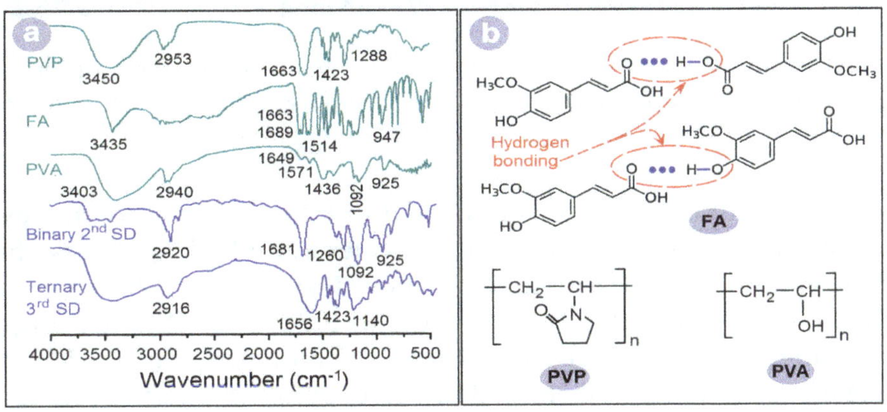

Figure 6. (**a**) FTIR spectra; (**b**) The molecular formula of the raw materials, ferulic acid (FA), polyvinylpyrrolidone (PVP), and poly(vinyl alcohol) (PVA).

In the spectra of binary 2nd SDs, there is, only one, sharp peak at 1681 cm^{-1} due to the stretching vibration of C=O groups, suggesting that FA lost its original crystal state in the binary nanocomposites with PVA. In the spectra of binary 3rd SDs, the large peak at 1656 cm^{-1} was a combined result from the stretching vibration of C=O groups both in the FA and also PVP molecules, similarly suggesting that FA was amorphous in the ternary nanocomposites. Meanwhile, the intensities of several sharp peaks in the fingerprint region of FA spectra were greatly decreased or had totally disappeared, giving hints about the formation of amorphous composites between FA and PVA in the binary 2nd SDs and between PVA and PVP in the ternary 3rd SDs.

3.4. Property and Functional Performance

PVA is a highly water-soluble polymer. Both types of electrospun nanofibers were highly hydrophilic. The water droplets rapidly receded after they were placed on the fibers' surfaces. Thus, to differentiate the hydrophilicity of SDs, WCA was recorded after a water droplet was placed on their surface for 2 s. Average Water Contact Angle (WCA) values ($n = 6$) and typical images are shown in Figure 7a. The 3rd SDs had an average value of 31.7° ± 5.2°, smaller than that of 2nd SDs, which had an average value of 53.3° ± 7.8°. This difference suggests that the 3rd SDs had better hydrophilicity than their counterpart due to the third additive PVP K10 and also their smaller diameter.

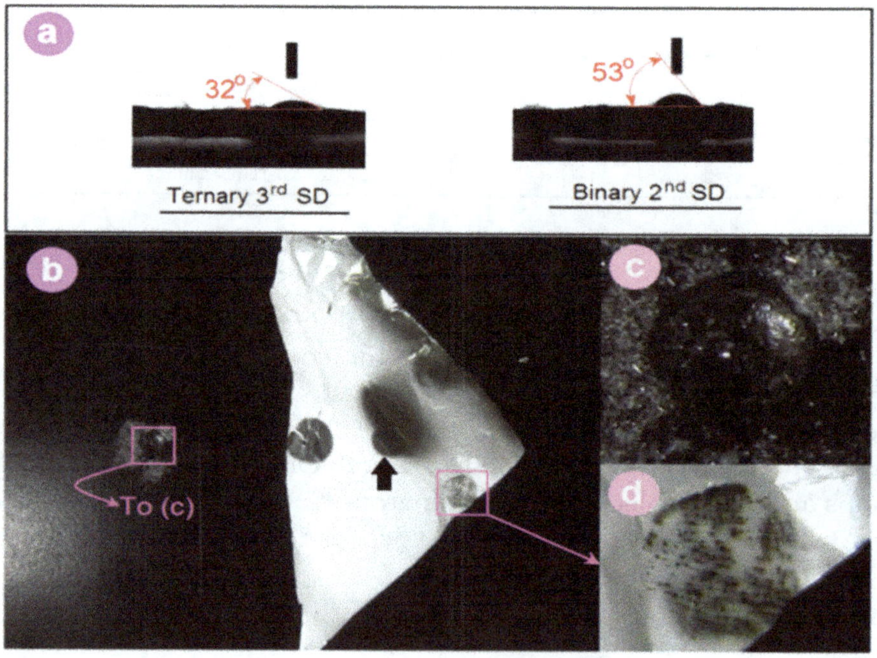

Figure 7. (**a**) Water contact angles (WCA). (**b**) Digital images when water droplet was dripped on the FA powders and the electrospun ternary SDs; (**c**) An enlarged image of the drop of water on the powder; (**d**) A fingermark on the electrospun nanofibers due to moisture.

Figure 7b shows an intuitive impression on the hydrophilic properties of the raw FA powders and the FA-loaded ternary nanofiber film. FA is a poorly water-soluble drug. Thus, the droplet of water stood on the powders without any discernible dissolution (Figure 7c). In sharp contrast, the FA-loaded film was dissolved at once, as indicated by the arrow in Figure 7b. When a finger was pressed on the fiber film, a clear fingermark appeared because of the moisture (Figure 7d). These phenomena demonstrate that the electrospun nanofibers had fine hydrophilicity, and the ternary SDs were better than the binary SDs.

Figure 8 shows the in vitro drug release profiles of raw FA powders and the 2nd and 3rd SDs. After 5 min, only 5.7 ± 2.4% of the raw FA powders were freed into the dissolution media. The 2nd

SDs released all their cargoes after 220 s, whereas the 3rd SDs needed only 60 s. Although both of them were amorphous and monolithic electrospun nanofibers, their functional applications in enhancing drug dissolution significantly differed. This could be attributed to the fact that the 3rd SDs had better hydrophilicity than their counterparts and they also had a smaller diameter.

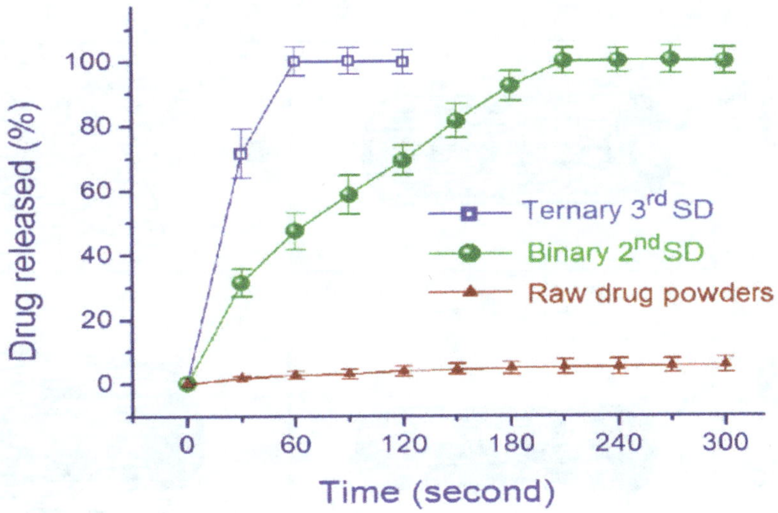

Figure 8. Drug-release profiles of the raw FA powders, the 2nd SDs and 3rd SDs.

Figure 9 is a schematic of the nanostructures of the two SDs and their dissolution processes. The 2nd and 3rd SDs had average diameters of 560 and 220 nm, respectively. For the nanofibers with a cylindrical shape, their volume (V) can be achieved according to the equation of $V = r^2\pi L$, where L and r are the length of fiber and the radius of its cross-section. The nanofiber's surface area (S) can be obtained by the equation $S = 2\pi rL$. Based on the same volume of nanofibers of 2nd SDs ($V_1 = r_1{}^2\pi L_1$) and 3rd SDs ($V_4 = r_4{}^2\pi L_4$), the following relationship can be deduced: $r_2{}^2\pi L_2 = r_3{}^2\pi L_3$, i.e., $L_3/L_2 = r_2{}^2/r_3{}^2$. Thus, the surface area ratio of 3rd SDs to 2nd SDs can be calculated as follows:

$$S_3/S_2 = (2\pi r_3 L_3)/(2\pi r_2 L_2)$$

$$= r_3/r_2 \cdot L_3/L_2$$

$$= r_3/r_2 \cdot r_2{}^2/r_3{}^2 = r_2/r_3$$

$$= 560/220 = 2.5$$

This is to say that the reduction in nanofiber diameter from 560 nm for 2nd SDs to 220 nm for 3rd SDs resulted in a significant increase in the fiber's total surface area by 2.5-fold. The smaller diameter meant double nano effects for drug dissolution, one was a larger surface area and the other was a shorter distance for the water/drug molecules to diffuse in/out of the bulk dissolution media.

However, the most important reason should be the presence of PVP in the PVA matrix, which effectively promoted the disintegration of PVA gels owing to PVP's relatively small molecular weight, high solubility in water, and high permeation ability. The dissolution of a polymer always experiences water absorbance, swelling, and disentanglement of the polymer chains before the polymeric molecules enter the dissolution media. Shown in Figure 9, the PVP K10 molecules completely revised the dissolution processes of PVA molecules. It made the 3rd SDs nanofibers swell more quickly than the 2nd SDs nanofibers. Meanwhile, it promoted the 3rd SDs to dissolve in a disintegration manner, getting rid of the traditional layer-by-layer dissolution model that happens in the 2nd SDs. Certainly, during these processes, the water and also the drug molecules were able to diffuse more easily into and out of the gel regions formed by the PVA matrix within the 3rd SDs than the 2nd SDs.

The generation of electrospun nanofibers on a large scale is drawing increasing attention in both the scientific research and industrial fields [43]. The ternary amorphous nanocomposites hold great promises for further developing fast dissolution drug delivery systems, which is popular for the administration of many active ingredients [44]. In future, these medicated nanofibers can be converted into different kinds of dosage forms, such as tablets, membranes, and also capsules [45].

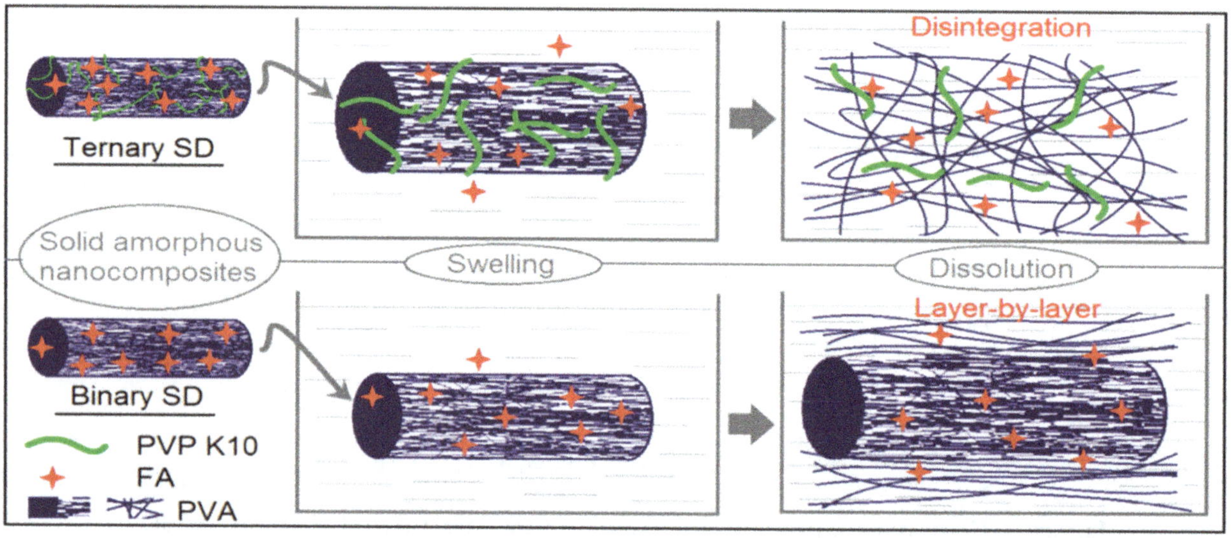

Figure 9. A diagram comparing the dissolution process of the 2nd SDs and 3rd SDs.

4. Conclusions

We successfully prepared 2nd and 3rd SDs by a one-fluid blending electrospinning process and a two-fluid coaxial process, respectively. Both processes were conducted smoothly and continuously, and the resulting nanofibers had fine linear morphology without any discernible bead or spindle. Although XRD patterns demonstrated that both SD types were monolithic and amorphous nanoproducts, 3rd SDs showed over three times faster drug-release rate than 2nd SDs. The added third component PVP, the smaller diameter and corresponding larger surface, the shorter water/drug molecule diffusion distance, and the improved hydrophilicity exerted a combined effect to result in the better performance of 3rd SDs. This study has provided a new protocol for designing and developing new kinds of functional biomaterials as an alternative solution to the problem of insoluble drugs.

Author Contributions: X.-L.L. and D.-G.Y. conceived and designed the experiments; W.H., Y.Y., B.Z., G.L. and S.L. performed the experiments and analyzed the data; W.H. and D.-G.Y. wrote the paper.

References

1. Singh, A.; Van den Mooter, G. Spray drying formulation of amorphous solid dispersions. *Adv. Drug Deliv. Rev.* **2016**, *100*, 27–50. [CrossRef] [PubMed]
2. Lauer, M.E.; Maurer, R.; Paepe, A.T.; Stillhart, C.; Jacob, L.; James, R.; Kojima, Y.; Rietmann, R.; Kissling, T.; van den Ende, J.A.; et al. A miniaturized extruder to prototype amorphous solid dispersions: Selection of plasticizers for hot melt extrusion. *Pharmaceutics* **2018**, *10*, 58. [CrossRef] [PubMed]
3. Feng, D.; Peng, T.; Huang, Z.; Singh, V.; Shi, Y.; Wen, T.; Lu, M.; Quan, G.; Pan, X.; Wu, C. Polymer-surfactant system based amorphous solid dispersion: Precipitation inhibition and bioavailability enhancement of itraconazole. *Pharmaceutics* **2018**, *10*, 53. [CrossRef] [PubMed]
4. Chen, L.; Okuda, T.; Lu, X.Y.; Chan, H.K. Amorphous powders for inhalation drug delivery. *Adv. Drug Deliv. Rev.* **2016**, *100*, 102–115. [CrossRef] [PubMed]

5. Ponnammal, P.; Kanaujia, P.; Yani, Y.; Ng, W.K.; Tan, R.B.H. Orally disintegrating tablets containing melt extruded amorphous solid dispersion of tacrolimus for dissolution enhancement. *Pharmaceutics* **2018**, *10*, 35. [CrossRef] [PubMed]
6. Ousset, A.; Chavez, P.F.; Meeus, J.; Robin, F.; Schubert, M.A.; Somville, P.; Dodou, K. Prediction of phase behavior of spray-dried amorphous solid dispersions: Assessment of thermodynamic models, standard screening methods and a novel atomization screening device with regard to prediction accuracy. *Pharmaceutics* **2018**, *10*, 29. [CrossRef] [PubMed]
7. Huang, S.; Mao, C.; Williams, R.O.; Yang, C.Y. Solubility advantage (and disadvantage) of pharmaceutical amorphous solid dispersions. *J. Pharm. Sci.* **2016**, *105*, 3549–3561. [CrossRef] [PubMed]
8. Li, J.; Patel, D.; Wang, G. Use of spray-dried dispersions in early pharmaceutical development: Theoretical and practical challenges. *AAPS J.* **2016**, *2016*, 1–13. [CrossRef] [PubMed]
9. Chiou, W.L.; Riegelman, S. Pharmaceutical applications for solid dispersion systems. *J. Pharm. Sci.* **1971**, *60*, 1281–1302. [CrossRef] [PubMed]
10. Mishra, J.; Rades, T.; Löbmann, K.; Grohganz, H. Influence of solvent composition on the performance of spray-dried co-amorphous formulations. *Pharmaceutics* **2018**, *10*, 47. [CrossRef] [PubMed]
11. Saleh, A.; McGarry, K.; Chaw, C.S.; Elkordy, A.A. Feasibility of using gluconolactone, trehalose and hydroxy-propyl gamma cyclodextrin to enhance bendroflumethiazide dissolution using lyophilisation and physical mixing techniques. *Pharmaceutics* **2018**, *10*, 22. [CrossRef] [PubMed]
12. Balogh, A.; Farkas, B.; Pálvölgyi, Á.; Domokos, A.; Démuth, B.; Marosi, G.; Nagy, Z.K. Novel alternating current electrospinning of hydroxypropylmethylcellulose acetate succinate (HPMCAS) nanofibers for dissolution enhancement: The importance of solution conductivity. *J. Pharm. Sci.* **2017**, *106*, 1634–1643. [CrossRef] [PubMed]
13. Balogh, A.; Farkas, B.; Domokos, A.; Farkas, A.; Démuth, B.; Borbás, E.; Nagy, B.; Marosi, G.; Nagy, Z.K. Controlled-release solid dispersions of Eudragit® FS 100 and poorly soluble spironolactone prepared by electrospinning and melt extrusion. *Eur. Polym. J.* **2017**, *95*, 406–417. [CrossRef]
14. Borbás, E.; Nagy, Z.K.; Nagy, B.; Balogh, A.; Farkas, B.; Tsinman, O.; Tsinman, K.; Sinkó, B. The effect of formulation additives on in vitro dissolution-absorption profile and in vivo bioavailability of telmisartan from brand and generic formulations. *Eur. J. Pharm. Sci.* **2018**, *114*, 310–317. [CrossRef] [PubMed]
15. Van Duong, T.; Van den Mooter, G. The role of the carrier in the formulation of pharmaceutical solid dispersions. Part II: Amorphous carriers. *Expert Opin. Drug Deliv.* **2016**, *13*, 1681–1694. [CrossRef] [PubMed]
16. Vasconcelos, T.; Sarmento, B.; Costa, P. Solid dispersions as strategy to improve oral bioavailability of poor water soluble drugs. *Drug Discov. Today* **2007**, *12*, 1068–1075. [CrossRef] [PubMed]
17. Kenawy, E.R.; Abdel-Hay, F.I.; El-Newehy, M.H.; Wnek, G.E. Controlled release of ketoprofen from electrospun poly (vinyl alcohol) nanofibers. *Mater. Sci. Eng. A* **2007**, *459*, 390–396. [CrossRef]
18. Le-Ngoc Vo, C.; Park, C.; Lee, B.J. Current trends and future perspectives of solid dispersions containing poorly water-soluble drugs. *Eur. J. Pharm. Biopharm.* **2013**, *85*, 799–813.
19. Zhang, Z.; Li, W.; Wang, G.; Qu, Y.; Yu, D.G. Electrospun 4th generation solid dispersions of poorly water-soluble drug utilizing two different processes. *J. Nanomater.* **2018**, *2018*, 2012140. [CrossRef]
20. Hallouard, F.; Mehenni, L.; Lahiani-Skiba, M.; Anouar, Y.; Skiba, M. Solid dispersions for oral administration: An overview of the methods for their preparation. *Curr. Pharm. Des.* **2016**, *22*, 4942–4958. [CrossRef] [PubMed]
21. Wang, K.; Wen, H.F.; Yu, D.G.; Yang, Y.; Zhang, D.F. Electrosprayed hydrophilic nanocomposites coated with shellac for colon-specific delayed drug delivery. *Mater. Des.* **2018**, *143*, 248–255. [CrossRef]
22. Yang, Y.; Zhang, M.; Wang, K.; Yu, D.G. pH-sensitive polymer nanocoating on hydrophilic composites fabricated using modified coaxial electrospraying. *Mater. Lett.* **2018**, *227*, 93–96. [CrossRef]
23. Liu, Z.P.; Zhang, L.L.; Yang, Y.Y.; Wu, D.; Jiang, G.; Yu, D.G. Preparing composite nanoparticles for immediate drug release by modifying electrohydrodynamic interfaces during electrospraying. *Powder Technol.* **2018**, *327*, 179–187. [CrossRef]
24. Yang, Y.Y.; Zhang, M.; Liu, Z.P.; Wang, K.; Yu, D.G. Meletin sustained-release gliadin nanoparticles prepared via solvent surface modification on blending electrospray. *Appl. Surf. Sci.* **2018**, *434*, 1040–1047. [CrossRef]
25. Liu, X.K.; Shao, W.Y.; Luo, M.Y.; Bian, J.Y.; Yu, D.G. Electrospun blank nanocoating for improved sustained release profiles from medicated gliadin nanofibers. *Nanomaterials* **2018**, *8*, 184.

26. Xu, Y.; Li, J.J.; Yu, D.G.; Williams, G.R.; Yang, J.H.; Wang, X. Influence of the drug distribution in electrospun gliadin fibers on drug-release behavior. *Eur. J. Pharm. Sci.* **2017**, *106*, 422–430. [CrossRef] [PubMed]
27. Li, X.Y.; Zheng, Z.B.; Yu, D.G.; Liu, X.K.; Qu, Y.L.; Li, H.L. Electrosprayed sperical ethylcellulose nanoparticles for an improved sustained-release profile of anticancer drug. *Cellulose* **2017**, *24*, 5551–5564. [CrossRef]
28. Liu, Z.P.; Zhang, Y.Y.; Yu, D.G.; Wu, D.; Li, H.L. Fabrication of sustained-release zein nanoparticles via modified coaxial electrospraying. *Chem. Eng. J.* **2018**, *334*, 807–816. [CrossRef]
29. Yu, D.G.; Li, X.Y.; Wang, X.; Yang, J.H.; Annie Bligh, S.W.; Williams, G.R. Nanofibers fabricated using triaxial electrospinning as zero order drug delivery systems. *ACS Appl. Mater. Interfaces* **2015**, *7*, 18891–18897. [CrossRef] [PubMed]
30. Yu, D.G.; Li, J.J.; Zhang, M.; Williams, G.R. High-quality janus nanofibers prepared using three-fluid electrospinning. *Chem. Commun.* **2017**, *53*, 4542–4545. [CrossRef] [PubMed]
31. Wang, Q.; Yu, D.G.; Zhang, L.L.; Liu, X.K.; Deng, Y.C.; Zhao, M. Electrospun hypromellose-based hydrophilic composites for rapid dissolution of poorly water-soluble drug. *Carbohydr. Polym.* **2017**, *174*, 617–625. [CrossRef] [PubMed]
32. Yang, Y.Y.; Liu, Z.P.; Yu, D.G.; Wang, K.; Liu, P.; Chen, X.H. Colon-specific pulsatile drug release provided by electrospun shellac nanocoating on hydrophilic amorphous composites. *Int. J. Nanomed.* **2018**, *13*, 2395–2404. [CrossRef] [PubMed]
33. Wang, K.; Liu, X.K.; Chen, X.H.; Yu, D.G.; Yang, Y.Y.; Liu, P. Electrospun hydrophilic janus nanocomposites for the rapid onset of therapeutic action of helicid. *ACS Appl. Mater. Interfaces* **2018**, *10*, 2859–2867. [CrossRef] [PubMed]
34. Agarwal, S.; Greiner, A.; Wendorff, J.H. Functional materials by electrospinning of polymers. *Prog. Polym. Sci.* **2013**, *38*, 963–991. [CrossRef]
35. Wang, Q.; Yu, D.G.; Zhou, S.Y.; Li, C.; Zhao, M. Fabrication of amorphous electrospun medicated-nanocomposites using a Teflon-based concentric spinneret. *e-Polymer* **2018**, *18*, 3–11. [CrossRef]
36. Tang, C.; Saquing, C.D.; Harding, J.R.; Khan, S.A. In situ cross-linking of electrospun poly (vinyl alcohol) nanofibers. *Macromolecules* **2009**, *43*, 630–637. [CrossRef]
37. Li, X.; Kanjwal, M.A.; Lin, L.; Chronakis, I.S. Electrospun polyvinyl-alcohol nanofibers as oral fast-dissolving delivery system of caffeine and riboflavin. *Colloid Surf. B* **2013**, *103*, 182–188. [CrossRef] [PubMed]
38. Démuth, B.; Galata, D.L.; Szabó, E.; Nagy, B.; Farkas, A.; Balogh, A.; Hirsch, E.; Pataki, H.; Rapi, Z.; Bezúr, L.; et al. Investigation of deteriorated dissolution of amorphous itraconazole: Description of incompatibility with magnesium stearate and possible solutions. *Mol. Pharm.* **2017**, *14*, 3927–3934. [CrossRef] [PubMed]
39. Gately, N.M.; Kennedy, J.E. The development of a melt-extruded shellac carrier for the targeted delivery of probiotics to the colon. *Pharmaceutics* **2017**, *9*, 38. [CrossRef] [PubMed]
40. Barone, E.; Calabrese, V.; Mancuso, C. Ferulic acid and its therapeutic potential as a hormetin for age-related diseases. *Biogerontology* **2009**, *10*, 97–108. [CrossRef] [PubMed]
41. Yu, D.G.; Yang, J.M.; Branford-White, C.; Lu, P.; Zhang, L.; Zhu, L.M. Third generation solid dispersions of ferulic acid in electrospun composite nanofibers. *Int. J. Pharm.* **2010**, *400*, 158–164. [CrossRef] [PubMed]
42. Yu, D.G.; Zhu, L.M.; Branford-White, C.; Yang, J.H.; Wang, X.; Li, Y.; Qian, W. Solid dispersions in the form of electrospun core-sheath nanofibers. *Int. J. Nanomed.* **2011**, *6*, 3271–3280. [CrossRef] [PubMed]
43. Szabó, E.; Démuth, B.; Nagy, B.; Molnár, K.; Farkas, A.; Szabó, B.; Balogh, A.; Hirsch, E.; Marosi, G.; Nagy, Z.K. Scaled-up preparation of drug-loaded electrospun polymer fibres and investigation of their continuous processing to tablet form. *Express Polym. Lett.* **2018**, *12*, 436–451. [CrossRef]
44. Ono, A.; Ito, S.; Sakagami, S.; Asada, H.; Saito, M.; Quan, Y.S.; Kamiyama, F.; Hirobe, S.; Okada, N. Development of novel faster-dissolving microneedle patches for transcutaneous vaccine delivery. *Pharmaceutics* **2017**, *9*, 59. [CrossRef] [PubMed]
45. Démuth, B.; Nagy, Z.K.; Balogh, A.; Vigh, T.; Marosi, G.; Verreck, G.; Van Assche, I.; Brewster, M.E. Downstream processing of polymer-based amorphous solid dispersions to generate tablet formulations. *Int. J. Pharm.* **2015**, *486*, 268–286. [CrossRef] [PubMed]

11

Application of Permeation Enhancers in Oral Delivery of Macromolecules

Sam Maher [1,*], David J. Brayden [2], Luca Casettari [3] and Lisbeth Illum [4]

1 School of Pharmacy, Royal College of Surgeons in Ireland, St. Stephens Green, Dublin 2, Ireland
2 School of Veterinary Medicine and UCD Conway Institute, University College Dublin, Belfield, Dublin 4, Ireland; david.brayden@ucd.ie
3 Department of Biomolecular Sciences, University of Urbino Carlo Bo, Piazza del Rinascimento 6, 61029 Urbino (PU), Italy; luca.casettari@uniurb.it
4 IDentity, 19 Cavendish Crescent North, The Park, Nottingham NG7 1BA, UK; lisbeth.illum@illumdavis.com
* Correspondence: sammaher@rcsi.com

Abstract: The application of permeation enhancers (PEs) to improve transport of poorly absorbed active pharmaceutical ingredients across the intestinal epithelium is a widely tested approach. Several hundred compounds have been shown to alter the epithelial barrier, and although the research emphasis has broadened to encompass a role for nanoparticle approaches, PEs represent a key constituent of conventional oral formulations that have progressed to clinical testing. In this review, we highlight promising PEs in early development, summarize the current state of the art, and highlight challenges to the translation of PE-based delivery systems into safe and effective oral dosage forms for patients.

Keywords: permeation enhancer; oral delivery; formulation; permeability; safety; simulated intestinal fluid; hydrophobization; epithelium

---

1. Introduction

Since the early 1990s, the pharmaceutical industry has gradually reduced attrition related to non-optimal pharmacokinetics (PK) and low bioavailability (BA) of drugs in development [1]. A combination of tools that predict sub-optimal physicochemical properties, as well as technologies that address impediments to translation from in vitro/preclinical studies to successful clinical trials (e.g., low aqueous solubility, short plasma half-life ($t^1/_2$)) has led to a shift in overall attrition from PK to safety. Despite this, non-optimal PK characteristics continue to rank amongst the most common cause of attrition [2]. The shift towards the development of more lipophilic compounds that are less likely to suffer from sub-optimal PK has however been associated with low solubility and increased toxicity [3,4]. A cohort of macromolecules that can exhibit desirable safety and efficacy are large hydrophilic compounds with greater molecular complexity (e.g., oligomeric peptide backbones), but such properties inevitably confer low intestinal epithelial permeability. In theory, poorly permeable drugs may be administered orally at higher doses to offset low absorption, but this is usually impractical for formulation and cost reasons. Low permeability might be acceptable if a safe and consistent therapeutic effect can be achieved with a molecule that has a long $t^1/_2$, even in the context of high variability in BA, otherwise poorly permeable drugs are typically formulated in injectable dosage forms or in dosage forms using other routes of delivery with higher membrane permeability than the intestine, such as the nasal route.

A paucity of delivery technologies that address low intestinal epithelial permeability for macromolecules has left pharmaceutical manufacturers with little option but to limit screening of these complex hydrophilic macromolecules or default to parenteral formulation. Delivery systems that enable poorly permeable molecules to be efficiently delivered across the intestine may diversity the type of compounds screened in discovery and may permit reformulation of selected injectable macromolecules. There is debate as to whether medicinal chemists in the discovery field should solely focus on safety and efficacy of the active, and rely on formulation and delivery scientists to address sub-optimal solubility, ADME (absorption, distribution, metabolism and excretion), and stability characteristics—or whether medicinal chemists should focus on all of the aforementioned properties to rely less on delivery and formulation scientists [5]. Recent advances highlight the importance of dual focus early in development: optimizing the molecule and the formulation [6,7]. The key challenge with focusing on delivery platforms is the current lack of proven technologies that can significantly improve intestinal permeability in humans.

2. Permeation Enhancer (PE) Categories

The potential of improving the oral BA of macromolecules has been extensively researched, but the majority of delivery systems have failed to progress beyond preliminary animal model evaluation. The inclusion of an excipient that facilitates transport across the intestinal epithelial barrier is a desirable approach. Proprietary formulations that attempt to improve oral absorption of macromolecules in humans usually include permeation enhancers (PEs). However, failure of these PE-based formulations to translate into commercial products has led academic investigators to prioritize development of more technologically advanced drug delivery systems rather than address impediments to translation of PEs. Several hundred compounds have been shown to alter permeability in oral, nasal, buccal, pulmonary, vaginal, and corneal delivery models. These compounds are broadly categorized as paracellular or transcellular PEs.

Paracellular PEs can be sub-categorized into first and second generation [8]. The older first generation paracellular PEs open tight junctions (TJs) through intracellular signaling mechanisms, while the second sub-category act via direct disruption of homophilic interactions at cell adhesion recognition (CAR) sequences. Major targets to afford TJ opening include: the cytoskeleton, claudins, occludin, and E-cadherin and Ca^{2+} [9]. Toxins and their derivatives are one of the largest sources of paracellular PEs, irrespective of sub-category (e.g., *zonula occludins* toxin, *clostridium perfringens* enterotoxin (CPE) [10]). Despite extensive preclinical assessment of microbial toxins and derived motifs, clinical trials with paracellular PEs are dominated by older agents with broader mechanisms of action, one example being ethylenediaminetetraacetic acid (EDTA) (POD™, Oramed, Israel [11]).

Transcellular PEs alter epithelial permeability by two contrasting mechanisms, (i) reversible perturbation of the epithelial plasma membrane [9], or (ii) physical interaction with the active to improve passive transcellular permeation (e.g., hydrophobization [12]). Surfactant-based PEs are a widely tested category that alter membrane integrity. Included in this category are medium chain fatty acids, acylcarnitines, acylated amino acids, bile salts, and a variety of non-ionic surfactants (e.g., polyoxyethylene-8 lauryl ether ($C_{12}E_8$), sucrose laurate, macrogol-8 glycerides [13,14]). A number of surfactants have been evaluated clinically in oral delivery systems for macromolecules: lauroylcarnitine chloride (Peptilligence™, Enteris Biopharma, Boonton, NJ, USA [15]) sodium caprate (C_{10}) (GIPET™, Merrion Pharma, Dublin, Ireland [16]), sodium caprylate (TPE™ Chiasma, Ness Ziona, Israel [17]), and sodium cholate (Biocon, Bangalore, India [18]). Soluble and insoluble surfactants are also constituents of complex lipoidal systems including oily suspensions [17] and emulsions [19]. At low test concentrations in reductionist cell and tissue based delivery models, transcellular perturbants (i) activate plasma membrane receptors and enzymes, (ii) modulate intracellular mediators, (iii) selectively remove TJ proteins from fluidic regions of the membrane, and (iv) initiate repair mechanisms related to opening of TJs [20]. In some cases, these actions are uncoupled from membrane perturbation [21]. This has led investigators to suggest that some perturbants may in part act indirectly via a paracellular mode of action. However, low concentrations of such agents that do not induce transcellular perturbation cause only modest increases on permeability in vitro [21].

Transcellular permeation may also be improved by physical complexation, either by hydrophobic ion pairing (HIP) or dipole–dipole interaction [9]. HIP involves electrostatic-based complexation of an ionizable lead (usually a peptide) with an amphiphilic counterion. The hydrophobic moiety of the counter ion confers a lower capacity for solvation than conventional counterions typically used in the preparation of pharmaceutical salts to address low aqueous solubility. HIP reduces the solubility of several peptides including insulin [22], desmopressin [23], octreotide [24], and exenatide [25]. Hydrophobization via dipole–dipole interactions between the poorly permeable macromolecule and acylated amino acids (the so-called Eligen® carriers of Emisphere, Roseland, NJ, USA [26]) is a more widely studied approach than HIP, although the less well understood. Emisphere have assessed the clinical potential of Eligen carriers most notably SNAC (sodium salcaprozate) and 5-CNAC (N-(5-chlorosalicyloyl)-8-aminocaprylic acid) over a 20-year period. In that time, Emisphere discontinued development of SNAC for oral delivery of heparin and insulin. SNAC has however been successfully used in a marketed oral vitamin B_{12} supplement (Eligen B_{12}) [27], and more recently was shown to improve oral absorption of semaglutide in Phase II trials [28]. Development of an oral salmon calcitonin (sCT) using 5-CNAC failed to meet primary endpoints in two Phase III trials [29].

Several non-surfactant PEs have also been tested in pre-clinical studies. These include chitosan and its derivatives, cell penetrating peptides (CPPs), solvents (e.g., ethanol), salicylates, and enamines. CPPs such as penetratin and its analog, PentraMax™, continue to be researched for oral peptide delivery. There is evidence that these CPPs act by altering membrane barrier integrity [30], endocytosis [30], and physical complexation [31]. Although a few CPPs have progressed to clinical evaluation, the majority relate to the intracellular delivery of small molecules and not to oral delivery of macromolecules [32]. It remains to be seen if CPPs will eventually advance to clinical testing in oral delivery of anti-diabetic peptides [33].

3. Targets for Intestinal Permeation Enhancement: Beyond Insulin

Development of delivery platforms that improve epithelial permeability was historically associated with creating non-invasive formulations of insulin. Insulin represents an inexpensive and available prototype peptide with established analytical methods for PK and pharmacodynamic assays. In justifying the use of insulin, it can be argued that a prototype that can improve permeation of this large peptide (5.8 kDa) could be even more effective with smaller peptides (1–4 kDa), so it is a high bar. While there is some merit to the development of an oral insulin dosage, the focus on insulin has restricted effort to develop oral delivery systems for other macromolecules with more favourable physicochemical properties. Additionally, the emphasis on oral delivery of insulin and the lack of success in that pursuit during the hype of the 1990s has led to a largely negative view in the pharmaceutical industry and with journal editors of novel strategies to improve intestinal permeability.

Table 1 shows a selection of licensed peptides marketed via oral or injectable routes. This table shows that dose (potency), $t_{1/2}$, Mw, lipophilicity (LogP) and target action site are important factors that influence whether a peptide is commercially successful via oral or injectable routes. There are currently nine peptides on the market as oral products [34], although only two desmopressin and cyclosporin are intended to act on systemic targets; the properties of which are shown in Table 1. All other peptides in Table 1, except the regionally acting vancomycin, are marketed in injectable formulations and BA values are considered negligible (<0.1%).

All peptides marketed via the oral route are assigned low permeability within the Biopharmaceutics Classification System (BCS). Marketed injectable peptides are not formally assigned a BCS Class, although all peptides in Table 1 are considered BCS Class III. It is evident from Table 1 that while peptides exhibit low and variable BA (apart from cyclosporin), an optimal balance between potency, size/complexity, and apparent plasma $t_{1/2}$ can facilitate the development of a successful oral form (e.g., desmopressin) (Table 1). The extent to which chemical modification and the delivery system can compensate for peptides that do not exhibit an optimal balance between potency, size/complexity, and apparent plasma half-life is not clear. Structural modifications can reduce demand on delivery systems for peptides that are larger and more complex. A recent example being the very long $t_{1/2}$ GLP-1 analog, semaglutide [35], which has demonstrated promising results in clinical trials in an oral formulation containing SNAC, a PE that failed with macromolecules that did not have such favorable features.

In atypical cases where peptides are lipophilic and stable to proteolytic degradation, oral BA can be significantly higher than equivalent hydrophilic peptides (e.g., cyclosporin). The downside of high lipophilicity is low aqueous solubility, which has been addressed using lipid-based formulations [36]. Clinical evaluation of the cyclosporin (Sandimmune® Neoral, Novartis) has shown that 86% of the intact peptide permeates the intestinal epithelium [37]. While brush border and hepatic metabolism reduce BA of cyclosporin to 27%, oral BA is far higher than equivalent hydrophilic peptides such as desmopressin and octreotide. Chemical modification has been less successful in addressing low permeability, for example, in the case of insulin [38], although there is emerging evidence that physical modification of peptides using hydrophobizing agents may improve passive permeation (Section 4.7) [9,12,39]. A key area of development, therefore, is the combined development of hydrophobized peptides with a suitable lipid-based delivery system.

Table 1. Properties of selected approved peptides and their routes of delivery (source of information: Health Products Regulatory Authority (HPRA) summary of product characteristics (SPC), Drugbank, PubChem, and Welcome Compound Report Card).

Active	Mw	Dose	Frequency	Route	$t_{1/2}$	LogP †	BCS	Oral BA
Desmopressin	1069 Da	1–4 mcg	Daily	sc	~2.8 h	−4	III	0.17%
Octreotide	1019 Da	200 mcg	Thrice daily	sc	~1.7 h	−1.4	—	Phase 3
Cyclosporin	1203 Da	280 mg	Daily	iv inf.	~8.4 h	7.5	II	27%
Vancomycin	1449 Da	1500 mg	Twice daily	iv inf.	~7.2 h	−2.6	III	Local
Salmon calcitonin	3432 Da	16.7 mcg	Daily	sc	~1.3 h	−16.6	—	Phase 3
Semaglutide	4114 Da	500 mcg *	Weekly	sc	~168 h	−5.8	—	Phase 3
Exenatide	4186 Da	10 mcg	Daily	sc	~2.4 h	−21	—	Phase 1
Insulin degludec	6108 Da	350 mcg	Daily	sc	~25 h	−4.9	—	—
Insulin aspart	5832 Da	1.8 mg **	—	sc	~1.4 h	—	—	—

* oral dose in clinical testing [28]; ** estimated daily dose; † estimated logP (XLogP3-AA [40]); BCS: Biopharmaceutics classification system; $t_{1/2}$: plasma half-life; LogP: octanol water partition coefficient.

4. Recent Highlights

4.1. Oral Semaglutide Reduces HBA1c in Type 2 Diabetics by over 1.5% in Phase II Trials

Novo Nordisk (Bagsværd, Denmark) has adopted an integrated approach to enabling oral peptide delivery, combining structural engineering and formulation optimization [6]. Semaglutide is a long-acting acylated GLP-1 agonist (Ozempic® once weekly, s.c.) that also has greater stability to enzymatic degradation in the gastrointestinal (GI) tract. A once-a-day oral formulation of semaglutide in an immediate release formulation with SNAC is likely to have a significant effect on the management of diabetes. In a Phase II randomised controlled trial of 632 patients, daily administration of oral semaglutide (2.5–40 mg) lowered HbA1c by 0.7% to 1.9% [28]. Although there was a 280-fold difference in the cumulative dose relative to the once weekly sub-cutaneous (sc) injection (1 mg), the long plasma $t_{1/2}$, high potency, and improved stability reduces the need for a high-performing PE. Induction of high local pH in the immediate vicinity of the semaglutide/SNAC tablet in the stomach to increase solubility is considered a central aspect of the technology [41], where the contemporaneous release of SNAC and semaglutide to fasting patients enables co-localisation in high concentration at the site of enhancement. In gamma scintigraphy studies in healthy volunteers, the anatomical location for tablet erosion was confirmed as the stomach irrespective of whether participants ingested the formulation with 50 mL or 240 mL water [42]. The time to complete tablet erosion was 95 min (50 mL water) and 66.2 min (240 mL). Slow erosion of tablets (<54% in 1 h) was associated with higher plasma semaglutide levels and a longer T_{max} compared to fast eroding tablets. It is unclear why gastric emptying does not occur in patients receiving oral semaglutide, although it is possible that the peptide could slow gastric emptying [43]. It is not clear if the slow progressive release of semaglutide in the stomach may necessitate a longer delay before ingestion of a meal. The unusual gastric pH mechanism advocated for semaglutide/SNAC seems to be highly specific for this peptide. This topic is discussed in detail in the current special issue review by Twarog et al.

4.2. The Ionic Liquid Choline Geranate (CAGE) Has a Major Effect on Oral BA of Insulin

Ionic liquids are salt-like materials that are liquids below 100 °C. There has been renewed interest in the use of ionic liquids primarily due to their solvent properties. A recent study showed that intestinal co-instillation of a relatively low dose of insulin with choline geranate (CAGE) led to a dramatic lowering in blood sugar levels in non-diabetic rats [44]. The decrease in blood sugar compared favourably with the s.c. delivered insulin. The oral BA of insulin (10 IU) in rats was 45% following delivery with CAGE (80 mg) in enteric coated capsules in rodents, one of the highest values ever recorded for an insulin formulation in a rat PK study, albeit relative to 2 IU (s.c.) as against 1IU (s.c.) in most studies. CAGE increased the fluidity of mucous, reduced epithelial barrier integrity and protected insulin from degradation by trypsin. There was no apparent histological damage to the intestinal mucosa of rats. However, CAGE caused a partial reduction in Caco-2 cell viability, a decrease in transepithelial electrical resistance (TEER) and evidence of intracellular insulin-fluorescein isothiocyanate (FITC) in fluorescence microscopy, suggesting some transcellular perturbation. It is noteworthy that choline-based ionic liquids were amongst the least cytotoxic in a screen assessing the effect of a panel on the viability of Caco-2 and HT29 cells [45]. Moreover, insulin was stable in CAGE for four months at 4 °C. It is noteworthy that peptide stability concerns have been overcome in non-aqueous polyprotic solvents [46]. It will be interesting to see if these results translate to large animal models with a dosage form that can translate to human trials.

4.3. Mode of Action Studies on the PE, PIP 640

Permeant inhibitor of phosphatase (PIP) peptide 640 (PIP 640) is a decapeptide that transiently opens TJs. PIP640 inhibits myosin light chain phosphatase (MLCP), which in turn inhibits dephosphorylation of myosin light chain (MLC) [47]. This is achieved by binding to a subunit complex of protein phosphatase 1 (PP1) and MYPT1 (myosin phosphatase target subunit) in the same manner as CPI-17 (C-kinase-activated protein phosphatase-1 (PP1) inhibitor-17kDa). PIP-640 increased fluorescein isothiocyanate dextran 4 kDa (FD4) permeation across Caco-2 monolayers and improved BA of insulin to 4% in rat intestinal instillations [47]. More recently, a structure–activity assessment of PIP 640 showed that residues of glutamic acid and tyrosine are requisite for binding to MYPT1 subunit of the MLCP complex, while substitution of aspartic acid for arginine led to more specific targeting of PP1 subunit, which was associated with greater cytotoxicity [48]. In a follow-on study, PIP 640 was shown to selectively increase total levels of claudin 2 (both the cytoplasm and at the membrane) [49]. This increment was attributed to the preserved stability of existing claudin 2 rather than increased expression. Alteration of Caco-2 monolayer permeability by PIP 640 was biased towards paracellular transport of positively-charged diethylaminoethyl dextran compared to neutral dextran or carboxymethyl dextran, in keeping with data showing that claudin-2 is responsible for the formation of a channel that is selective for cations. A similar effect was observed in the comparison of sCT (cationic at the pH in the small intestine) and exenatide (anionic at the pH in the small intestine). PIP640 caused a greater increase on permeation of sCT over exenatide in both Caco-2 monolayers and rat intestinal instillations. Together these data highlight a potential for development of new chemical entity PEs that show bias towards permeation of cationic actives. These studies are noteworthy due the molecular biology and rational screening approaches taken to produce a PE molecule. Increasing the potency of PIP 640 is however likely to be required in order to allow a translatable oral dosage formulation to be developed.

4.4. Application of Nanoparticles to Co-Localise Active and PE

Nanotechnology has several potential applications in the science of oral delivery including protecting payload, targeting epithelial receptors in GI regions, and improving permeability [50]. The original working hypothesis for application in oral delivery of peptides was that nanoencapsulation would protect labile actives from pre-systemic degradation and shuttle cargo across the intestinal epithelium [51]. While this is the desired outcome, low and variable transmucosal uptake of nanoparticles and formulation complexity continue to impede progression. Investigators have attempted to improve transmucosal flux of drug-loaded nanoparticles using PEs, but it is difficult to envisage a PE improving uptake of colloids when uptake of peptides is inherently low and variable. An evolving view of nanoencapsulation is their potential to permeate mucus and to co-localise release of the macromolecule and PE at the intestinal epithelial wall, a key requirement for effective permeation enhancement [52,53]. It remains to be seen whether PE-macromolecule loaded nanoparticles, either passive or receptor-targeted, can be an effective strategy for delivering payloads across the intestine.

4.5. Application of PEs in Delivery of Nutraceuticals

Bioactive molecules in foodstuffs may have potential health benefits beyond their basic nutritional value. Many of these are complex natural substances that have low aqueous solubility and/or low intestinal permeability. These include peptides, carbohydrates, lipids, and complex organic phytochemicals. There is considerable overlap in the approaches to enable oral delivery of pharmaceutical and nutraceutical products [54], although development considerations related to safety, efficacy, and cost-effectiveness vary between the two.

Application of PEs to improve the oral BA of nutraceuticals is an emerging area. Safety concerns related to additives that might alter intestinal barrier integrity may outweigh any health benefits derived from selected nutraceuticals. PEs that are likely to be useful in oral delivery of nutraceuticals are substances that have food additive status, GRAS status, or can be made to food grade, so this limits the range for selection. These include medium and long chain fatty acids, bile salts (e.g., sodium chloeate [13]), chitosan and its derivatives [55] and certain non-ionic surfactants (e.g., sucrose esters [56], lactose esters [57], polysorbates [58]). Although most PEs are tested with transport markers of poorly permeable drugs, recent studies have evaluated oral delivery of antihypertensive tripeptides derived from milk and chicken muscle. Co-delivery of C_{10} (180 mM) with isoleucine-proline-proline (IPP) and leucine-lysine-proline (LKP) from milk did not improve oral absorption any further in rats in part because basal permeability seemed to be already high [59]. C_{10} reversed the effect of the Pep-T1 inhibitor (glycyl sarcosine) on oral absorption of these tripeptides. Other PEs have been shown to act in part via solubilization (bile salts [60]), inhibition of transporters (piperine [61]), or alteration to pre-systemic metabolism (genistein [62]). There are questions as to whether PEs can be effective as part of food matrices, and it may, therefore, be necessary to deliver bioactives as nutritional supplements in capsules or tablets. The relatively lower potency of nutraceutical versus therapeutic peptides is a challenge to the use of PEs. On the other hand, bioactive nutraceutical peptides are likely to be cheap to manufacture and exhibit intrinsically low toxicity. Thus it may be possible to offset lower potency with a higher amount of peptide and PE.

4.6. Can Non-Ionic Surfactants be More Effective than Ionizable Surfactants?

Surfactant-based PEs have long been the leading candidates to improve oral absorption of poorly permeable actives. The most prominent surfactant categories include medium chain fatty acids (anionic), acylcarnitines (amphoteric), alkyl sulfates (anionic), and bile salts (anionic). A structurally diverse group of non-ionic surfactants have been shown to alter epithelial barrier integrity including fatty alcohol ethoxylates, ethoxylated sugar esters, alkylphenol ethoxylates, alkyl maltosides/glucosides, macrogol glycerides, and sucrose/lactose esters. Most non-ionic surfactants in this category are liquid or unctuous semi-solids at room temperature, which limits their formulation potential. Small quantities of liquid PE can be incorporated into solid dosage forms using adsorbent. However, it is more challenging to prepare powders that have acceptable properties for capsule filling or compaction into tablets (such as flowability, disintegration, dissolution, desorption). For example, solidification of Labrasol® (Gattefosse, Saint Priest, Lyon, France) was achieved using relatively low quantities of silica (e.g., Neusilin® US2, Fuji Chemicals, Nakaniikawa-gun, Toyama, Japan) (Figure 1). Tablets prepared using a Labrasol® (50%), and Neusilin® US2 had poor disintegration times, but this was corrected by inclusion of a disintegrant (Table 2). Use of additional excipients lowers the quantity by weight of PE that can be incorporated into the formulation. This approach is more therefore likely to be only useful for the most potent non-ionic surfactants (e.g., $C_{12}E_8$), where less PE is required to improve permeation.

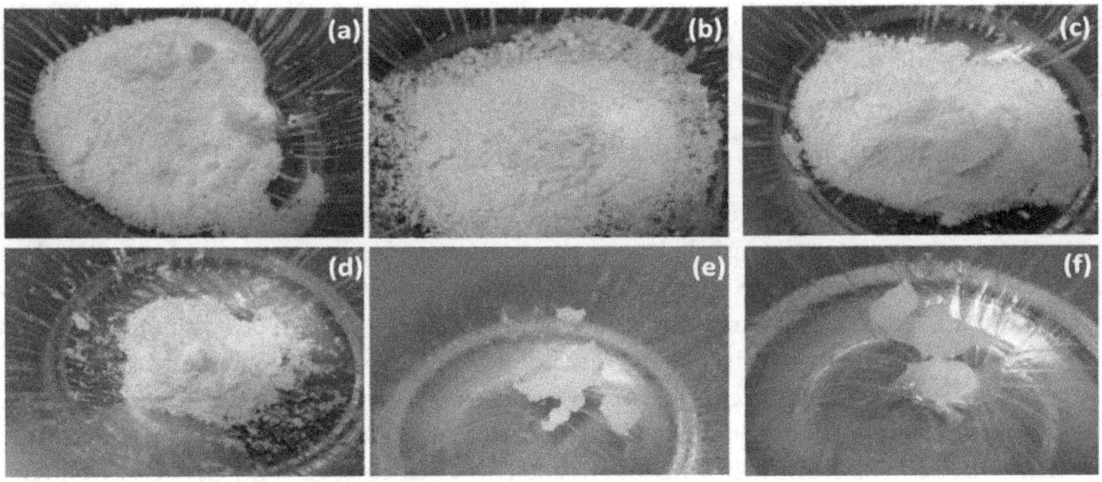

Figure 1. Visual effect of Neusilin® US2 on physical state of Labrasol®. Ratio of Neusilin® US2 to Labrasol® are (**a**) 1:0, (**b**) 0.75:0.25, (**c**) 0.67:0.33, (**d**) 0.5:0.5, (**e**) 0.33:0.67, (**f**) 0.25:0.75 (Maher unpublished).

Table 2. Disintegration times and break strength values for a panel of formulations containing Labrasol®, Neusilin® US2 and a disintegrant (Croscarmellose Sodium).

Formulation Additives	Disintegrant (% w/w)	Tableting Pressure (psi)	Disintegration Time (min)	Break Strength (N)
Labrasol and Neusilin® US2 (1:1)	0	1000	>60	29.1 ± 2.9
Labrasol and Neusilin® US2 (1:1)	0	2000	>60	68.8 ± 3.2
Labrasol and Neusilin® US2 (1:1)	5	1000	5.5 ± 0.2	49.8 ± 6.2
Labrasol and Neusilin® US2 (1:1)	5	2000	4.9 ± 0.3	72.4 ± 2.7

Some non-ionic surfactants are solids at room temperature (e.g., sucrose and lactose esters) although a low melting point makes it challenging to incorporate into tablets. Growth in the number of poorly soluble drugs administered in lipid-based formulations (LBFs) has led investigators to assess delivery of macromolecules in non-aqueous vehicles in soft or hard gelatin capsules. An underpinning question is what are the advantages of non-ionic surfactants versus ionizable surfactants, salts of which are easier to formulate into solid dosage forms? In general, non-ionic surfactants are safer and more widely used as excipients and food additives, primarily as emulsifiers. Sucrose laurate is an excipient included in some marketed formulations, and, although it is present in low amounts, its status as an excipient reduces risks in development. In a recent head-to-head, sucrose laurate and Labrasol® (Gattefosse, France) improved the flux of transmucosal marker molecules to a similar level to C_{10} and sodium undecylenate ($C_{11:1}$) at comparable concentrations across isolated rat intestinal tissue mucosae [13]. Sucrose laurate caused less damage to isolated rat colonic mucosae compared with C_{10} at similar concentrations [63]. In intestinal instillations, sucrose laurate improved permeation of insulin in the absence of histological damage [64]. It is noteworthy that other sugar esters have recently been shown to exhibit permeation enhancement. For example, the enhancement action of lactose laurate was comparable to sucrose laurate [65]. Although sucrose laurate and other sucrose esters can be synthesized as monoesters and have demonstrated enhancement action in their pure forms, food and excipient grades are typically supplied as mixtures containing the soluble mono-ester assigned a hydrophilic lipophilic balance (HLB) of 15 and a significant proportion of insoluble di-, tri-, and polyesters (HLB < 5). Thus, dispersions formed by mixed sucrose esters are not simple micellar systems; they comprise mixed micelles and/or micro/nanoemulsions. There is a requirement for safe and selective methods for production and material separation.

Labrasol® is another example of a complex blend of soluble and insoluble surfactants containing a large proportion of macrogol glycerides and 10% medium chain glycerides. Although Labrasol® caused perturbation of isolated rat intestinal mucosae, there was a degree of separation between the enhancement action and the histology damage score [13]. The effect of the difference in dispersion properties has not yet been fully elucidated, although there is emerging evidence that the extent of the monomeric surfactant that is free to interact with the mucosal surface plays a role in permeation enhancement [66,67]. The effect of free surfactant on enhancement action is discussed further in Section 4.9.

4.7. Can Physical Hydrophobization Improve Passive Intestinal Flux?

The majority of PEs act by altering epithelial barrier integrity. In recent years, investigators have attempted to improve the lipophilicity of the active to facilitate passive intestinal permeation. Hydrophobisation can be achieved by chemical conjugation (prodrugs [68]) or physical complexation [9] (Section 2). Chemical modification is not ideal for large ionizable peptides as it is not practical to mask several amino acid side chains within a macromolecule. The reversible formation of a salt between the peptide and a complexing agent can lead to a more dramatic increase in lipophilicity. This occurs through a combination of charge neutralization, exposure of hydrophobic domains within the peptide and/or the introduction of lipophilic moieties via the counterion. The process of HIP, therefore, leads to extensive lowering of aqueous solubility, which can be addressed through encapsulation in nanoparticles (e.g., poly(lactic-co-glycolic acid [69]), solubilization in lipid-based formulations [70], and non-aqueous solvents [22,71]. Incorporation of HIP complexes in the non-aqueous vehicle may prevent enzymatic degradation, limit pH dependent complex destabilization, and counterions may also perform as PEs [72]. Given the successful application of lipoidal vehicles in oral delivery of cyclosporin, there is research effort assessing the factors that impact loading in LBFs [70]. There are cases where HIP does not result in loss of aqueous solubility [73] and do not immediately breakdown at high pH values where deprotonation of cationic functional groups is known to occur [74]. However, further investigation is required to understand the permeability of soluble HIP complexes. Other considerations require kinetic and thermodynamic assessment of the dissociation of the hydrophobized peptide complex during permeation.

4.8. Mode of Action Studies are Required to Provide Evidence for a Paracellular Effect

The mechanism by which PEs alter the intestinal barrier has implications for safety and approval of PE-containing oral macromolecule formulations. In general, few PEs solely act via a paracellular mode of action, and it is necessary to distinguish paracellular and transcellular pathways across intestinal epithelia. Reduction in TEER for example or an increase in flux of paracellular transport markers is not direct proof of a paracellular mode of action, as transcellular perturbation can also reduce TEER and increase such fluxes. The absence of cytotoxicity in common cell viability assays (e.g., MTT) at concentrations that cause alteration to TEER and marker transport favour an interpretation relating to paracellular pathways. However, cytotoxicity assays based on mitochondrial enzymes may not represent the first sign of membrane perturbation. In this case, it may be appropriate to combine the use of MTT assay and techniques that directly evaluate membrane perturbation (e.g., lactate dehydrogenase (LDH) release assay). Two-path impedance spectroscopy has been used to show that C_{10} acts via a paracellular mode of action in vitro at low concentrations [75]. However, this method requires strict verification that the PE does not cause intracellular uptake of a paracellular dye [76], and applications that do not assess membrane integrity can overestimate the contribution of the paracellular route [75]. A recent study showed restoration of barrier integrity and a parallel decrease in absorption of a model peptide following cessation of intra-duodenal perfusion of C_{10} in rats [77]. This reversible action was equated to a paracellular mode of action, the rationale being that, had the effect been related to mucosal perturbation, the absorption of peptide would have continued to remain high. This conclusion does not, however, take into account the capacity of the GI tract to undergo rapid repair following perturbation [78]. Overall, more direct mode of action studies are required to confirm a paracellular mode of action.

4.9. Growing Need for Simulated Intestinal Fluid in PE Experiments

Over the last 30 years, there has been extensive effort to predict the behaviour of oral formulations in humans from solubility and release characteristics in vitro. This has given rise to important topics in biopharmaceutics including bioequivalence testing and in vitro/in vivo correlations. Solubility enhancement strategies highlighted the importance of replicating in vivo fasted and fed state conditions in order to predict release characteristics in humans, however there has not been the same emphasis on how constituents of intestinal luminal fluids affect intestinal permeability and in vivo absorption in preclinical models (including cell culture monolayers grown on Transwell® supports, isolated tissues mounted in Ussing chambers, everted and non-everted intestinal sacs, open/closed loop instillations, tablet insertion into gut loop, single-pass intestinal perfusion, infusion via intubation, oral administration as liquid or solid dosage forms).

Gastrointestinal fluid contains a complex mixture of endogenous secretions (including gastric, pancreatic, luminal, and biliary secretions, sloughed cells) and dietary substances (nutrients, drugs, microorganisms). This heterogeneous milieu consists of a cocktail of ions, bicarbonate, enzymes, mucin, bile acids, phospholipids, carbohydrates, proteins, amino acids, lipids, fatty acids, indigestible solid particles, and lysates from sloughed epithelial cells and non-viable microorganisms. In principle, the luminal milieu can modulate enhancement action of PEs. In the simplest example, PEs that are peptides/proteins may be degraded by proteolytic enzymes. Not all protein-based PEs are inactivated by luminal fluid as evident from the fact that many protein-based toxins stimulate electrogenic chloride secretion and TJ openings [79]. It remains to be seen whether peptide-based PEs can consistently modulate epithelial permeability or whether these additives must be chemically-modified to increase stability (e.g., cyclisation, synthesis of all D-forms, amino acid substitutions) or mixed with excipients that prevent enzymatic degradation of the therapeutic peptide (e.g., citric acid, soybean trypsin inhibitor). Other structural PEs categories can also be enzymatically degraded in the small intestine. Macrogol glycerides (e.g., Labrasol®, Gattefosse, France) are substrates of digestive lipase [80], although the degradation products in this instance are free medium chain fatty acids which may contribute to permeation enhancement [81].

It is not only chemical degradation that can attenuate the enhancement action. PEs that have demonstrated the most significant effect on epithelial permeability are soluble surfactants. This surfactant type exists in the monomeric form up to threshold concentration above which they form micelles. This critical micelle concentration (CMC) is both a measure of the solubility of the monomeric surfactant form and a direct measure of when surfactants begin to form micelles. Ionic surfactants with high CMC values are generally good detergents because it is the monomeric form of the surfactant that is responsible. As detergent-like membrane perturbation caused by surfactants is largely driven by the monomeric form of the surfactant, any physiological factor that reduces the CMC can potentially reduce efficacy. The CMC of ionizable surfactants such as medium chain fatty acids, acylcarnitines, and alkyl sulfates can be decreased by increasing the ionic strength of the medium, as the addition of counterions reduces repulsion between anionic hydrophilic head groups, which makes micellization favorable at low concentrations [82]. Recently, enhancement action of C_{10} and sodium dodecyl sulphate (SDS) was increased in hypotonic conditions (achieved with NaCl) in a single-pass intestinal perfusion in rats [83], an effect that could relate to a reduction in the CMC. In the case of ionizable surfactants that contain weakly acidic or weakly basic hydrophilic head groups, alteration to pH can transform a surfactant from its soluble form to its insoluble form, which although still capable of lowering surface tension, has reduced capacity to act as a detergent.

Divalent cations such as calcium found in milk can decrease the permeation enhancement of anionic surfactants through precipitation of inactive salts [84]. On the other hand, alteration to pH may increase permeation enhancement. For example, reduction in the regional pH with an amphoteric surfactant may increase the proportion of the surfactant in the cationic form, which is likely to have a greater affect. Additionally, it has been proposed that co-solvents that increase the solubility of insoluble surfactants can improve aqueous solubility and enable greater interaction with the cell membrane [66]. Several other factors may modulate the free surfactant concentration within the small intestine. These include adsorption to undigested solid particles and oil droplets and incorporation into colloidal structures (e.g., mixed micelles with free fatty acids and bile salts). Depending on the quantity and type of materials within the GI tract, free surfactant monomers may be efficiently replenished from micelles, but as the window for efficient enhancement can be shortened by dilution, spreading, and absorption of the PE itself, the availability of surfactant within that window may be quickly diluted. Phospholipid and bile salt constituents of simulated intestinal media can attenuate the effects of alkyl maltopyranosides through the formation of mixed micelles [67]. Fasted state simulated intestinal media (FaSSIF) containing taurocholate, phosphatidylcholine in buffered isosmotic buffer salt solution (pH 7.1) also attenuated the permeation enhancement of palmitoylcarnitine and hexyphosphocholine surfactants in Caco-2 monolayers [85]. In the same study, FaSSIF did not affect the enhancement action of non-surfactant PEs, EDTA and 3-nitrocoumarin. In some cases, mixing surfactants can increase enhancement action still further [86]. Combinations of medium chain fatty acids with PEG-8 glycerides increased permeation of FD4 across isolated rat intestinal tissue by 10-fold over the respective individual agents [87].

A recent study assessed the effect of FaSSIF and fed state simulated intestinal fluid (FeSSIF on the absorption of BCS Class I, II and III drugs in a single pass intestinal perfusion (Roos et al., submitted). Even in the absence of PEs, there was a significant difference in the absorption of atenolol, enalaprilat, ketoprofen, and metoprolol between FaSSIF and FeSSIF. This result was not surprising as an analysis of 92 clinical datasets found that 67% of BCS Class I drugs had no food effect, 71% of Class II had a positive food effect, and 61% of BCS Class III had an adverse food effect [88]. Additionally, there is evidence of reduced drug absorption in rats when metoprolol was perfused in aspirated fed state intestinal fluids compared to fasted state aspirates [89]. Absorption of selected PE active combinations were reduced in FeSSIF, which the authors attributed to the presence of colloidal structures formed by lecithin and bile acids in FeSSIF (Roos et al., submitted). Surfactant PEs have potential to emulsify dietary lipids and can form mixed micelles with both soluble (e.g., bile salts, ionized free fatty acids) and insoluble surfactant (glycerides, phospholipids), and as the CMC of these mixed micelles is typically lower than the native surfactant, these structures are capable of lowering the sufficient quantity of free monomeric surfactant that is available to perturb membranes. A conclusion is that luminal surfactants can exert a protective effect against mucosal perturbation by ionizable surfactants. It is noteworthy that the presence of a luminal surfactant does not change the CMC of the PE, so if there is a large excess of PE over the luminal surfactants, it will exist in the molecular form at its CMC and will therefore be available to exhibit transcellular perturbation.

Further work is required to determine the effect of luminal composition on the absorption of soluble macromolecules and the enhancement action of PEs. A question arising from studies showing the effect of luminal constituents on PE actions is what constitutes the typical composition within the GI tract? Given the variability in free fatty acid, lipids, and bile salts in human intestinal fluid [90], it may be difficult to precisely identify the type and amount of substances that must be included in the SIF for permeability studies. Additionally, it remains unclear whether there is a substantial difference in the concentration and type of constituents in bulk luminal fluid and local extrinsic mucus gel layer.

Therefore, it is also unclear if SIF for permeability testing should represent bulk luminal fluid (and hence mirror dissolution media), or whether it should mirror the composition of the extrinsic mucus gel layer. In addition, it is difficult to use SIFs designed for dissolution testing [91] in cell- or tissue-based in vitro assays, as several constituents of intestinal fluid (e.g., bile acids, phospholipids, and free fatty acids) are themselves capable of altering permeability and causing local perturbation. There have been efforts to develop biorelevant media that do not alter the viability or barrier integrity of Caco-2 monolayers over short periods [92]. By necessity there are reductions in the concentrations of bile salts in the SIF used in vitro compared to intestinal aspirates (e.g., free fatty acids). Other investigators have opted to use full biorelevant media and overcome damage to Caco-2 monolayers using overlying biosimilar mucus [93,94]. It may be that studies with SIF should begin with more robust in situ models such as the rat single pass intestinal perfusion [83,95,96]. More research assessing the effect of PEs in SIF would also help investigators understand how a growing number of lipoidal dispersions improve intestinal permeability (e.g., TPE™, Chiasma, Ness Ziona, Israel [17]).

4.10. Improving PE Action in the Dynamic GI Tract

Of those PE that have been assessed in oral formulation of macromolecules in clinical trials, only a modest single digit increase in oral BA has ever been observed. The majority of PEs are effective in static delivery models, where the PE and active are co-delivered in liquid dosage forms to cells, isolated tissues or tied intestinal loops for extended periods. In these models, the PE and active are typically presented to the epithelial surface above a threshold concentration for an extended period of several hours. This provides the PE sufficient time to alter barrier integrity in the presence of a high concentration gradient of both macromolecule and PE. These optimal conditions do not prevail in the human GI tract following oral delivery of a solid dosage form (Figure 2).

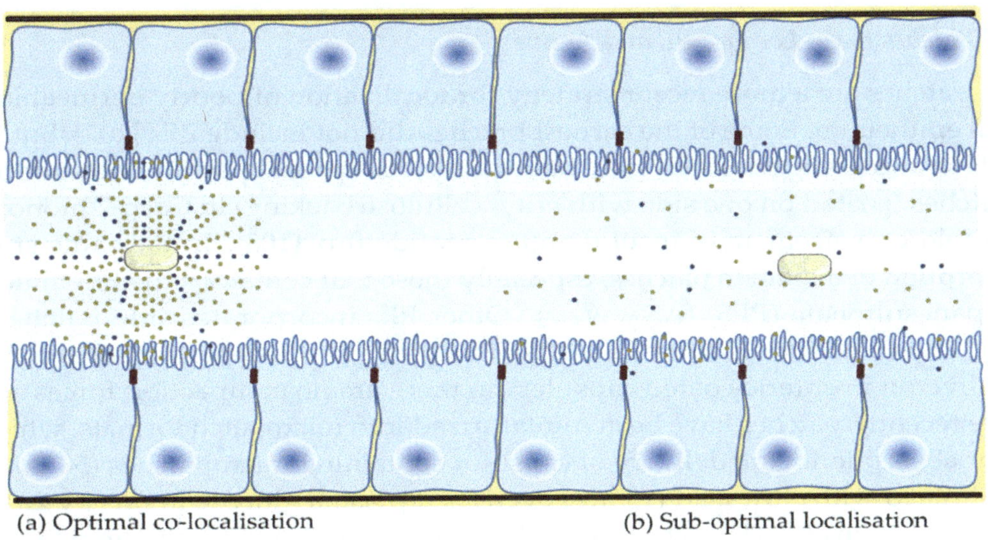

(a) Optimal co-localisation (b) Sub-optimal localisation

Figure 2. Presentation of PE and active at the small intestinal mucosa. (**a**) Co-localization of PE and active at the intestinal epithelium ensures that the PE is present at a high concentration and is present for long enough to alter barrier integrity. (**b**) A high local concentration of active provides the drive force for intestinal flux. A low release rate and more gradual dissolution of PE dosage forms, fast transit, spreading and dilution in luminal fluid and interaction with constituents of luminal fluid will impede optimal co-localization because the concentration of both are ultimately not high enough.

Few published studies assess the effect of PEs in oral dosage forms. The majority of oral peptide dosage forms in clinical development are enteric coated, and so that active and PE are co-released in the small intestine. Relatively quick transit along the small intestine attenuates enhancement in the GI lumen as the PE requires time at a focal point within the lumen to alter integrity and facilitate permeation of the macromolecule, while not being too rapidly absorbed itself (as is the case with C_{10}

and SNAC). This is problematic for all PEs, in particular, those that do not cause a rapid decrease in barrier integrity. Investigators have shown that confining PE and macromolecule over a focussed area [97] and the synchronous co-release of both in high concentration in a short period [78,98,99] can improve enhancement. The fluid volume within the stomach and small intestine is another potential variable. Intestinal fluid is not homogeneously spread across the small intestine, it forms fluid-filled pockets of varying number and volume [100], which may give rise to variable absorption. This is because dissolution of PE in a small volume will lead to greater enhancement action than if the PE is dissolved in a larger fluid volume. As there has been little research assessing the effect of release metrics on permeability, it follows that few delivery technologies have been developed to improve localization of PE and active at the intestinal epithelium. Initial experimental strategies tested include mucoadhesives, superporous hydrogels [101], electronic capsules (e.g., IntelliCap™ [102]), controlled release of PE [98,103,104], intestinal patches (Section 4.11) and pharmacological motility (e.g., loperamide). Overall, the goal of optimizing co-presentation aims to create a diffusion gradient to improve the rate and extent of enhancement action and all PEs to reach and sustain a threshold concentration required to improve intestinal flux.

Dissolution of the PE and active is another factor that must be considered for effective translation. Peptides often exhibit their lowest solubility at the isoelectric point (pI) and greatest solubility at pH values below the pI owing to ionization of basic side chains in acidic conditions. Insulin (pI 5.5) for example, dissolves well in acidic media, but has low solubility at neutral pH. Peptides with low potency and low intrinsic solubility may dissolve more slowly in the small intestine, which may lower the concentration gradient that drives flux. Gradual dissolution may prevent a PE from reaching and sustaining a threshold local concentration for enhancement (e.g., chitosan [105], medium chain fatty acids [106]). Investigators have attempted to improve release through the inclusion of disintegrants [97], or via formulation as liquids [46].

4.11. Intestinal Patches to Co-Localise PE and Active

Intestinal patches are a more recent strategy for localization of poorly permeable solutes at the small intestinal epithelium. Some of the earliest patches did not include PEs [107], but their inclusion in more recent iterations suggests they may be required for optimal patch performance. Assessment of a 13 mm patches (coated on one side with ethyl cellulose backing) in Caco-2 monolayers showed a modest two-fold enhancement of insulin and exenatide flux [108]. In the same study, there was significant absorption of insulin in patches, especially those that contained the PE, dimethyl palmitoyl ammonio propanesulfonate (PPS) (0.5% w/v). Other PEs incorporated into patches include SDS, polyoxyethylene hydrogenated castor oil 60 [109], thiolated polycarbophils [110] and Labrasol® [111]. Patches are delivered in enteric-coated capsules, so there are no compaction forces associated with tableting. More recently, patches have been miniaturized into micropatch formats, which offer a large surface area for absorption. Oral delivery of capsules containing micropatches (50 U/kg insulin and 0.2 mg PPS) admixed with citric acid (15 mg) decreased plasma glucose in rats by 22% compared to a drop of 54% with free insulin (1 U/kg, s.c.) [112]. Further optimization is required to ensure adequate adhesion within the GI tract and optimal retention at the mucosal surface.

4.12. Is Safety of PEs a Real Impediment to Translation?

Safety is a widely held concern to the application of PEs in oral delivery (reviewed in [113]). This concern can be sub-categorized into those related to individual or sub-classes of compounds and concerns relating to modulation of intestinal barrier integrity on a chronic basis. Over 250 compounds have been shown to alter intestinal permeability, but only about a dozen of these are realistic candidate PEs for clinical trials. The reversible modulation of TJ opening might be viewed as a safer approach to improving permeation relative to transcellular membrane perturbation.

The first-generation TJ modulators acted via intracellular cell signaling pathways which alter TJ architecture from within epithelial cells. There are risks related to PEs that alter permeability through ubiquitous cell signaling processes such as protein kinase C [114]. Although additional pharmacological effects observed with currently 'allowed' excipients, this is secondary to a primary action, examples including depression of the CNS (e.g., ethyl alcohol), inhibition of metabolic enzymes and transporters (D-alpha-tocopherol polyethylene glycol 1000 succinate [115], and Cremophor EL [116]) and interference with metabolic enzymes [116]. Most second-generation paracellular PEs selectively disrupt the interaction between TJ proteins in adjacent cells [8], although the consequences of modulating TJ at other barriers is not yet entirely clear [9].

The alternative is to use surfactant-based PEs that increase permeation via transcellular perturbation. High concentrations of these additives often cause temporary mild local mucosal injury, but when diluted are less likely to reach the high concentrations required for cell perturbation at other sites within the body even if absorbed. Additionally, some leading candidates in this category have food additive (e.g., C_{10}) or GRAS status (e.g., SNAC) or are pharmaceutical excipients (e.g., sucrose esters). There may be a relatively low risk of systemic toxicity for such surfactants, although there are ongoing concerns related to local mucosal perturbation. The majority of evidence to date suggests that surfactant PEs do not possess a discrete mechanism of action; instead they act by directly compromising the integrity of enterocyte plasma membranes. This category of PE has been assessed extensively in clinical trials over the last 20 years, and while there have been no major adverse events reported, there has also been only a modest effect on oral BA in most trials. It remains to be seen if new technologies designed to improve residence of PE and active at a focal point within the intestinal lumen may result in more histological damage. It is difficult to determine if PEs cause histological damage at the site of release in the human GI tract, owing to difficulty pinpointing the site of release and performing a biopsy within the enhancement window and before epithelial repair. In one of the few clinical trials assessing the effect of PEs on histology score within the GI tract, administration of Doktacillin™ suppositories (ampicillin (250 mg), C_{10} (25 mg) and hard fat (950 mg, Pharmasol™ B-105, NOF Corp. Shibuya-ku, Tokyo, Japan)) improved rectal BA of ampicillin from 13 to 23% [117]. Doktacillin™ suppositories caused a significant increase in the average histology score from 0.62 in the control group (before administration) to a score of 1.94 after administration of the suppository (25 min). The average histology score measured three hours after administration of Doktacillin™ was 0.96, suggesting the barrier can repair from mucosal perturbation. The authors note that C_{10} itself and hyperosmolarity of the rectal fluid contribute to the histological damage score. Irrespective of whether C_{10} causes hyperosmolarity, exposure time in the rectum is longer than any equivalent segment of the small intestine owing to longer residence time. There is also a higher concentration of PE due to a lower amount of rectal fluid than in other intestinal segments. To allay fears over chronic daily use of PEs, some may be confined to administrations with a different dosing regimen. Some PE formulations tested in trials include for example, a once-weekly tablet zoledronic acid with C_{10} (Orazol®, Merrion Pharma, Ireland [118]), which would provide time for recovery of barrier integrity. Nonetheless, time to recovery from PEs that cause mild mucosal perturbation does not seem to be a problem in clinical trials so far (e.g., daily administration of semaglutide with SNAC [28]). To date, there has been no evidence of intestinal problems that are unrelated to the GLP-1 class in any oral semaglutide trials performed.

It is tempting to justify the use of PEs that cause mild reversible mucosal damage by citing precedence for the use of substances that cause GI disturbances. Regarding medicines approval, it is not possible to justify the use of PEs that act to improve flux via transcellular perturbation by citing the side effects of drugs, excipients or food additives. However, a PE may not be listed as such in any given formulation, and therefore their use may be more comparable to other additives that have been shown to cause membrane perturbation in vitro (e.g., surfactants [119]). Comparison of PEs to established excipients does help to show that mild mucosal perturbation may be common.

There is concern that altering the integrity of the intestinal epithelium, irrespective of mode of action, may facilitate colonization of epithelial cells and invasion of deeper tissues by opportunistic pathogens. While there is no evidence to date that oral PE-macromolecule dosage forms cause infections in clinical trials, it is important to mention that if this is true risk, then potential clinical manifestations range from asymptomatic infection to diarrhea, to more serious infections depending on the micro-organism and host genetic variability [120]. This concern would seem to be more plausible for PEs that cause reversible mucosal damage, and not TJ modulators, because the maximum opening of the TJ is far smaller than the diameter of a bacterium [121]. Compromising the integrity of the intestinal mucosae is more likely to facilitate the translation of microorganisms. In Caco-2 monolayers, co-incubation of octyl phenol ethoxylate (Triton X-100) with *E. coli* increased translocation, although whether such translocation occurs in vivo has not been assessed [118].

There is the additional concern that other luminal bystanders may be translocated within the enhancement window. There is evidence that ischemia can increase levels of plasma lipopolysaccharide (LPS) [122] which may contribute to septic shock [123]. Given that PEs cause only a modest uptake of small peptides co-localised in the formulation, it seems unlikely that large luminal xenobiotics (such as LPS or LPS fragments) that are spread diffusely across the GI lumen would be appreciably absorbed. Again, this potential issue may be less likely for PEs that act via the opening of TJs, as the diameter of an open junction within the small intestine is estimated to be 10 nm [84]. It is noteworthy however, that altered expression of the TJ protein claudin is associated with intestinal bowel disorders [124]. The surfactants hexadecylphosphocholine and octylphenol ethoxylate increase permeation of LPS across Caco-2 monolayers [125]. Co-delivery of C_{10} (154 mM) or penetratin (2 mM) with LPS to mice for seven consecutive days did not cause LPS induced hepatic damage, as measured by plasma levels of alanine aminotransferase (ALT) and aspartate aminotransferase (AST) which are both released during hepatic necrosis [126]. A significant elevation in those enzymes was observed when LPS was co-delivered with taurodeoxycholate (96 mM) in the same study. However, as there was no control treatment in the absence of LPS it remains unclear whether elevated levels of hepatic necrosis markers relate to LPS or PE only. There is also evidence from a controversial study that prolonged exposure of two common emulsifiers (polysorbate 80 and carboxymethyl cellulose) causes low-grade inflammation in healthy mice and colitis in predisposed mice via altering the microbiome [127]. It is not known if these findings have any relevance for human exposure to excipients.

4.13. Convergence between Delivery Concepts, Intestinal Physiology, and Formulation Science

In order to address the hurdles to translation, there must be convergence between delivery concepts, intestinal physiology, and formulation. The material and physicochemical properties of the PE must be considered more; especially as PEs can be a significant proportion of the formulations. As noted in Section 4.6, it can be challenging to incorporate liquid or semi-solid PEs into oral dosage forms. Salts of ionizable surfactants are more readily incorporated into tablets. However, there remains the likely requirement for other excipients in the formulation, which in some instances may require a reduction in the quantity of PE to accommodate these additives. The type of formulation and process additives and their quantity in the final manufacturable scalable dosage form are important considerations as delivery researchers begin to assess optimal luminal presentation, be it for immediate release or controlled release. There are also practical considerations in the progression of PEs to clinical testing, such as availability of GMP grade material or a specification. There is the requirement for extensive information in any regulatory submission, including details of manufacture and purification procedures, extensive physical and chemical properties of any new PE and provision of supporting safety data (non-clinical/clinical).

Reliable animal models are prerequisite for identification of promising macromolecule drug delivery systems that have potential to translate to humans. There is variability between key anatomical and physiological parameters in humans and those observed in rats, pigs and dogs (Table 3). These include differences in gastric emptying time, gastric retention time, absolute water content, transit time, local pH, gut length, mucous thickness, and average stomach capacity [128,129]. It is possible to purchase minicapsules and manufacture minitablets for oral delivery to rats, but there are additional challenges. In the case of minicapsules it can be difficult to load sufficient levels of PE into the capsule shell without prior granulation (e.g., by roll compaction) and these formulations are difficult to enteric coat by manual dip coating (thus necessitating the use of specialist coating equipment). It is possible to purchase single- or multi-tip tooling for the preparation of minitablets, although this requires specialist tableting equipment (granulator, spray coater, and tablet press) and expertise in formulation and process development. There are very few studies where complete dosage forms are administered to rodents, and therefore the formulation factors that impact translation are rarely assessed in this widely used animal model. There is the argument that formulations administered to rats have little relevance to formats tested in larger animals and humans, and there is therefore a need for studies in more representative animals and humans. Nevertheless, if the impediments to translation of PE dosage forms can be partially optimized in rodent models, this could better inform development of formulations in humans. Oral peptide research in rodents typically involves oral gavage of liquid mixtures and not dosage forms tested in humans. This is the same for rat in situ static intestinal instillations, which help identify PEs in ad-mixtures with payloads, but do not offer information on transit time, fluid volume, pH conditions within the small intestine nor do they adequately model dissolution of PE dosage forms. Hence, translation of results from rats to humans is limited by fundamental anatomical and physiological differences in intestinal length (1.8 m versus 5.9 m [128]), transit time in the fed (20 h versus 4 h [130]) and water volume (0.06 g/cm gut length versus 0.58 g/cm [130]).

Dosage forms of similar dimensions to those used in humans are amenable to administration in dogs and pigs. However, as there are longer gastric emptying times in these animals, immediate release PE dosage forms intended to increase flux within the stomach (e.g., semaglutide) could be more effective in dogs and pigs owing to greater residence time (localization of PE and active), although such data may not be replicated in humans due to shorter residence times. In the case of enteric coated macromolecule formulations, longer gastric emptying times in pigs and dogs may result in a longer delay to onset of drug absorption compared to humans. The pH in the stomach of healthy fasted dogs is highly variable (pH 1–8) [129,131], leading some investigators to pre-administer an acidic solution containing 0.1 M HCl and 0.1 M KCl [132] or the hormone pentagastrin to stimulate endogenous acid secretion [133]. Both approaches aim to standardize the pH prior to oral administration to animals. In the absence of pH adjustment, the stomach of dogs may not adequately model release of enteric-coated oral peptide formulations. In the small intestine, transit time is shorter by half in dogs compared to humans and pigs. Faster transit reduces the absorption window for drugs, which gives rise to differences in oral BA. As the importance of local GI retention of PE and macromolecule is requisite for efficient enhancement, study of PEs in dogs may underestimate the action of these additives. Further interspecies divergence is observed at the intestinal epithelium, where mucous thickness is appreciably larger in dogs compared to humans. The anatomy physiology and diet of pigs closely aligns to humans [134], and in some aspects (but not all aspects, e.g., gastric residence time) pigs are considered an appropriate model to assess GI permeability [133]. The composition of enterocyte membranes in different animal models [128] could also play a role in different susceptibility to surfactant PEs [9]. It is also worth emphasizing that there can be differences in GI physiology in different disease states [135], which could also influence the action of PEs.

Interspecies differences highlight that the best model of human is human [136], nevertheless combinations of animal models are still relevant for optimization of oral PE macromolecule formulations and ultimately translation into effective dosage forms in man. Although most oral peptide formulations fail to progress to clinical evaluation, poor translation between animal models and humans is likely to be one of many reasons. There is nearly always higher BA in open- and closed-loop instillations and single pass intestinal perfusion compared to oral dosage forms, but these models still provide a necessary first hurdle with a relatively low bar; it is then the challenge for formulation and delivery researchers to develop technologies that recreate such presentation in appropriate oral dosage forms.

Table 3. Potential effects of GI physiology in different animals on the action of PEs.

Anatomical/Physiological Property	Species	Influence on PE Action
Gastric emptying time (h)	Human: 1 h [130] Rat: 0.7–2.1 h [130] Dog: 3.9–5.3 h [130] Pig: 1.5–6 h [130]	For immediate release dosage forms, slower gastric emptying in pig and dog than in humans may increase gastric residence time of PE and payload, thus overestimating enhancement. For enteric dosage forms, slower gastric emptying, may delay dissolution in the GI tract and ultimately increase Tmax in these species versus humans.
Gastric fluid volume (mL)	Human: 118 mL [137] Rat: 2.29 [137] Dog: 500–1000 mL [137] Pig: 278 mL [137]	For immediate release dosage forms, the larger volume in dogs may result in greater dilution of PE to below a threshold for enhancement action, thereby underestimating enhancement.
Stomach pH	Human: 1.7 [128] Rat: 3.9 [138] Dog: 1.5 [128] Pig: 1.7 [128]	As many PEs that have progressed to clinical testing in oral formulations are weak acid surfactants, differences in solubility can be observed if there is variation in gastric pH. This gives rise to differences in enhancement as acidic surfactants are more effective in their ionizable form at high pH.
Small intestine transit time (Fasted state) (time (h) and length (m))	Human: 3–4 h [139] Human: 6.25 m [137] Rat: 4–5 h [128] Rat: 0.34 m [137] Dog: 1.5 h [137] Dog: 2.48 m [137] Pig: 3–4 h [137] Pig: 14.2 m [137]	Faster transit may reduce the exposure of PE and payload at the epithelium, thereby reducing enhancement, and potentially underestimating the effects of the PE. A short transit time does not strictly mean faster movement, as length of the small intestine is different in different species.
Small intestine fluid volume (total and g/cm)	Human: 212 mL [137] Human: 0.6 g/cm [130] Rat: 3.9 mL [137] Rat: 0.06 g/cm [130] Dog: 300 mL [137] Dog: 0.9 [130] Pig: 476 mL [137] Pig: 0.62 [130]	Differences in fluid volume, or more specifically the volume and number of intestinal fluid pockets in the small intestine could lead to differences in the regional concentration of PE and payload, as well as differences in dissolution rate. This could lead to under- or overestimation of enhancement.
Duodenal mucus thickness (μm)	Human: 15.5 μm [137] Rat: 30.6 μm [137] Dog: — Pig: 25.6 μm [137]	Difference in the thickness of the protective mucus gel layer overlying the epithelium has potential to modulate enhancement.
Small intestine diameter	Human: 5 cm [137] Rat: 2.5–3 mm [137] Dog: — Pig: —	The diameter of the intestinal lumen may impact the proximity of enteric formulations to the epithelium and ultimately impact co-localization of PE and payload.
Plasma membrane phospholipid composition of intestinal epithelium	Human: — Rat: — Dog: — Pig: —	There are differences in phospholipid composition in different species [128], which may impact sensitivity to perturbation by surfactant PEs

5. Conclusions

Discovery of safe, effective, and formulation-compatible PEs for oral delivery of macromolecules has been a priority for investigators. Research on PEs has branched into the discovery of agents that target opening of TJs [47] or using substances with established use in humans [106]. Recent studies have examined (i) the behavior of PEs and acidifiers in the intestinal lumen, (ii) factors that impact enhancement within the dynamic environment in the GI tract in vivo (e.g., intestinal fluid, tonicity, exposure time), (iii) physiochemical properties of PEs that give rise to enhancement, (iv) effect of PE combinations, and (v) learnings from clinical investigations [140,141]. These studies have highlighted the need for greater emphasis on the hurdles to translation, in particular, development of concepts to optimize the co-presentation of PE and macromolecule payload in high concentration for as long as possible at the intestinal wall. Greater focus on this area may improve the likelihood of translation.

Acknowledgments: The research performed in Figure 1 and Table 2 was performed by an Erasmus Exchange student (Ninon Chardon).

References

1. Kola, I.; Landis, J. Can the pharmaceutical industry reduce attrition rates? *Nat. Rev. Drug Discov.* **2004**, *3*, 711. [CrossRef] [PubMed]
2. Waring, M.J.; Arrowsmith, J.; Leach, A.R.; Leeson, P.D.; Mandrell, S.; Owen, R.M.; Pairaudeau, G.; Pennie, W.D.; Pickett, S.D.; Wang, J.; et al. An analysis of the attrition of drug candidates from four major pharmaceutical companies. *Nat. Rev. Drug Discov.* **2015**, *14*, 475–486. [CrossRef] [PubMed]
3. Barton, P.; Riley, R.J. A new paradigm for navigating compound property related drug attrition. *Drug Discov. Today* **2016**, *21*, 72–81. [CrossRef]
4. Leeson, P.D. Molecular inflation, attrition and the rule of five. *Adv. Drug Deliv. Rev.* **2016**, *101*, 22–33. [CrossRef] [PubMed]
5. Crew, M.; Lipinski, C. Where to Invest? The Drug or the Delivery System? American Association of Pharmaceutical Scientists Blog. 2016. Available online: https://aapsblog.aaps.org/2016/11/05/where-to-invest-the-drug-or-the-delivery-system/#more-9226 (accessed on 17 January 2019).
6. Buckley, S. Oral Semaglutide: Delivering new possibilities in the treatment of diabetes. In Proceedings of the Annual Meeting and Exposition of the Controlled Release Society (Oral Peptide Workship), New York, NY, USA, 22–24 July 2018.
7. Maher, S. An Outlook on Oral Peptide Delivery. AAPS Blog. 2017. Available online: https://aapsblog.aaps.org/2017/02/08/an-outlook-on-oral-peptide-delivery/#more-9531 (accessed on 17 January 2019).
8. Kondoh, M.; Yoshida, T.; Kakutani, H.; Yagi, K. Targeting tight junction proteins-significance for drug development. *Drug Discov. Today* **2008**, *13*, 180–186. [CrossRef] [PubMed]
9. Maher, S.; Mrsny, R.J.; Brayden, D.J. Intestinal Permeation Enhancers for Oral Peptide Delivery. *Adv. Drug Deliv. Rev.* **2016**, *106*, 277–319. [CrossRef] [PubMed]
10. Eichner, M.; Protze, J.; Piontek, A.; Krause, G.; Piontek, J. Targeting and alteration of tight junctions by bacteria and their virulence factors such as Clostridium perfringens enterotoxin. *Pflügers Arch. Eur. J. Physiol.* **2017**, *469*, 77–90. [CrossRef] [PubMed]
11. Eldor, R.; Arbit, E.; Corcos, A.; Kidron, M. Glucose-reducing effect of the ORMD-0801 oral insulin preparation in patients with uncontrolled type 1 diabetes: A pilot study. *PLoS ONE* **2013**, *8*, e59524. [CrossRef]
12. Zupančič, O.; Bernkop-Schnürch, A. Lipophilic peptide character—What oral barriers fear the most. *J. Control. Release* **2017**, *255*, 242–257. [CrossRef]
13. Maher, S.; Heade, J.; McCartney, F.; Waters, S.; Bleiel, S.B.; Brayden, D.J. Effects of surfactant-based permeation enhancers on mannitol permeability, histology, and electrogenic ion transport responses in excised rat colonic mucosae. *Int. J. Pharm.* **2018**, *539*, 11–22. [CrossRef]
14. Perinelli, D.R.; Cespi, M.; Casettari, L.; Vllasaliu, D.; Cangiotti, M.; Ottaviani, M.F.; Giorgioni, G.; Bonacucina, G.; Palmieri, G.F. Correlation among chemical structure, surface properties and cytotoxicity of N-acyl alanine and serine surfactants. *Eur. J. Pharm. Biopharm.* **2016**, *109*, 93–102. [CrossRef] [PubMed]
15. Lee, Y.-H.; Sinko, P.J. Oral delivery of salmon calcitonin. *Adv. Drug Deliv. Rev.* **2000**, *42*, 225–238. [CrossRef]
16. Leonard, T.W.; Lynch, J.; McKenna, M.J.; Brayden, D.J. Promoting absorption of drugs in humans using medium-chain fatty acid-based solid dosage forms: GIPET. *Expert Opin. Drug Deliv.* **2006**, *3*, 685–692. [CrossRef]
17. Tuvia, S.; Pelled, D.; Marom, K.; Salama, P.; Levin-Arama, M.; Karmeli, I.; Idelson, G.H.; Landau, I.; Mamluk, R. A novel suspension formulation enhances intestinal absorption of macromolecules via transient and reversible transport mechanisms. *Pharm. Res.* **2014**, *31*, 2010–2021. [CrossRef] [PubMed]
18. Khedkar, A.; Iyer, H.; Anand, A.; Verma, M.; Krishnamurthy, S.; Savale, S.; Atignal, A. A dose range finding study of novel oral insulin (IN-105) under fed conditions in type 2 diabetes mellitus subjects. *Diabetes Obes. Metab.* **2010**, *12*, 659–664. [CrossRef] [PubMed]
19. Cilek, A.; Celebi, N.; Tirnaksiz, F. Lecithin-based microemulsion of a peptide for oral administration: Preparation, characterization, and physical stability of the formulation. *Drug Deliv.* **2006**, *13*, 19–24. [CrossRef]
20. Blikslager, A.T.; Moeser, A.J.; Gookin, J.L.; Jones, S.L.; Odle, J. Restoration of barrier function in injured intestinal mucosa. *Physiol. Rev.* **2007**, *87*, 545–564. [CrossRef]

21. Brayden, D.J.; Gleeson, J.; Walsh, E.G. A head-to-head multi-parametric high content analysis of a series of medium chain fatty acid intestinal permeation enhancers in Caco-2 cells. *Eur. J. Pharm. Biopharm.* **2014**, *88*, 830–839. [CrossRef]
22. Matsuura, J.; Powers, M.E.; Manning, M.C.; Shefter, E. Structure and stability of insulin dissolved in 1-octanol. *J. Am. Chem. Soc.* **1993**, *115*, 1261–1264. [CrossRef]
23. Zupancic, O.; Leonaviciute, G.; Lam, H.T.; Partenhauser, A.; Podricnik, S.; Bernkop-Schnurch, A. Development and in vitro evaluation of an oral SEDDS for desmopressin. *Drug Deliv.* **2016**, *23*, 2074–2083. [CrossRef]
24. Bonengel, S.; Jelkmann, M.; Abdulkarim, M.; Gumbleton, M.; Reinstadler, V.; Oberacher, H.; Prufert, F.; Bernkop-Schnurch, A. Impact of different hydrophobic ion pairs of octreotide on its oral bioavailability in pigs. *J. Control. Release* **2018**, *273*, 21–29. [CrossRef] [PubMed]
25. Menzel, C.; Holzeisen, T.; Laffleur, F.; Zaichik, S.; Abdulkarim, M.; Gumbleton, M.; Bernkop-Schnurch, A. In vivo evaluation of an oral self-emulsifying drug delivery system (SEDDS) for exenatide. *J. Control. Release* **2018**, *277*, 165–172. [CrossRef] [PubMed]
26. Goldberg, M.; Gomez-Orellana, I. Challenges for the oral delivery of macromolecules. *Nat. Rev. Drug Discov.* **2003**, *2*, 289–295. [CrossRef] [PubMed]
27. Castelli, M.C.; Friedman, K.; Sherry, J.; Brazzillo, K.; Genoble, L.; Bhargava, P.; Riley, M.G.I. Comparing the Efficacy and Tolerability of a New Daily Oral Vitamin B12 Formulation and Intermittent Intramuscular Vitamin B12 in Normalizing Low Cobalamin Levels: A Randomized, Open-Label, Parallel-Group Study. *Clin. Ther.* **2011**, *33*, 358–371. [CrossRef] [PubMed]
28. Davies, M.; Pieber, T.R.; Hartoft-Nielsen, M.L.; Hansen, O.K.H.; Jabbour, S.; Rosenstock, J. Effect of Oral Semaglutide Compared With Placebo and Subcutaneous Semaglutide on Glycemic Control in Patients With Type 2 Diabetes: A Randomized Clinical Trial. *JAMA* **2017**, *318*, 1460–1470. [CrossRef] [PubMed]
29. Karsdal, M.A.; Byrjalsen, I.; Alexandersen, P.; Bihlet, A.; Andersen, J.R.; Riis, B.J.; Bay-Jensen, A.C.; Christiansen, C. Treatment of symptomatic knee osteoarthritis with oral salmon calcitonin: Results from two phase 3 trials. *Osteoarthr. Cartil.* **2015**, *23*, 532–543. [CrossRef] [PubMed]
30. Lindgren, M.E.; Hallbrink, M.M.; Elmquist, A.M.; Langel, U. Passage of cell-penetrating peptides across a human epithelial cell layer in vitro. *Biochem. J.* **2004**, *377*, 69–76. [CrossRef]
31. Kamei, N.; Shigei, C.; Hasegawa, R.; Takeda-Morishita, M. Exploration of the Key Factors for Optimizing the in Vivo Oral Delivery of Insulin by Using a Noncovalent Strategy with Cell-Penetrating Peptides. *Biol. Pharm. Bull.* **2018**, *41*, 239–246. [CrossRef]
32. Guidotti, G.; Brambilla, L.; Rossi, D. Cell-Penetrating Peptides: From Basic Research to Clinics. *Trends Pharmacol. Sci.* **2017**, *38*, 406–424. [CrossRef]
33. Rehmani, S.; Dixon, J.E. Oral delivery of anti-diabetes therapeutics using cell penetrating and transcytosing peptide strategies. *Peptides* **2018**, *100*, 24–35. [CrossRef]
34. Lewis, A.L.; Richard, J. Challenges in the delivery of peptide drugs: An industry perspective. *Ther. Deliv.* **2015**, *6*, 149–163. [CrossRef] [PubMed]
35. Dhillon, S. Semaglutide: First Global Approval. *Drugs* **2018**, *78*, 275–284. [CrossRef] [PubMed]
36. Feeney, O.M.; Crum, M.F.; McEvoy, C.L.; Trevaskis, N.L.; Williams, H.D.; Pouton, C.W.; Charman, W.N.; Bergström, C.A.S.; Porter, C.J.H. 50 years of oral lipid-based formulations: Provenance, progress and future perspectives. *Adv. Drug Deliv. Rev.* **2016**, *101*, 167–194. [CrossRef] [PubMed]
37. Benet, L.Z.; Cummins, C.L. The drug efflux-metabolism alliance: Biochemical aspects. *Adv. Drug Deliv. Rev.* **2001**, *50* (Suppl. 1), S3–S11. [CrossRef]
38. Maher, S.; Ryan, B.; Duffy, A.; Brayden, D.J. Formulation strategies to improve oral peptide delivery. *Pharm. Pat. Anal.* **2014**, *3*, 313–336. [CrossRef]
39. Mahmood, A.; Bernkop-Schnurch, A. SEDDS: A game changing approach for the oral administration of hydrophilic macromolecular drugs. *Adv. Drug Deliv. Rev.* **2018**. [CrossRef] [PubMed]
40. Cheng, T.; Zhao, Y.; Li, X.; Lin, F.; Xu, Y.; Zhang, X.; Li, Y.; Wang, R.; Lai, L. Computation of Octanol−Water Partition Coefficients by Guiding an Additive Model with Knowledge. *J. Chem. Inf. Model.* **2007**, *47*, 2140–2148. [CrossRef]
41. Buckley, S.T.; Bækdal, T.A.; Vegge, A.; Maarbjerg, S.J.; Pyke, C.; Ahnfelt-Rønne, J.; Madsen, K.G.; Schéele, S.G.; Alanentalo, T.; Kirk, R.K.; et al. Transcellular stomach absorption of a derivatized glucagon-like peptide-1 receptor agonist. *Sci. Transl. Med.* **2018**, *10*, eaar7047. [CrossRef]

42. Novo Nordisk AS. Tablet Formulation Comprising Semaglutide and a Delivery Agent. U.S. Patent US9993430B2, 12 June 2018.
43. Hjerpsted, J.B.; Flint, A.; Brooks, A.; Axelsen, M.B.; Kvist, T.; Blundell, J. Semaglutide improves postprandial glucose and lipid metabolism, and delays first-hour gastric emptying in subjects with obesity. *Diabetes Obes. Metab.* **2018**, *20*, 610–619. [CrossRef]
44. Banerjee, A.; Ibsen, K.; Brown, T.; Chen, R.; Agatemor, C.; Mitragotri, S. Ionic liquids for oral insulin delivery. *Proc. Natl. Acad. Sci. USA* **2018**, *115*, 7296–7301. [CrossRef]
45. Frade, R.F.M.; Matias, A.; Branco, L.C.; Afonso, C.A.M.; Duarte, C.M.M. Effect of ionic liquids on human colon carcinoma HT-29 and CaCo-2 cell lines. *Green Chem.* **2007**, *9*, 873–877. [CrossRef]
46. Novo Nordisk AS. Stable Non-Aqueous Pharmaceutical Compositions. U.S. Patent US20100190706, 29 July 2010.
47. Taverner, A.; Dondi, R.; Almansour, K.; Laurent, F.; Owens, S.E.; Eggleston, I.M.; Fotaki, N.; Mrsny, R.J. Enhanced paracellular transport of insulin can be achieved via transient induction of myosin light chain phosphorylation. *J. Control. Release* **2015**, *210*, 189–197. [CrossRef]
48. Almansour, K.; Taverner, A.; Eggleston, I.M.; Mrsny, R.J. Mechanistic studies of a cell-permeant peptide designed to enhance myosin light chain phosphorylation in polarized intestinal epithelia. *J. Control. Release* **2018**, *279*, 208–219. [CrossRef] [PubMed]
49. Almansour, K.; Taverner, A.; Turner, J.R.; Eggleston, I.M.; Mrsny, R.J. An intestinal paracellular pathway biased toward positively-charged macromolecules. *J. Control. Release* **2018**, *288*, 111–125. [CrossRef] [PubMed]
50. Date, A.A.; Hanes, J.; Ensign, L.M. Nanoparticles for oral delivery: Design, evaluation and state-of-the-art. *J. Control. Release* **2016**, *240*, 504–526. [CrossRef] [PubMed]
51. Maher, S.; Ryan, K.B.; Ahmad, T.; O'Driscoll, C.M.; Brayden, D.J. Chapter 2.1 Nanostructures Overcoming the Intestinal Barrier: Physiological Considerations and Mechanistic Issues. In *Nanostructured Biomaterials for Overcoming Biological Barriers*; The Royal Society of Chemistry: London, UK, 2012; pp. 39–62. [CrossRef]
52. Brayden, S. Oral Peptide Delivery: The Potential of Combining Nanoparticle Constructs with Permeation Enhancers. In Proceedings of the Annual Meeting and Exposition of the Controlled Release Society, New York City, NY, USA, 22–24 July 2018.
53. Alonso, J.M. Learning from the EU TRANS-INT consortium: Oral peptide formulations using nanotechnologies. In Proceedings of the Annual Meeting and Exposition of the Controlled Release Society, New York City, NY, USA, 22–24 July 2018.
54. Gonçalves, R.F.S.; Martins, J.T.; Duarte, C.M.M.; Vicente, A.A.; Pinheiro, A.C. Advances in nutraceutical delivery systems: From formulation design for bioavailability enhancement to efficacy and safety evaluation. *Trends Food Sci. Technol.* **2018**, *78*, 270–291. [CrossRef]
55. Thanou, M.; Verhoef, J.C.; Junginger, H.E. Chitosan and its derivatives as intestinal absorption enhancers. *Adv. Drug Deliv. Rev.* **2001**, *50* (Suppl. 1), S91–S101. [CrossRef]
56. Onishi, H.; Imura, Y.; Uchida, M.; Machida, Y. Enhancement potential of sucrose laurate (L-1695) on intestinal absorption of water-soluble high molecular weight compounds. *Curr. Drug Deliv.* **2012**, *9*, 487–494. [CrossRef]
57. Lucarini, S.; Fagioli, L.; Campana, R.; Cole, H.; Duranti, A.; Baffone, W.; Vllasaliu, D.; Casettari, L. Unsaturated fatty acids lactose esters: Cytotoxicity, permeability enhancement and antimicrobial activity. *Eur. J. Pharm. Biopharm.* **2016**, *107*, 88–96. [CrossRef]
58. Dimitrijevic, D.; Shaw, A.J.; Florence, A.T. Effects of some non-ionic surfactants on transepithelial permeability in Caco-2 cells. *J. Pharm. Pharmacol.* **2000**, *52*, 157–162. [CrossRef]
59. Gleeson, J.P.; Frías, J.M.; Ryan, S.M.; Brayden, D.J. Sodium caprate enables the blood pressure-lowering effect of Ile-Pro-Pro and Leu-Lys-Pro in spontaneously hypertensive rats by indirectly overcoming PepT1 inhibition. *Eur. J. Pharm. Biopharm.* **2018**, *128*, 179–187. [CrossRef] [PubMed]
60. Moghimipour, E.; Ameri, A.; Handali, S. Absorption-Enhancing Effects of Bile Salts. *Molecules* **2015**, *20*, 14451–14473. [CrossRef] [PubMed]
61. Shoba, G.; Joy, D.; Joseph, T.; Majeed, M.; Rajendran, R.; Srinivas, P.S. Influence of piperine on the pharmacokinetics of curcumin in animals and human volunteers. *Planta Med.* **1998**, *64*, 353–356. [CrossRef] [PubMed]

62. Lambert, J.D.; Kwon, S.J.; Ju, J.; Bose, M.; Lee, M.J.; Hong, J.; Hao, X.; Yang, C.S. Effect of genistein on the bioavailability and intestinal cancer chemopreventive activity of (−)-epigallocatechin-3-gallate. *Carcinogenesis* **2008**, *29*, 2019–2024. [CrossRef] [PubMed]
63. McCartney, F.; Rosa, M.; Coulter, I.; Brayden, D.J. A sucrose ester is a novel permeation enhancer using isolated rat colonic mucosae mounted in Ussing chambers. In Proceedings of the Annual Meeting and Exposition of the American Association of Pharmaceutical Scientists (Poster Presentation), San Antonio, TX, USA, 10–14 November 2013.
64. McCartney, F.; Rosa, M.; Coulter, I.; Brayden, D.J. Sucrose laurate is an effective permeation enhancer for insulin: Rat intestinal instillations. In Proceedings of the Annual meeting and Exposition of the Controlled Release Society (Oral Presentation), Boston, MA, USA, 16–19 July 2017.
65. Casettari, L. Ex-vivo evaluation of intestinal permeability-enhancing effects of mono-esterified sugar based surfactants. In Proceedings of the 11th World Meeting on Pharmaceutics, Biopharmaceutics, and Pharmaceutical Technology (Oral Presentation), Granada, Spain, 19–22 March 2017.
66. Maher, S.; Medani, M.; Carballeira, N.N.; Winter, D.C.; Baird, A.W.; Brayden, D.J. Development of a Non-Aqueous Dispersion to Improve Intestinal Epithelial Flux of Poorly Permeable Macromolecules. *AAPS J.* **2017**, *19*, 244–253. [CrossRef] [PubMed]
67. Gradauer, K.; Nishiumi, A.; Unrinin, K.; Higashino, H.; Kataoka, M.; Pedersen, B.L.; Buckley, S.T.; Yamashita, S. Interaction with Mixed Micelles in the Intestine Attenuates the Permeation Enhancing Potential of Alkyl-Maltosides. *Mol. Pharm.* **2015**, *12*, 2245–2253. [CrossRef] [PubMed]
68. Rautio, J.; Kumpulainen, H.; Heimbach, T.; Oliyai, R.; Oh, D.; Jarvinen, T.; Savolainen, J. Prodrugs: Design and clinical applications. *Nat. Rev. Drug Discov.* **2008**, *7*, 255–270. [CrossRef] [PubMed]
69. Sun, S.; Liang, N.; Kawashima, Y.; Xia, D.; Cui, F. Hydrophobic ion pairing of an insulin-sodium deoxycholate complex for oral delivery of insulin. *Int. J. Nanomed.* **2011**, *6*, 3049–3056. [CrossRef]
70. Griesser, J.; Hetenyi, G.; Moser, M.; Demarne, F.; Jannin, V.; Bernkop-Schnurch, A. Hydrophobic ion pairing: Key to highly payloaded self-emulsifying peptide drug delivery systems. *Int. J. Pharm.* **2017**, *520*, 267–274. [CrossRef]
71. Li, P.; Nielsen, H.M.; Fano, M.; Mullertz, A. Preparation and characterization of insulin-surfactant complexes for loading into lipid-based drug delivery systems. *J. Pharm. Sci* **2013**, *102*, 2689–2698. [CrossRef]
72. Hintzen, F.; Laffleur, F.; Sarti, F.; Müller, C.; Bernkop-Schnürch, A. In vitro and ex vivo evaluation of an intestinal permeation enhancing self-microemulsifying drug delivery system (SMEDDS). *J. Drug Deliv. Sci. Technol.* **2013**, *23*, 261–267. [CrossRef]
73. Meyer, J.D.; Manning, M.C. Hydrophobic Ion Pairing: Altering the Solubility Properties of Biomolecules. *Pharm. Res.* **1998**, *15*, 188–193. [CrossRef] [PubMed]
74. Günday Türeli, N.; Türeli, A.E.; Schneider, M. Counter-ion complexes for enhanced drug loading in nanocarriers: Proof-of-concept and beyond. *Int. J. Pharm.* **2016**, *511*, 994–1001. [CrossRef] [PubMed]
75. Krug, S.M.; Amasheh, M.; Dittmann, I.; Christoffel, I.; Fromm, M.; Amasheh, S. Sodium caprate as an enhancer of macromolecule permeation across tricellular tight junctions of intestinal cells. *Biomaterials* **2013**, *34*, 275–282. [CrossRef] [PubMed]
76. Krug, S.M.; Fromm, M.; Günzel, D. Two-Path Impedance Spectroscopy for Measuring Paracellular and Transcellular Epithelial Resistance. *Biophys. J.* **2009**, *97*, 2202–2211. [CrossRef] [PubMed]
77. Koeplinger, K.A. Oral peptide-protein interaction inhibitors (PPI): Excited about cycling. In Proceedings of the Annual meeting and Exposition of the Controlled Release Society (Oral Presentation, Oral Peptide Workshop), New York, NY, USA, 22–24 July 2018.
78. Wang, X.; Maher, S.; Brayden, D.J. Restoration of rat colonic epithelium after in situ intestinal instillation of the absorption promoter, sodium caprate. *Ther. Deliv.* **2010**, *1*, 75–82. [CrossRef] [PubMed]
79. Fasano, A.; Nataro, J.P. Intestinal epithelial tight junctions as targets for enteric bacteria-derived toxins. *Adv. Drug Deliv. Rev.* **2004**, *56*, 795–807. [CrossRef] [PubMed]
80. Fernandez, S.; Jannin, V.; Rodier, J.D.; Ritter, N.; Mahler, B.; Carriere, F. Comparative study on digestive lipase activities on the self emulsifying excipient Labrasol, medium chain glycerides and PEG esters. *Biochim. Biophys. Acta* **2007**, *1771*, 633–640. [CrossRef]
81. Sadhukha, T.; Layek, B.; Prabha, S. Incorporation of lipolysis in monolayer permeability studies of lipid-based oral drug delivery systems. *Drug Deliv. Transl. Res.* **2018**, *8*, 375–386. [CrossRef]

82. Shaw, D.J. *Introduction to Colloid and Surface Chemistry*; Butterworth-Heinemann: Oxford, UK, 1992.
83. Dahlgren, D.; Roos, C.; Lundqvist, A.; Tannergren, C.; Sjoblom, M.; Sjogren, E.; Lennernas, H. Effect of absorption-modifying excipients, hypotonicity, and enteric neural activity in an in vivo model for small intestinal transport. *Int. J. Pharm.* **2018**, *549*, 239–248. [CrossRef]
84. Anderberg, E.K.; Lindmark, T.; Artursson, P. Sodium Caprate Elicits Dilatations in Human Intestinal Tight Junctions and Enhances Drug Absorption by the Paracellular Route. *Pharm. Res.* **1993**, *10*, 857–864. [CrossRef]
85. Tippin, T.K.; Thakker, D.R. Biorelevant refinement of the Caco-2 cell culture model to assess efficacy of paracellular permeability enhancers. *J. Pharm. Sci.* **2008**, *97*, 1977–1992. [CrossRef] [PubMed]
86. Whitehead, K.; Karr, N.; Mitragotri, S. Discovery of synergistic permeation enhancers for oral drug delivery. *J. Control. Release* **2008**, *128*, 128–133. [CrossRef] [PubMed]
87. Heade, J.; Maher, S.; Bleiel, S.B.; Brayden, D.J. Labrasol((R)) and Salts of Medium-Chain Fatty Acids Can Be Combined in Low Concentrations to Increase the Permeability of a Macromolecule Marker Across Isolated Rat Intestinal Mucosae. *J. Pharm. Sci.* **2018**, *107*, 1648–1655. [CrossRef] [PubMed]
88. Gu, C.-H.; Li, H.; Levons, J.; Lentz, K.; Gandhi, R.B.; Raghavan, K.; Smith, R.L. Predicting Effect of Food on Extent of Drug Absorption Based on Physicochemical Properties. *Pharm. Res.* **2007**, *24*, 1118–1130. [CrossRef] [PubMed]
89. Stappaerts, J.; Wuyts, B.; Tack, J.; Annaert, P.; Augustijns, P. Human and simulated intestinal fluids as solvent systems to explore food effects on intestinal solubility and permeability. *Eur. J. Pharm. Sci.* **2014**, *63*, 178–186. [CrossRef] [PubMed]
90. Riethorst, D.; Mols, R.; Duchateau, G.; Tack, J.; Brouwers, J.; Augustijns, P. Characterization of Human Duodenal Fluids in Fasted and Fed State Conditions. *J. Pharm. Sci.* **2016**, *105*, 673–681. [CrossRef]
91. Jantratid, E.; Janssen, N.; Reppas, C.; Dressman, J.B. Dissolution media simulating conditions in the proximal human gastrointestinal tract: An update. *Pharm. Res.* **2008**, *25*, 1663–1676. [CrossRef]
92. Markopoulos, C.; Thoenen, F.; Preisig, D.; Symillides, M.; Vertzoni, M.; Parrott, N.; Reppas, C.; Imanidis, G. Biorelevant media for transport experiments in the Caco-2 model to evaluate drug absorption in the fasted and the fed state and their usefulness. *Eur. J. Pharm. Biopharm.* **2014**, *86*, 438–448. [CrossRef]
93. Birch, D.; Diedrichsen, R.G.; Christophersen, P.C.; Mu, H.; Nielsen, H.M. Evaluation of drug permeation under fed state conditions using mucus-covered Caco-2 cell epithelium. *Eur. J. Pharm. Sci.* **2018**, *118*, 144–153. [CrossRef]
94. Wuyts, B.; Riethorst, D.; Brouwers, J.; Tack, J.; Annaert, P.; Augustijns, P. Evaluation of fasted state human intestinal fluid as apical solvent system in the Caco-2 absorption model and comparison with FaSSIF. *Eur. J. Pharm. Sci.* **2015**, *67*, 126–135. [CrossRef] [PubMed]
95. Dahlgren, D.; Roos, C.; Lundqvist, A.; Tannergren, C.; Sjoblom, M.; Sjogren, E.; Lennernas, H. Time-dependent effects on small intestinal transport by absorption-modifying excipients. *Eur. J. Pharm. Biopharm.* **2018**, *132*, 19–28. [CrossRef] [PubMed]
96. Roos, C.; Dahlgren, D.; Sjogren, E.; Tannergren, C.; Abrahamsson, B.; Lennernas, H. Regional Intestinal Permeability in Rats: A Comparison of Methods. *Mol. Pharm.* **2017**, *14*, 4252–4261. [CrossRef] [PubMed]
97. Thanou, M.; Verhoef, J.C.; Verheijden, J.H.M.; Junginger, H.E. Intestinal Absorption of Octreotide Using Trimethyl Chitosan Chloride: Studies in Pigs. *Pharm. Res.* **2001**, *18*, 823–828. [CrossRef] [PubMed]
98. Baluom, M.; Friedman, M.; Assaf, P.; Haj-Yehia, A.I.; Rubinstein, A. Synchronized release of sulpiride and sodium decanoate from HPMC matrices: A rational approach to enhance sulpiride absorption in the rat intestine. *Pharm. Res.* **2000**, *17*, 1071–1076. [CrossRef] [PubMed]
99. Sutton, S.C.; LeCluyse, E.L.; Engle, K.; Pipkin, J.D.; Fix, J.A. Enhanced Bioavailability of Cefoxitin Using Palmitoylcarnitine. II. Use of Directly Compressed Tablet Formulations in the Rat and Dog. *Pharm. Res.* **1993**, *10*, 1516–1520. [CrossRef] [PubMed]
100. Schiller, C.; Fröhlich, C.-P.; Giessmann, T.; Siegmund, W.; Mönnikes, H.; Hosten, N.; Weitschies, W. Intestinal fluid volumes and transit of dosage forms as assessed by magnetic resonance imaging. *Aliment. Pharmacol. Ther.* **2005**, *22*, 971–979. [CrossRef]
101. Dorkoosh, F.A.; Verhoef, J.C.; Verheijden, J.H.M.; Rafiee-Tehrani, M.; Borchard, G.; Junginger, H.E. Peroral Absorption of Octreotide in Pigs Formulated in Delivery Systems on the Basis of Superporous Hydrogel Polymers. *Pharm. Res.* **2002**, *19*, 1532–1536. [CrossRef]

102. Koziolek, M.; Grimm, M.; Becker, D.; Iordanov, V.; Zou, H.; Shimizu, J.; Wanke, C.; Garbacz, G.; Weitschies, W. Investigation of pH and Temperature Profiles in the GI Tract of Fasted Human Subjects Using the Intellicap® System. *J. Pharm. Sci.* **2015**, *104*, 2855–2863. [CrossRef]
103. Baluom, M.; Friedman, M.; Rubinstein, A. The importance of intestinal residence time of absorption enhancer on drug absorption and implication on formulative considerations. *Int. J. Pharm.* **1998**, *176*, 21–30. [CrossRef]
104. Tillman, L.G.; Geary, R.S.; Hardee, G.E. Oral delivery of antisense oligonucleotides in man. *J. Pharm. Sci.* **2008**, *97*, 225–236. [CrossRef] [PubMed]
105. Junginger, H. Excipients as Absorption Enhancers. In *Biopharmaceutics Applications in Drug Development*; Krishna, R., Yu, L., Eds.; Springer: New York, NY, USA, 2008; pp. 139–174. [CrossRef]
106. Brayden, D.J.; Walsh, E. Efficacious intestinal permeation enhancement induced by the sodium salt of 10-undecylenic acid, a medium chain fatty acid derivative. *AAPS J.* **2014**, *16*, 1064–1076. [CrossRef] [PubMed]
107. Whitehead, K.; Shen, Z.; Mitragotri, S. Oral delivery of macromolecules using intestinal patches: Applications for insulin delivery. *J. Control. Release* **2004**, *98*, 37–45. [CrossRef] [PubMed]
108. Gupta, V.; Hwang, B.H.; Doshi, N.; Banerjee, A.; Anselmo, A.C.; Mitragotri, S. Delivery of Exenatide and Insulin Using Mucoadhesive Intestinal Devices. *Ann. Biomed. Eng.* **2016**, *44*, 1993–2007. [CrossRef] [PubMed]
109. Eiamtrakarn, S.; Itoh, Y.; Kishimoto, J.; Yoshikawa, Y.; Shibata, N.; Murakami, M.; Takada, K. Gastrointestinal mucoadhesive patch system (GI-MAPS) for oral administration of G-CSF, a model protein. *Biomaterials* **2002**, *23*, 145–152. [CrossRef]
110. Grabovac, V.; Foger, F.; Bernkop-Schnurch, A. Design and in vivo evaluation of a patch delivery system for insulin based on thiolated polymers. *Int. J. Pharm.* **2008**, *348*, 169–174. [CrossRef] [PubMed]
111. Venkatesan, N.; Uchino, K.; Amagase, K.; Ito, Y.; Shibata, N.; Takada, K. Gastro-intestinal patch system for the delivery of erythropoietin. *J. Control. Release* **2006**, *111*, 19–26. [CrossRef]
112. Banerjee, A.; Wong, J.; Gogoi, R.; Brown, T.; Mitragotri, S. Intestinal micropatches for oral insulin delivery. *J. Drug Target.* **2017**, *25*, 608–615. [CrossRef]
113. McCartney, F.; Gleeson, J.P.; Brayden, D.J. Safety concerns over the use of intestinal permeation enhancers: A mini-review. *Tissue Barriers* **2016**, *4*, e1176822. [CrossRef]
114. Fasano, A.; Fiorentini, C.; Donelli, G.; Uzzau, S.; Kaper, J.B.; Margaretten, K.; Ding, X.; Guandalini, S.; Comstock, L.; Goldblum, S.E. Zonula occludens toxin modulates tight junctions through protein kinase C-dependent actin reorganization, in vitro. *J. Clin. Investig.* **1995**, *96*, 710–720. [CrossRef]
115. Bogman, K.; Zysset, Y.; Degen, L.; Hopfgartner, G.; Gutmann, H.; Alsenz, J.; Drewe, J. P-glycoprotein and surfactants: Effect on intestinal talinolol absorption. *Clin. Pharmacol. Ther.* **2005**, *77*, 24–32. [CrossRef] [PubMed]
116. Tomaru, A.; Takeda-Morishita, M.; Maeda, K.; Banba, H.; Takayama, K.; Kumagai, Y.; Kusuhara, H.; Sugiyama, Y. Effects of Cremophor EL on the absorption of orally administered saquinavir and fexofenadine in healthy subjects. *Drug Metab. Pharmacokinet.* **2015**, *30*, 221–226. [CrossRef] [PubMed]
117. Lindmark, T.; Soderholm, J.D.; Olaison, G.; Alvan, G.; Ocklind, G.; Artursson, P. Mechanism of absorption enhancement in humans after rectal administration of ampicillin in suppositories containing sodium caprate. *Pharm. Res.* **1997**, *14*, 930–935. [CrossRef] [PubMed]
118. Maher, S.; Leonard, T.W.; Jacobsen, J.; Brayden, D.J. Safety and efficacy of sodium caprate in promoting oral drug absorption: From in vitro to the clinic. *Adv. Drug Deliv. Rev.* **2009**, *61*, 1427–1449. [CrossRef]
119. Kiss, L.; Walter, F.R.; Bocsik, A.; Veszelka, S.; Ozsvari, B.; Puskas, L.G.; Szabo-Revesz, P.; Deli, M.A. Kinetic analysis of the toxicity of pharmaceutical excipients Cremophor EL and RH40 on endothelial and epithelial cells. *J. Pharm. Sci.* **2013**, *102*, 1173–1181. [CrossRef] [PubMed]
120. Ribet, D.; Cossart, P. How bacterial pathogens colonize their hosts and invade deeper tissues. *Microbes Infect.* **2015**, *17*, 173–183. [CrossRef] [PubMed]
121. Gunzel, D.; Yu, A.S. Claudins and the modulation of tight junction permeability. *Physiol. Rev.* **2013**, *93*, 525–569. [CrossRef] [PubMed]
122. Drewe, J.; Beglinger, C.; Fricker, G. Effect of ischemia on intestinal permeability of lipopolysaccharides. *Eur. J. Clin. Investig.* **2001**, *31*, 138–144. [CrossRef]
123. Tomlinson, J.E.; Blikslager, A.T. Interactions between lipopolysaccharide and the intestinal epithelium. *J. Am. Vet. Med Assoc.* **2004**, *224*, 1446–1452. [CrossRef]
124. Barmeyer, C.; Schulzke, J.D.; Fromm, M. Claudin-related intestinal diseases. *Semin. Cell Dev. Boil.* **2015**, *42*, 30–38. [CrossRef]

125. Tippin, T.K.; Thakker, D.R. Novel Approaches to Assess the Efficacy and Toxicity of Intestinal Absorption Enhancers. Ph.D. Thesis, ProQuest, Ann Arbor, MI, USA, 2006.
126. Nielsen, E.J.; Kamei, N.; Takeda-Morishita, M. Safety of the cell-penetrating peptide penetratin as an oral absorption enhancer. *Boil. Pharm. Bull.* **2015**, *38*, 144–146. [CrossRef] [PubMed]
127. Chassaing, B.; Koren, O.; Goodrich, J.K.; Poole, A.C.; Srinivasan, S.; Ley, R.E.; Gewirtz, A.T. Dietary emulsifiers impact the mouse gut microbiota promoting colitis and metabolic syndrome. *Nature* **2015**, *519*, 92–96. [CrossRef]
128. Kararli, T.T. Comparison of the gastrointestinal anatomy, physiology, and biochemistry of humans and commonly used laboratory animals. *Biopharm. Drug Dispos.* **1995**, *16*, 351–380. [CrossRef] [PubMed]
129. Dressman, J.B. Comparison of canine and human gastrointestinal physiology. *Pharm. Res.* **1986**, *3*, 123–131. [CrossRef] [PubMed]
130. Tyagi, P.; Pechenov, S.; Anand Subramony, J. Oral peptide delivery: Translational challenges due to physiological effects. *J. Control. Release* **2018**, *287*, 167–176. [CrossRef] [PubMed]
131. Lui, C.Y.; Amidon, G.L.; Berardi, R.R.; Fleisher, D.; Youngberg, C.; Dressman, J.B. Comparison of gastrointestinal pH in dogs and humans: Implications on the use of the beagle dog as a model for oral absorption in humans. *J. Pharm. Sci.* **1986**, *75*, 271–274. [CrossRef]
132. Polentarutti, B.; Albery, T.; Dressman, J.; Abrahamsson, B. Modification of gastric pH in the fasted dog. *J. Pharm. Pharmacol.* **2010**, *62*, 462–469. [CrossRef] [PubMed]
133. Henze, L.J.; Koehl, N.J.; O'Shea, J.P.; Kostewicz, E.S.; Holm, R.; Griffin, B.T. The pig as a preclinical model for predicting oral bioavailability and in vivo performance of pharmaceutical oral dosage forms: A PEARRL review. *J. Pharm. Pharmacol.* **2018**. [CrossRef]
134. Sjogren, E.; Abrahamsson, B.; Augustijns, P.; Becker, D.; Bolger, M.B.; Brewster, M.; Brouwers, J.; Flanagan, T.; Harwood, M.; Heinen, C.; et al. In vivo methods for drug absorption—Comparative physiologies, model selection, correlations with in vitro methods (IVIVC), and applications for formulation/API/excipient characterization including food effects. *Eur. J. Pharm. Sci.* **2014**, *57*, 99–151. [CrossRef]
135. Hatton, G.B.; Madla, C.M.; Rabbie, S.C.; Basit, A.W. Gut reaction: Impact of systemic diseases on gastrointestinal physiology and drug absorption. *Drug Discov. Today* **2018**. [CrossRef]
136. Davis, S.S.; Wilding, I.R. Oral drug absorption studies: The best model for man is man! *Drug Discov. Today* **2001**, *6*, 127–130. [CrossRef]
137. Hatton, G.B.; Yadav, V.; Basit, A.W.; Merchant, H.A. Animal Farm: Considerations in Animal Gastrointestinal Physiology and Relevance to Drug Delivery in Humans. *J. Pharm. Sci.* **2015**, *104*, 2747–2776. [CrossRef] [PubMed]
138. McConnell, E.L.; Basit, A.W.; Murdan, S. Measurements of rat and mouse gastrointestinal pH, fluid and lymphoid tissue, and implications for in-vivo experiments. *J. Pharm. Pharmacol.* **2008**, *60*, 63–70. [CrossRef]
139. Bak, A.; Ashford, M.; Brayden, D.J. Local delivery of macromolecules to treat diseases associated with the colon. *Adv. Drug Deliv. Rev.* **2018**, *136–137*, 2–27. [CrossRef]
140. Karsdal, M.A.; Henriksen, K.; Bay-Jensen, A.C.; Molloy, B.; Arnold, M.; John, M.R.; Byrjalsen, I.; Azria, M.; Riis, B.J.; Qvist, P.; et al. Lessons learned from the development of oral calcitonin: The first tablet formulation of a protein in phase III clinical trials. *J. Clin. Pharmacol.* **2011**, *51*, 460–471. [CrossRef] [PubMed]
141. Karsdal, M.A.; Riis, B.J.; Mehta, N.; Stern, W.; Arbit, E.; Christiansen, C.; Henriksen, K. Lessons learned from the clinical development of oral peptides. *Br. J. Clin. Pharmacol.* **2015**, *79*, 720–732. [CrossRef] [PubMed]

12

Chitosan-Coated Nanoparticles: Effect of Chitosan Molecular Weight on Nasal Transmucosal Delivery

Franciele Aline Bruinsmann [1,2], Stefania Pigana [2], Tanira Aguirre [3], Gabriele Dadalt Souto [1], Gabriela Garrastazu Pereira [1], Annalisa Bianchera [2], Laura Tiozzo Fasiolo [2,4], Gaia Colombo [4], Magno Marques [5], Adriana Raffin Pohlmann [1,6], Silvia Stanisçuaski Guterres [1] and Fabio Sonvico [2,*]

1 Programa de Pós-Graduação em Ciências Farmacêuticas, Universidade Federal do Rio Grande do Sul, Porto Alegre 90610-000, Brazil; fbruinsmann@gmail.com (F.A.B.); gabrieledadalt@gmail.com (G.D.S.); garrastazugp@gmail.com (G.G.P.); adriana.pohlmann@ufrgs.br (A.R.P.); silvia.guterres@ufrgs.br (S.S.G.)
2 Food and Drug Department, University of Parma, Parco Area delle Scienze 27/a, 43124 Parma, Italy; stefania.pigana@studenti.unipr.it (S.P.); annalisa.bianchera@unipr.it (A.B.); laura.tiozzofasiolo@studenti.unipr.it (L.T.F.)
3 Programa de Pós-Graduação em Biociências, Universidade Federal de Ciências da Saúde de Porto Alegre, Porto Alegre RS 900500-170, Brazil; tanira@ufcspa.edu.br
4 Department of Life Sciences and Biotechnology, University of Ferrara, Via Fossato di Mortara 17/19, 44121 Ferrara, Italy; clmgai@unife.it
5 Programa de Pós-Graduação em Ciências Fisiológicas, Universidade Federal do Rio Grande, Rio Grande RS 96203-000, Brazil; magnomarques@aol.com
6 Departamento de Química Orgânica, Instituto de Química, Universidade Federal do Rio Grande do Sul, Porto Alegre 91501-970, Brazil
* Correspondence: fabio.sonvico@unipr.it

Abstract: Drug delivery to the brain represents a challenge, especially in the therapy of central nervous system malignancies. Simvastatin (SVT), as with other statins, has shown potential anticancer properties that are difficult to exploit in the central nervous system (CNS). In the present work the physico–chemical, mucoadhesive, and permeability-enhancing properties of simvastatin-loaded poly-ε-caprolactone nanocapsules coated with chitosan for nose-to-brain administration were investigated. Lipid-core nanocapsules coated with chitosan (LNC_{chit}) of different molecular weight (MW) were prepared by a novel one-pot technique, and characterized for particle size, surface charge, particle number density, morphology, drug encapsulation efficiency, interaction between surface nanocapsules with mucin, drug release, and permeability across two nasal mucosa models. Results show that all formulations presented adequate particle sizes (below 220 nm), positive surface charge, narrow droplet size distribution (PDI < 0.2), and high encapsulation efficiency. Nanocapsules presented controlled drug release and mucoadhesive properties that are dependent on the MW of the coating chitosan. The results of permeation across the RPMI 2650 human nasal cell line evidenced that LNC_{chit} increased the permeation of SVT. In particular, the amount of SVT that permeated after 4 hr for nanocapsules coated with low-MW chitosan, high-MW chitosan, and control SVT was 13.9 ± 0.8 μg, 9.2 ± 1.2 μg, and 1.4 ± 0.2 μg, respectively. These results were confirmed by SVT ex vivo permeation across rabbit nasal mucosa. This study highlighted the suitability of LNC_{chit} as a promising strategy for the administration of simvastatin for a nose-to-brain approach for the therapy of brain tumors.

Keywords: nasal permeability; nose-to-brain; simvastatin; nanocapsules; mucoadhesion; CNS disorders; chitosan

---

1. Introduction

Statins are potent inhibitors of the hydroxymethyl glutaryl coenzyme A (HMG-CoA) reductase, and they are commonly administered for the treatment of cardiovascular disease [1]. However, in recent years, it has been suggested that the statin therapeutic indications might expand, due to their pleiotropic effects [2]. These non-cholesterol-related effects include their modulation of immune responses, the enhancement of endothelial function, the reduction of oxidative stress, and checking of inflammation processes [3,4]. The majority of pleiotropic effects are mediated by preventing the synthesis of isoprenoids, and the subsequent inhibition of small signaling proteins [5,6]. Among the diseases that could benefit from statin's pleiotropic effects are multiple sclerosis, rheumatoid arthritis, systemic lupus erythematosus, chronic obstructive pulmonary disease, neurodegenerative disorders, bacterial infections, and cancer [3].

In the field of cancer therapy, statins showed pro-apoptotic effects against various tumor cell lines [7,8], and numerous studies have examined their potential chemopreventive action [9]. Due to the inhibition of the enzyme HMG-CoA reductase, statins decrease the levels of mevalonate, the precursor of dolichol, geranylpyrophosphate (GPP), and farnesyl-pyrophosphate (FPP). Dolichol enhances DNA synthesis and is associated with several proteins found in tumor cells [10]. GPP and FPP are post-translational modifications of intracellular proteins as the G-proteins Ras and Rho, which regulate the signal transduction of several membrane receptors, and which are critical for the transcription of genes involved in cell proliferation, differentiation, and apoptosis. Ras and Rho gene mutations are found in a variety of tumor cells [7,11]. Furthermore, statins show apoptotic effects in human glioblastoma cell lines that induce the depletion of geranylgeranylated proteins, which is important for the transition to cell cycle phases [12]. Statins have also shown to play a role in the prevention of tumor metastases by the inhibition of epithelial growth factor–induced tumor cell invasion [13]. Moreover, statins, inducing the inactivation of nuclear factor kB, reduce urokinase and matrix metalloproteinase-9 expression, which are pivotal for tumor metastatic processes [7,14].

In the case of glioma cell lines, simvastatin (SVT) showed a suppression of cell proliferation and the induction of apoptosis [15,16]. However, when evaluated in an in vivo orthotopic model of the glioblastoma multiform model, simvastatin did not show tumor-inhibitory effects [17]. As in this experiment, the major factor for the failure of chemotherapies against central nervous system (CNS) tumors has been attributed to limited brain-blood barrier (BBB) permeability [18]. In addition, after oral administration statins are extensively metabolized in the liver, their hydrophilic metabolites are prevented from crossing the BBB [19].

Some new strategies have been proposed to deal with such limitations in order to increase the distribution of drugs in the CNS, such as the use of nose-to-brain route [20,21] and the development of nanocarriers [22–24]. In recent years, nose-to-brain delivery has attracted much attention as a means of delivering drugs more efficiently to the CNS bypassing the BBB. This is because the nasal cavity is anatomically connected to the CNS via the olfactory system [25]. Moreover, it offers advantages such as non-invasiveness, the avoidance of hepatic first-pass metabolism, practicality and the convenience of administration [26]. However, due to the presence of the rapid mucociliary clearance mechanism, nasal delivery applications for brain delivery are hindered by the short residence time of conventional formulations. Moreover, the barrier of the nasal epithelium, nasal metabolism, and the limited volume of administration are limiting aspects for the development of nose-to-brain drug delivery systems [25,27].

To increase bioavailability after nasal delivery, polymeric nanocapsules have been investigated [28–30]. These nanocarriers are considered a type of reservoir drug delivery system [31], and can be obtained by the interfacial deposition of pre-formed polymers [32]. Their structure is characterized by an oil core surrounded by a polymeric shell stabilized by a surfactant system [31,33]. The lipid-core nanocapsules (LNCs), developed by our research group, are composed of a dispersion of sorbitan monostearate (solid lipid) and medium-chain triacylglycerols (liquid lipids) in the core, surrounded by poly(ε-caprolactone), an aliphatic polyester as a polymeric wall, and polysorbate 80 as a stabilizing surfactant [34]. The lipid core dispersion, i.e., sorbitan monostearate dispersed in oil, confers different properties to this system, such as controlling the drug release and increasing the encapsulation efficiency when compared to the core of the conventional nanocapsules containing only liquid lipids [34–36]. These nanocarriers showed efficient brain delivery of drugs as resveratrol [37] and curcumin [38] when administered orally and intraperitoneally, as well as the reduction of the side effects of the antipsychotic drug olanzapine [39]. Furthermore, they demonstrated improved the vitro and in vivo antitumor effectiveness of resveratrol, methotrexate, and acetyleugenol when compared to the free drugs [40–42].

Bender and co-authors [43], developed a two-step process to obtain modified LNC stabilized simultaneously with polysorbate 80, and lecithin and coated with chitosan. Chitosan is a cationic biopolymer obtained by the partial deacetylation of chitin under alkaline conditions [44]. Chitosan demonstrated several interesting properties for pharmaceutical application, such as biodegradability, biocompatibility, antibacterial activity, and the controlled release of drugs [45,46]. Furthermore, chitosan showed mucoadhesive and penetration-enhancing properties, which are particularly desirable for its application in drug nasal delivery [47,48]. These actions are mediated by the structural reorganization of the tight junctions of the nasal epithelium, increasing the paracellular transport of drugs [49].

In the present study, LNC stabilized with lecithin and coated with chitosan was obtained by an innovative one-pot technique. Moreover, the pharmaceutical properties of formulations with chitosans of different molecular weights (MW), intended for the nose-to-brain delivery of simvastatin, were evaluated.

2. Materials and Methods

2.1. Materials

Poly (ε-caprolactone) (PCL) (MW = 14,000) and Span 60® (sorbitan monostearate) were purchased from Sigma-Aldrich (Strasbourg, France). Caprylic/capric triglyceride was obtained from Delaware (Porto Alegre, Brazil), and simvastatin (SVT) was purchased from Pharma Nostra (Rio de Janeiro, Brazil). Chitosan low MW (21 kDa—viscosity 9 cP) and high MW (152 kDa—viscosity 114 cP) was provided by Primex (Chitoclear FG, deacetylation degree 95%, Siglufjordur, Iceland). Soybean lecithin (Lipoid S75) was kindly donated by Lipoid AG (Ludwigshafen, Germany). Minimum essential medium (MEM), fetal bovine serum (FBS), phosphate-buffered saline (PBS), and Hank's Balanced Salt Solution (HBSS) were supplied by Gibco (Carlsbad, CA, USA). Transwell® cell culture inserts (1.12 cm^2 surface area, polyester, 0.4 μm pore size) were supplied by Corning Costar (Lowell, MA, USA). All of the other chemicals and solvents used were of analytical or pharmaceutical grade.

2.2. Preparation of the Lipid-Core Nanocapsules Coated using a One-Pot Technique

Chitosan-coated simvastatin-loaded lipid-core nanocapsules were prepared according to the method of interfacial deposition of pre-formed polymers already reported in literature [35]. An organic phase (25 mL of acetone) containing the polymer (PCL, 0.04 g), sorbitan monostearate (0.016 g), and caprylic/capric triglyceride (0.048 mL) was kept under magnetic stirring at 40 °C. After complete dissolution of the components, an ethanolic solution (4 mL) containing lecithin (0.025 g) was added into the organic phase, and finally, simvastatin (0.010 g) was added and completely dissolved. The aqueous phase (50 mL) contained 0.1% (*w*/*v*) chitosan, prepared as a dilution from a 0.5% (*w*/*v*) of chitosan solution in 1% (*v*/*v*) acetic acid. The organic phase was injected using a funnel into the aqueous phase under moderate magnetic stirring. The solvents were eliminated at 40 °C to a final volume of 10 mL, by the use of a rotary evaporator, Büchi® R-114 (Flawill, Switzerland). The formulations obtained were named $LNC_{SVT\text{-}LMWchit}$ when low-MW chitosan (viscosity 9 cP) was used, and $LNC_{SVT\text{-}HMWchit}$ when high-MW chitosan (viscosity 114cP) was used. Blank nanocapsules ($LNC_{LMWchit}$ and $LNC_{HMWchit}$) were also prepared, omitting the simvastatin from the organic phase preparation.

2.3. Drug Content and Encapsulation Efficiency

SVT quantification was carried out by high performance liquid chromatography with detection in the ultraviolet range (HPLC-UV), using a previously validated method [30]. The analysis was performed with a Shimadzu HPLC system (Kyoto, Japan) with detection at 238 nm and using a column Phenomenex Lichrosphere® C18 (4.6 × 250 mm, 5 μm). The composition of the mobile phase was 65% acetonitrile and 35% sodium dihydrogen phosphate buffer (25 mM, pH 4.5), the flow rate was 1.0 mL·min^{-1}, with an injection volume of 100 μL. Calibration curves (n = 3) were prepared to determine the linearity ($R > 0.99$) in the concentration range from 0.1 to 20 μg·mL^{-1}. The drug content in the formulations was determined by diluting a precise volume of nanoparticle suspension (100 μL) in 10 mL of the mobile phase. The samples were then sonicated for 30 min and filtered through a 0.45 μm membrane (Millipore®, Billerica, MA, USA) before being assayed by HPLC-UV. Free simvastatin was determined in the ultrafiltrate after ultrafiltration–centrifugation (Ultrafree-MC, cut-off of 30 kDa, Millipore) at 2688× g (Scilogex D3024, Rocky Hill, CT, USA) for 15 min and quantification by HPLC-UV. Encapsulation efficiency (EE) as a percentage was calculated by the difference between the total and free, i.e., non-encapsulated, drug amount, divided by the total drug amount multiplied by 100. All analyses were performed for triplicate batches (n = 3).

2.4. Physicochemical Characterization

The nanoparticle formulations were characterized with multiple techniques, as described below. All analyses, with the exception of transmission electron microscopy (TEM) (n = 1), were performed for triplicate batches (n = 3).

2.4.1. Laser Diffraction

Particle size and the size distribution were determined by laser diffraction (Mastersizer® 2000, Malvern Instruments, Malvern, UK), with the aim of detecting the eventual presence of micrometric particles or aggregates. The sample was directly added to water in the wet dispersion accessory (Hydro 2000SM-AWM2002, Malvern Instruments) until an obscuration level of 2% was reached. The particle size was then expressed by using the volume-weighted mean diameter (D[4,3]), and the diameters calculated at the 10th, 50th, and 90th percentiles ($d_{0.1}$, $d_{0.5}$, and $d_{0.9}$, respectively) of the cumulative size distribution curve, by volume (v) and by the number (n) of particles. The width of the distribution (*Span*) was determined according to Equation (1):

$$Span = \frac{d_{0.9} - d_{0.1}}{d_{0.5}}, \quad (1)$$

2.4.2. Dynamic Light Scattering

The mean particle size (Z-average diameter) and the polydispersity index (PDI) of the nanocapsules were evaluated by dynamic light scattering (DLS) at 25 °C, using a Zetasizer® Nano ZS (Malvern Instruments). After dilution of the samples (500×) in purified and filtered (0.45 μm) water, the correlogram was obtained by allowing the instrument software to determine the optimal time of acquisition, and the Z-average diameter and PDI were calculated by the method of Cumulants, with the same software.

2.4.3. Nanoparticle Tracking Analysis

The nanoparticles tracking analysis (NTA) method was used to determine the mean diameter and the concentration of nanocapsules per volume, expressed as the particle number density (PND) (NanoSight LM10, Malvern Pananalytical, UK). The analysis was carried out by diluting the samples in ultrapure water (1000×) and introducing them into the instrument sample chamber cell by a syringe. The chamber is located on an optical microscope, where a laser diode (635 nm) illuminates the particles in suspension. The NTA 3.2 software tracks single particles, which are in Brownian motion, and it can relate this particle movement to a sphere equivalent hydrodynamic radius, as calculated using the Stokes–Einstein equation (Equation (2)). The samples were evaluated at room temperature for 60 s, with automatic detection. The results correspond to the arithmetic average of the calculated sizes of all particles analyzed:

$$\overline{(x,\ y)^2} = \frac{4\ Tk_B}{3\pi\eta d_h}, \tag{2}$$

where k_B is the Boltzmann constant, and $\overline{(x,\ y)^2}$ is the mean-squared displacement of a particle during time t at temperature T, in a medium of viscosity η, with a hydrodynamic diameter of d_h.

2.4.4. pH and Zeta Potential

The pH values of the nanocapsules suspensions were determined using a calibrated potentiometer (DM-22 Digimed, São Paulo, Brazil) via direct measurements of the formulations at 25 °C. The zeta potential values were determined by electrophoretic mobility after the samples were diluted in 10 mM NaCl aqueous solution (500×), previously filtered (0.45 μm, Millipore®, Billerica, USA). The zeta potentials of the nanoparticles suspensions were also measured at different pH values, using the MPT-2 autotitrator for the Zetasizer® Nano ZS (Malvern Instruments, Malvern, UK). The samples (10 mL) were placed in the titration cell and titrated over acid (0.1 M HCl) towards a basic (0.05 M NaOH) pH range in 1.0 pH unit intervals. This combination allowed for automated titration over a wide pH range, and thus, made it possible to determine the isoelectric point (IEP) of the nanoparticles.

2.4.5. Morphology

TEM was used to evaluate the morphology of the formulations. TEM samples were diluted in ultrapure water (10×, *v*/*v*), and then deposited (10 μL) onto specimen grids (Formvar-Carbon support film, Electron Microscopy Sciences, Hatfield, PA, USA) and negatively stained with uranyl acetate solution (2% (*w*/*v*), Sigma-Aldrich, St.Louis, MO, USA). Analyses were performed using a transmission electron microscope (JEM 2200-FS, Jeol, Tokyo, Japan) operating at 80 kV. The images were processed with Digital Micrograph (Gatan Inc., Pleasanton, CA, USA) software.

2.5. *In Vitro Evaluation of the Interaction between Nanocapsules and Mucin*

The mucoadhesive properties of the formulations were assessed by using mucin from porcine stomach (Type II, Sigma-Aldrich, St. Louis, MO, USA), as previously described [29,50]. The mucin was dispersed in ultrapure water (0.5% (*w*/*v*)) by magnetic stirring for 3 h at room temperature. The suspension was centrifuged at 4000× *g* for 30 min. The supernatant was collected and lyophilized. Then, mucin solutions were prepared in a simulated nasal electrolytic solution (SNES) [51] at predetermined weight ratios f, determined as:

$$f = \frac{W_{mucin}}{W_{mucin} + WNC}, \tag{3}$$

where W_{mucin} is the mucin mass and *WNC* is the LNC_{chit} nanocapsule mass.

The Z-average diameter and PDI before and after contact with mucin were measured by DLS as described above, after the dilution (500×) of the samples in mucin solutions. The mucoadhesive index values (MI) were determined as:

$$MI = \frac{d}{d_0}, \tag{4}$$

where d and d_0 are the diameters of the LNC_{chit} nanocapsules before and after their interaction with mucin, respectively.

Furthermore, changes in the zeta potential were measured after the nanocapsules were diluted (500×) in mucin solutions containing 10 mM NaCl.

2.6. *In Vitro Release Study*

The in vitro release profiles of SVT from the formulations were determined by using the dialysis bag method. Briefly, 1 mL of each sample was placed in a dialysis bag (14 kDa molecular weight cut-off, Sigma-Aldrich, St. Louis, MO, USA) and suspended into 100 mL of SNES containing 0.5% of polysorbate 80, to improve SVT solubility and to reach the sink conditions. A free drug solution was placed in the dialysis bag in the control experiment ($SVT_{solution}$, simvastatin dissolved in 1% ethanol and 0.5% polysorbate 80). The dialysis bags were maintained in the medium under stirring, and maintained in a temperature-constant water bath (37 °C). One milliliter of release medium was collected at predetermined time intervals (from 0.16 to 8 h) and filtered (0.45 µm, Millipore®). The volume was replaced by adding one milliliter of fresh release medium pre-heated at 37 °C. The samples were analyzed by HPLC–UV, and the cumulative drug release was determined.

2.7. *Transport Studies across an In Vitro Nasal Epithelial Cell Model*

RPMI 2650 human nasal cells (human nasal septum tumor, ECACC, Salisbury, UK) were cultured in MEM media supplemented with 10% (*v*/*v*) fetal bovine serum (FBS). Cells were grown at 37 °C in an atmosphere of 95% air/5% CO_2. Transwell® cell culture inserts were used to establish an air–liquid interface (ALI) nasal model, as previously reported [52]. Briefly, 200 uL of cell suspensions (2.5×10^6 cell/mL) were seeded onto Transwell® and after 24 h, the media from apical compartment was removed, resulting in an ALI culture configuration. After 14 days from seeding, the Transwell® was removed and transferred to a 12-well plate containing 1.5 mL of pre-warmed HBSS. Then, 200 µL of $LNC_{SVT\text{-}LMWchit}$, $LNC_{SVT\text{-}HMWchit}$, and $SVT_{suspension}$ were added to the upper compartment, and samples of 200 µL were collected from the baso-lateral chamber at pre-determined time points (1, 2, 3 and 4 h) and replaced with the same volume of fresh HBSS buffer. The samples were quantified for simvastatin content using HPLC–UV ($n = 4$). TEER measurements were performed with a Millicell-ers® (Millipore) at the beginning and at the end of experiment, in order to confirm that the integrity of the cell layer was maintained.

2.8. *Ex Vivo Transport Experiments across Rabbit Nasal Mucosa*

The transport of simvastatin across rabbit nasal tissue was evaluated by using Franz-type vertical diffusion cells with a receptor volume of 4.5 mL and a diffusional area of 0.58 cm^2. On the day of the experiment, nasal mucosae were freshly excised from rabbits obtained from a local slaughterhouse (Pola, Finale Emilia, Italy), and cleaned to remove the adhering submucosal tissue [53]. The rabbit nasal mucosa were placed between the donor and the receptor compartments of the diffusion cells. Then, in order to check the mucosa integrity, the donor compartment was filled with medium to confirm that no liquid leaked into the cell receptor compartment. If the nasal mucosa passed this test, the donor compartment received 200 µL of one of the three tested preparations, i.e., $LNC_{SVT\text{-}LMWchit}$, $LNC_{SVT\text{-}HMWchit}$, or $SVT_{suspension}$, equivalent to 200 µg of SVT. The Franz cells were maintained at 37 °C under mild magnetic stirring. At predetermined time intervals, 500 µL of the receptor medium, SNES containing 0.5% w/v of polysorbate 80, was withdrawn, and the receptor compartment was refilled with an equivalent volume of fresh medium. All samples were analyzed by HPLC-UV. In order to evaluate the retention of SVT in the nasal tissue, mucosa samples were placed in a volumetric flask (10 mL) containing a solvent of extraction (acetonitrile), and subjected to vortexing (2 min) and sonication (15 min). The solvent of extraction was then filtered (0.45 µm, Millipore®) and simvastatin was quantified using HPLC–UV. The experiments were conducted in triplicate for each formulation.

2.9. *Preliminary Nasal Toxicity Studies*

Nasal toxicity studies were performed by using rabbit nasal mucosa in a similar way to the ex vivo permeation study mentioned above, in order to evaluate any damage to the mucosa. Each mucosa piece of uniform thickness was treated with $LNC_{SVT\text{-}LMWchit}$, $LNC_{SVT\text{-}HMWchit}$, SVT, or PBS pH 6.4 (negative control) by placing 200 μL in the donor compartments of the Franz diffusion cells. The acceptor contained 4.5 mL of SNES containing 0.5% (*w*/*v*) of polysorbate 80. After 4 h, for each condition, the nasal mucosa was washed with PBS, fixed in 10% (*v*/*v*) buffered formalin for 6 h, and embedded in histological paraffin. A rotatory microtome was used to perform transverse cuts to obtain sections (5 μm) that were stained with hematoxylin–eosin. Images of mucosa samples were observed by using an Olympus BX51 optical microscope with an attached DP72 camera (Olympus, Tokyo, Japan) [54].

2.10. Statistical Analysis

Data are presented as the mean ± standard deviation (SD) of the analysis of at least triplicate batches ($n = 3$). Statistical analysis was performed using the Student's t-test for two groups, or one-way analysis of variance (ANOVA) followed by Tukey's test for multiple groups, using GraphPad Prism Software 5.0 (GraphPad Software, Inc., San Diego, CA, USA). Differences were considered significant at $p < 0.05$.

3. Results

SVT-nanocapsules were prepared by using the interfacial deposition of pre-formed polymer method, and coated with chitosan with a one-pot technique. The surfaces of the NPs were coated with two different chitosan grades, characterized by different molecular weights, and hence different viscosities, in order to evaluate the effect of chitosan molecular weight on the mucoadhesive properties and permeability enhancement of the nanocapsules obtained.

3.1. Characterization of Nanocapsules

SVT nanocapsules appeared macroscopically as an opalescent white homogeneous dispersion. The total SVT content in the formulations was found to be 0.94 ± 0.04 mg·mL^{-1} for $LNC_{SVT\text{-}LMWchit}$ and 0.96 ± 0.02 mg·mL^{-1} for $LNC_{SVT\text{-}HMWchit}$. Regarding the encapsulation efficiency (EE), SVT was not detected in the ultrafiltrate for both formulations, indicating almost complete encapsulation. The high EE achieved is probably linked to the high SVT distribution coefficient (log D) of 4.72, which confirms its great affinity for the lipophilic phase, and its concentration in the core of the nanocapsules [55]. Laser diffraction (LD) analysis showed D[4,3] of 150 ± 7 nm ($LNC_{LMWchit}$), 157 ± 6 nm ($LNC_{HMWchit}$), 163 ± 2 nm ($LNC_{SVT\text{-}LMWchit}$), and 161 ± 3 nm ($LNC_{SVT\text{-}HMWchit}$), with Span values of 1.3 ± 0.1, 1.3 ± 0.1, 1.4 ± 0.03, and 1.2 ± 0.2, respectively. According to the results obtained with this technique, there were no significant differences in terms of the particle diameter and polydispersity, between the formulations with and without SVT ($p > 0.05$). The shapes of the curves in the radar chart presented in Figure 1 are fingerprints of the formulations, which demonstrate the narrow size distributions and confirm their low polydispersities [56]. All of the formulations showed similar behaviors and they had $d_{0.9}$ calculated both for the cumulative distribution by number, and by a volume lower than 300 nm (Figure 1).

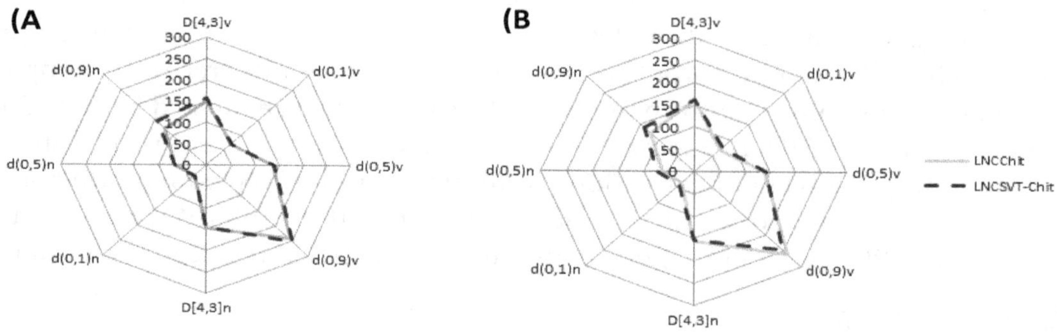

Figure 1. Radar chart presenting the volume-weighted mean diameters (D[4,3]) and the diameters at percentiles 10, 50, and 90 under the size distribution curves by volume and by the number of particles. Chitosan-coated simvastatin-loaded lipid-core nanocapsules developed with (**A**) low-MW chitosan and (**B**) high-MW chitosan.

The mean particle size was further confirmed by DLS and NTA analysis, as shown in Table 1. The DLS analysis showed a narrow particle size distribution for all of the formulations (PDI < 0.2). In particular, the encapsulation of SVT did not affect the particle size of the nanocapsules coated with low-MW chitosan. In fact, the diameters of $LNC_{LMWchit}$ and $LNC_{SVT\text{-}LMWchit}$ were not significantly different ($p > 0.05$).

Table 1. Physicochemical characterization of the nanocapsules ($n = 3$, Mean ± Standard Deviation).

Header	DLS		NTA		Zeta Potential (mV)	pH
	Z-Average (nm)	PDI	Mean (nm)	PND (Particles/mL)		
$LNC_{LMWchit}$	166 ± 5	0.13 ± 0.02	174 ± 5	$1.3 \pm 0.3 \times 10^{12}$	25.4 ± 4.1	4.1 ± 0.01
$LNC_{SVT\text{-}LMWchit}$	168 ± 5	0.12 ± 0.04	166 ± 7	$1.2 \pm 0.6 \times 10^{12}$	28.95 ± 2.1	4.1 ± 0.02
$LNC_{HMWchit}$	179 ± 14	0.13 ± 0.02	188 ± 7	$1.1 \pm 0.4 \times 10^{12}$	33.6 ± 3.9	4.1 ± 0.03
$LNC_{SVT\text{-}HMWchit}$	185 ± 7	0.16 ± 0.03	210 ± 10	$6.6 \pm 0.2 \times 10^{11}$	33.8 ± 5.5	4.4 ± 0.04

On the other hand, the presence of SVT led to a significant size increase ($p \leq 0.05$) in the case of $LNC_{SVT\text{-}HMWchit}$ (210 ± 10 nm) when compared with the blank nanocapsules ($LNC_{HMWchit}$, 188 ± 7 nm) according to the NTA analysis, but not according to the DLS data. This difference may be explained by the formation of a small number of particle agglomerates, compared to the formulation prepared without the drug. In addition, these agglomerates appeared to be detected more efficiently by the NTA technique compared to DLS. This is supported by the particle number density (PND) also measured by NTA, which evidenced, upon SVT encapsulation, almost a halving of the particle number density (PND), which was $1.1 \pm 0.4 \times 10^{12}$ particles/mL for $LNC_{HMWchit}$ and $6.6 \pm 0.2 \times 10^{11}$ particles/mL for $LNC_{SVT\text{-}HMWchit}$ (Table 1). Furthermore, in general, the nanocapsules coated with HMW chitosan showed a slightly higher mean diameter than those coated with LMW chitosan ($p > 0.05$), probably as a consequence of the higher molecular weight and higher viscosity of the chitosan in the water phase. In general, it has been reported that the higher the viscosity of the dispersion medium, the higher the mean diameter of the nanoparticles produced [57]. The zeta potentials of $LNC_{LMWchit}$ and $LNC_{HMWchit}$ were similar to those determined for the SVT-loaded nanocapsules. Therefore, the encapsulation of SVT did not significantly affect this parameter ($p > 0.05$). The pH value at which the nanoparticles do not exhibit any net charge is termed the isoelectric point (IEP). $LNC_{SVT\text{-}LMWchit}$ and $LNC_{SVT\text{-}HMWchit}$ showed an IEP at pH value 7.1 ± 0.2 and 7.2 ± 0.5, respectively. The positive zeta potential obtained for all the formulations prepared, and an IEP near the IEP of chitosan (IEP = 6.8) [58] is a good indicator that the chitosan was present at the external interface of the nanocapsules. $LNC_{SVT\text{-}LMWchit}$ and $LNC_{SVT\text{-}HMWchit}$ were further characterized in terms of their morphologies (Figure 2).

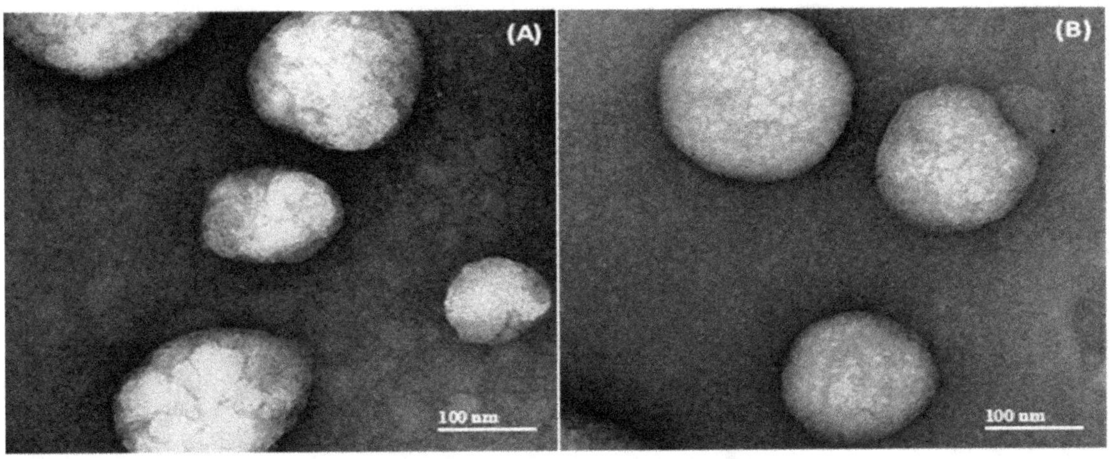

Figure 2. Transmission electron microscopy (TEM) micrographs (magnification 40,000×) of chitosan-coated lipid core nanocapsules: (**A**) $LNC_{SVT\text{-}LMWchit}$ and (**B**) $LNC_{SVT\text{-}HMWchit}$.

Concerning the nanocapsule morphology, TEM images clearly displayed spherical-shaped particles, with a core with low electron density, as expected for lipid nanocapsules. Also, from the results of the particle diameters, the images were in good agreement with the mean nanocapsule sizes determined with DLS, NTA, and LD.

3.2. Mucoadhesion Studies

To investigate the interaction between the formulations and mucin, a mucoadhesion index (MI), the PDI, and the zeta potentials of mixtures between the nanocapsules and mucin were determined for different mucin weight ratios f (Figure 3). For $LNC_{SVT\text{-}LMWchit}$ in the range of f values up to 0.3, particle sizes and MI values increased to a maximum of 474 ± 6 nm and 2.9 ± 0.1 (f = 0.3), respectively. Similarly, $LNC_{SVT\text{-}HMWchit}$ particle size and MI increased in the f range from 0 to 0.55, reaching a maximum of 557 ± 30 nm, 3.0 ± 0.3 (f = 0.55), respectively (Figure 3A). Despite the increase of the fraction by weight of mucin above f values of 0.3, for $LNC_{SVT\text{-}LMWchit}$, particle size and MI decreased to 318 ± 5 nm and 1.9 ± 0.1 for f values of 0.85. It has been hypothesized here that while at values of f of around 0.3, nanocapsules are able to form large agglomerates with mucin chains entangled and linked with more nanoparticles, above this value, the mucin is in such a large excess that almost all single particles are enrobed with mucins, leading to a decrease in the overall mean particle size. In fact, the MI values for f = 0.55 and 0.85 did not change significantly. On the other hand, for $LNC_{SVT\text{-}HMWchit}$ this decrease in the MI occurred only for f values above 0.55, with particle size and MI decreasing to 321 ± 7 nm, 1.7 ± 0.1 (f = 0.85). Therefore, the MI maximum was observed at lower f values (0.3) for $LNC_{SVT\text{-}LMWchit}$, and higher f values (0.55) for $LNC_{SVT\text{-}HMWchit}$, indicating a higher capacity to interact with larger quantities of mucin for nanoparticles coated with high MW chitosan, macroscopically translating to more efficient mucoadhesion.

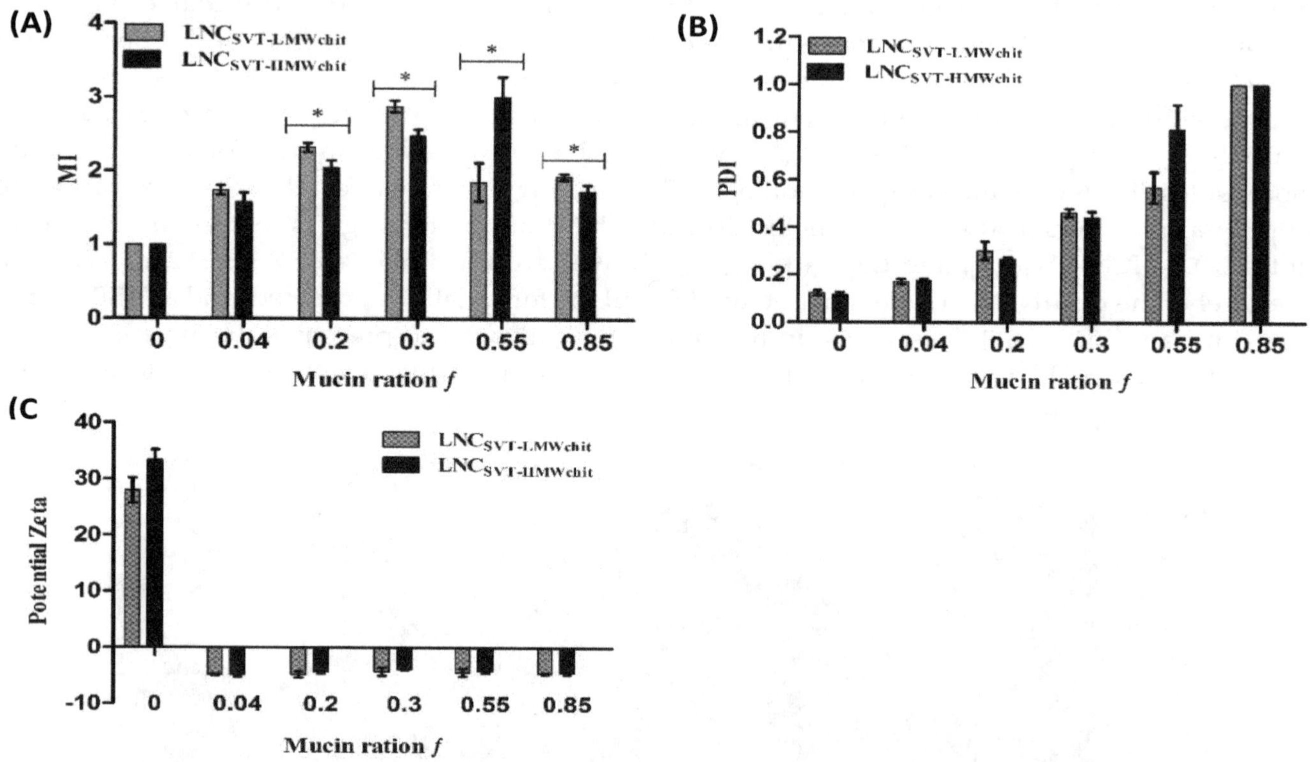

Figure 3. (**A**) Mucoadhesive index (MI) values, (**B**) PDI and (**C**) zeta potentials measured for various mixtures of mucin and nanocapsules. Values of the two formulations were obtained before (f = 0) and after incubation with different mucin weight ratios f.

The PDI before nanocapsule interaction with mucin was 0.12 ± 0.01 for $LNC_{SVT\text{-}LMWchit}$ and 0.11 ± 0.01 for $LNC_{SVT\text{-}HMWchit}$. After mixing the nanocapsules with mucin, PDI progressively increased for both formulations, up to 1 (f = 0.85), indicating the formation of agglomerates and the switch to highly polydispersed particle size distributions (Figure 3B). The zeta potentials of the formulations that were initially positive due to the chitosan coating immediately after interaction with even the smallest amount of mucin (f = 0.04), became negative for both formulations (−4.8 ± 0.1 mV for $LNC_{SVT\text{-}LMWchit}$ and −4.8 ± 0.7 mV for $LNC_{SVT\text{-}HMWchit}$) and remained roughly constant for both formulations, even with increasing f values (Figure 3C).

3.3. *In Vitro Drug Release*

The in vitro release profiles of the simvastatin-loaded chitosan coated lipid core nanocapsules were performed over 8 h (Figure 4). A solution of simvastatin was used as a control. It can be observed that 56.3 ± 2.5% of SVT diffused out from the dialysis bag when using the control simvastatin solution, within 8 h. On the other hand, the percentage of drug released from $LNC_{SVT\text{-}LMWchit}$ and $LNC_{SVT\text{-}HMWchit}$ after 8 h were 37.3 ± 1.5% and 31.0 ± 1.1%, respectively. These results show that nanocapsules provided a controlled release of simvastatin, and that the different types of chitosan affected the drug release rate. Indeed, the release of SVT from $LNC_{SVT\text{-}HMWchit}$ was slower in comparison to the $LNC_{SVT\text{-}LMWchit}$.

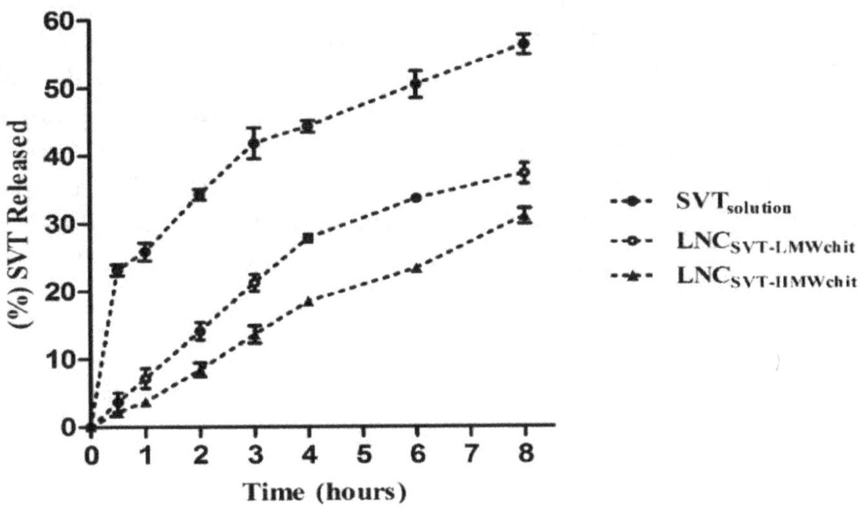

Figure 4. In vitro drug release profile from $LNC_{SVT\text{-}LMWchit}$, $LNC_{SVT\text{-}HMWchit}$ and from the control (SVT solution), using the dialysis bag method at 37 °C (n = 3, ± SD).

3.4. *Transport Studies in a Nasal Cell Model*

To confirm the potential permeability enhancement effects of the nanocapsules, the total amount of SVT transported across nasal mucosa model was determined by using RPMI2650 human nasal epithelial cells [52]. Figure 5 shows the amount of SVT transported when using the formulations, compared to a suspension of the raw material, over 4 h. After 1 h, the formulations already showed increased degrees of permeation compared to the control. However, no significant differences ($p > 0.05$) were observed at 1 h for the SVT permeation between $LNC_{SVT\text{-}LMWchit}$ and $LNC_{SVT\text{-}HMWchit}$. After the first hour however, each single time point showed an amount of SVT transported to be statistically different between the formulations ($p < 0.05$), confirming the greater permeation of $LNC_{SVT\text{-}LMWchit}$.

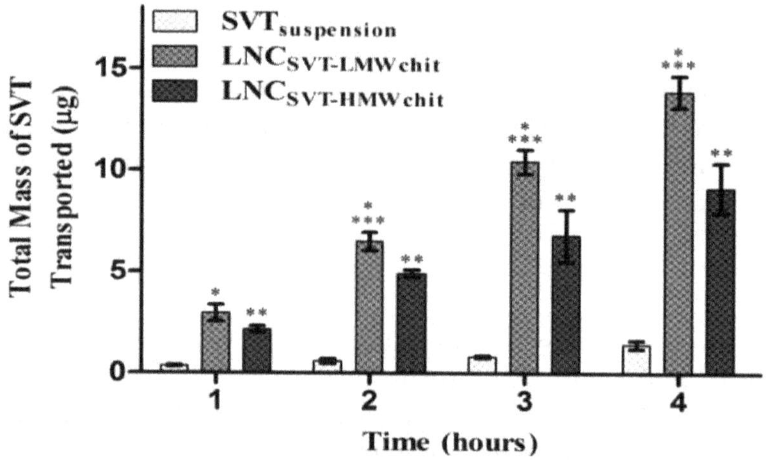

Figure 5. Amount (µg) of SVT transported across RPMI 2650 cells grown under air–liquid interface conditions (n = 4, ± SD). Significant difference ($p < 0.05$) is expressed considering the following comparisons: * SVT versus $LNC_{SVT\text{-}LMWchit}$, ** SVT versus $LNC_{SVT\text{-}HMWchit}$, *** $LNC_{SVT\text{-}LMWchit}$ versus $LNC_{SVT\text{-}HMWchit}$.

3.5. Ex Vivo Transport Experiments across Rabbit Nasal Mucosa

Figure 6A shows the SVT permeation across the excised rabbit nasal mucosa using Franz type vertical diffusion cells. The results of the ex vivo permeation studies on the rabbit nasal mucosa evidenced that the formulations significantly increased the permeation of SVT compared to the control. $LNC_{SVT\text{-}LMWchit}$ showed the highest percentage of SVT permeation after 4 h (19.2 ± 0.5%·cm^{-2}), followed by $LNC_{SVT\text{-}HMWchit}$ (11.0 ± 0.5%·cm^{-2}), while the control (SVT suspension) showed an extremely low degree of permeation (2.6 ± 0.2%·cm^{-2}). The results indicate that SVT permeation from $LNC_{SVT\text{-}LMWchit}$ was 1.74 and 7.4 times greater than $LNC_{SVT\text{-}HMWchit}$ and the SVT control, respectively.

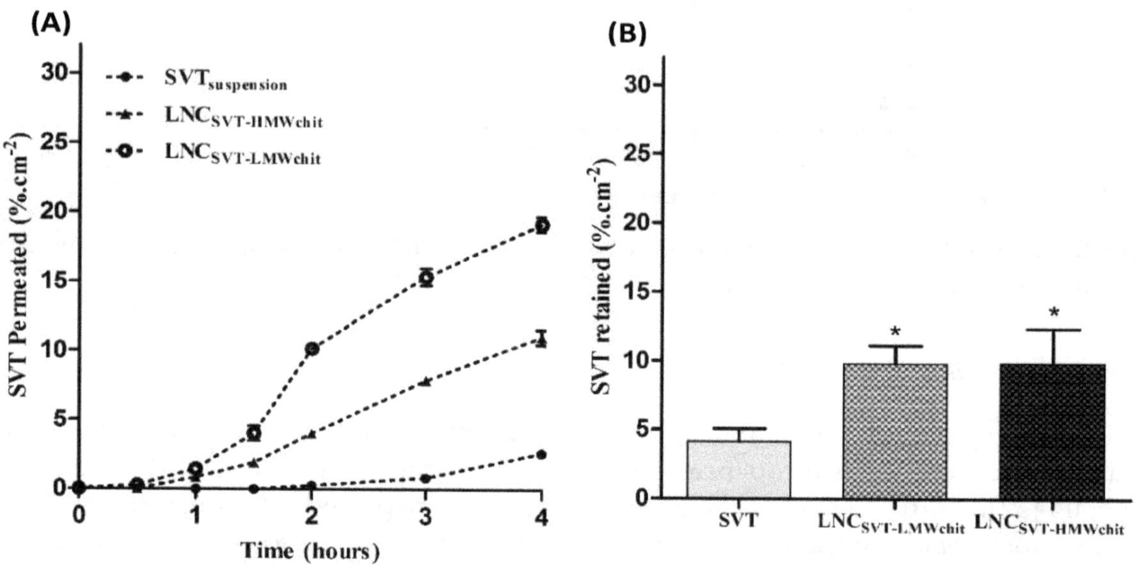

Figure 6. (**A**) Ex vivo SVT permeation across rabbit nasal mucosa up to 4 h in simulated nasal electrolytic solution (SNES) containing 0.5% of polysorbate 80 at 37 °C (n = 3, ± SD). (**B**) Percentage of SVT retained in nasal mucosa after 4 h of the permeation test in Franz-type diffusion cells (n = 3, ± SD). Asterisk (*) indicates significant differences between SVT versus $LNC_{SVT\text{-}LMWchit}$ and $LNC_{SVT\text{-}HMWchit}$.

The results of SVT retained in the mucosa tissue after 4 h experimental time are shown in Figure 6B. It can be seen that there was better retention of both formulations with respect to the control. The SVT fraction found in the tissue for the control was 4.2 ± 0.9%·cm^{-2}, while in the case of $LNC_{SVT\text{-}LMWchit}$ and $LNC_{SVT\text{-}HMWchit}$, the fraction of simvastatin found in the tissue was more than doubled, i.e., 9.8 ± 1.3 and 9.9 ± 2.5%·cm^{-2}, respectively. In this case, the difference between the amount of retained SVT from $LNC_{SVT\text{-}LMWchit}$ and $LNC_{SVT\text{-}HMWchit}$ was not statistically significant.

3.6. Preliminary Nasal Toxicity Studies

Nasal mucosa histopathology studies were performed to assess the integrity of the rabbit mucosa after 4 h of the permeation test. As shown in Figure 7, the mucosa treated with PBS pH 6.4 (negative control), SVT, $LNC_{SVT\text{-}LMWchit}$, and $LNC_{SVT\text{-}HMWchit}$ did not show any evident structural damage. The results from histological examinations indicated that the LNC nanocapsules did not cause any irritation or toxicity, and they can be considered to be biocompatible for nasal administration.

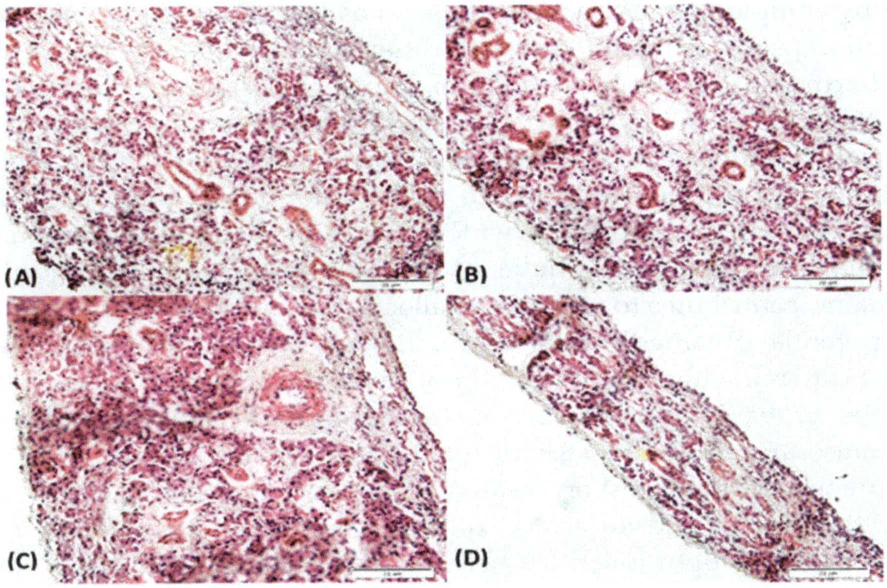

Figure 7. Histopathological sections of rabbit nasal mucosa after 4 h of permeation test in Franz-type diffusion cells treated with **(A)** PBS pH 6.4 (negative control), **(B)** SVT, **(C)** $LNC_{SVT\text{-}LMWchit}$, and **(D)** $LNC_{SVT\text{-}HMWchit}$. Sections are stained with hematoxylin and eosin.

4. Discussion

Over the past couple of decades, pharmaceutical nanotechnology has received considerable attention and demonstrated significant potential for the development of innovative medicinal products, both for the therapy and the diagnosis of severe diseases [59]. In this work, we report a new preparation method of lipid-core PCL nanocapsules, optimizing a two-step process (self-assembly step followed by a coating step) into a one-pot technique to develop chitosan-coated nanoparticles. Moreover, we compared the pharmaceutically relevant properties in terms of physicochemical characterization, mucoadhesive properties, drug release, and permeability studies of $LNC_{SVT\text{-}LMWchit}$ and $LNC_{SVT\text{-}HMWchit}$ coated by chitosan with low MW and high MW, in view of a nose-to-brain administration.

Polymeric nanocapsules containing poly(ϵ-caprolactone), capric/caprylic triglyceride, and sorbitan monostearate, and coated with chitosan, were developed. This formulation has the advantage of efficiently encapsulating lipophilic drugs such as simvastatin [34,35]. The production of positively-coated lipid-core nanocapsules in one step, avoiding the use of non-ionic surfactants in the aqueous phase, is the main novelty of this approach. Previously, we developed mucoadhesive amphiphilic nanocapsules based on a blend of PCL and poly(methyl methacrylate-b-2-(dimethylamino)ethyl methacrylate) for the nose-to-brain delivery of olanzapine. Nevertheless, the self-assembly of the nanocapsules by using this block copolymer (positive surface) avoids the use of sorbitan monostearate in the formulation. Indeed, the cores of those nanocapsules are composed exclusively of medium-chain triglycerides [29]. Sorbitan monostearate dispersed in core of the lipid-core nanocapsules has been demonstrated to provide an addition diffusional barrier to control the drug release, and an increase of the rigidity of the nanocapsules polymer wall [34,36]. Furthermore, a comparative study conducted with polymeric nanocapsules demonstrated that the presence of sorbitan monostearate instead of sorbitan monooleate in the core improved the anti-apoptotic and antioxidant effects of melatonin during bovine embryo development [60]. In the present development, it was possible to obtain in a one-step process, lipid-core nanocapsules incorporating sorbitan monostearate in the oily core, and decorated on the surface with chitosan, providing mucoadhesion and penetration-enhancing properties that appear to be fundamental for nose-to-brain delivery [21].

The combination between the composition and the interfacial deposition of the pre-formed polymer method produced nanocapsules with adequate particle sizes and narrow size distributions, as was confirmed by complementary techniques such as laser diffraction, DLS, and NTA. Besides that, coating the nanocapsules with chitosan with different molecular weights (21 kDa and 152 kDa) influenced their pharmaceutical properties. For example, chitosan molecular weight and viscosity in water affected the sizes of the nanoparticles. In fact, particle size could be reduced by using lower molecular weight chitosan [61,62]. Actually, for $LNC_{SVT\text{-}HMWchit}$, the higher mean particle hydrodynamic diameter could be attributed to the lengths of the chains of chitosan present on the particle surface, possibly expanding the water hydration shell of the nanoparticle. In addition, low-MW chitosan has been reported to have a higher aqueous solubility, and this, together with shorter polymer chains, contributes to forming smaller particles compared to high-MW chitosan [63]. The positive zeta potential obtained for all formulations is evidence of the polysaccharide coating. Furthermore, using different chitosan types did not cause significant changes in the zeta potentials of both formulations, probably due of a similar degree of deacetylation (95%) [64]. Mucoadhesive polymers such as chitosan represent a significant strategy for overcoming the nasal drug delivery limits of low membrane permeability, short residence time, and mucociliary clearance. The presence of polysaccharides on the nanocapsule surface is expected to prolong the permanence of the formulation in the nasal cavity, open the tight junctions between the nasal epithelial cells, and promote drug permeation through the biological barriers, granting access to the CNS [65–67]. For these reasons, the evaluation of the ability of nanocapsules to interact with mucin is of great interest for nasal administration. Mucous membranes internally delimit the body cavities (stomach, esophagus, cornea, oral cavity, reproductive and respiratory tracts), and are characterized by a superficial mucus layer with protective and lubricating functions [68]. The mucus is composed of water (approximately 95%), lipids, inorganic salts, and mucin, a glycoprotein composed of *N*-acetylgalactosamine, *N*-acetylglucosamine, fucose, galactose, and sialic acid, which is responsible for the adhesive properties and the viscosity of the mucus [66]. Lipophilic drugs show an affinity for mucus glycoproteins, reducing their adsorption and the bioavailability. This issue, together with the drugs' poor aqueous solubilities, are limiting factors for the nose-to-brain delivery of lipophilic drugs. To improve the transport of SVT through this barrier, we used nanoparticles as a drug delivery system [69].

Our results showed how, for both formulations, particle size and MI increased with the increase in the mucin weight ratio, to a critical point. A previous study [50] has led to the conclusion that the nanoparticles in mucin solution form agglomerates in which the nanoparticles are the points of contact between negatively charged mucin chains. Beyond the critical value of the mucin ratio, the repulsive forces among the mucin chains break these agglomerates. Our results support this theory; nevertheless it has to be stressed that the decrease of MI observed for high mucin weight ratio does not indicate a decrease in the mucoadhesive capacity of the formulations [50]. However, the results indicate how in mucin excess, smaller aggregates are formed in order to minimize the repulsive forces between the chains of mucin, and to maximize the points of contact between the positive charges of chitosan and the negative charges of the mucin chains. Moreover, it was noticed that the critical point of the formulations was different for the nanocapsules coated with chitosan with different characteristics ($LNC_{SVT\text{-}LMWchit}$ f = 0.3 and for $LNC_{SVT\text{-}HMWchit}$ f = 0.55). This difference could be attributed to the different chain lengths of the two chitosan batches [63]. Indeed, in a previous study conducted with a different method, Menchicchi and co-authors proposed that mucin interacts mostly with high molecular weight chitosan [70]. On the other hand, the results presented in this paper, compared to similarly uncoated LNC, demonstrate a large increase in the mucoadhesive capacity, due to the presence of chitosan. The uncoated LNC showed values of MI = 1.4, PDI = 0.51, and a zeta potential of −9.5 mV after contact with the maximum concentration of mucin (0.5% *w/v*) [71]. The PDI increase with the increase in the *f* mucin ratio corroborates the above-mentioned explanation. In fact, PDI results indicated that the heterogeneity of the distribution of the particle size in solution increased along with the mucin weight ratio, because of the formation of aggregates of different sizes. The oligosaccharide chains of mucin glycoproteins presenting terminal sialic acid residues confer a negative charge to the molecule; therefore, the variation of the particle zeta potential from positive to negative values demonstrates how the mucin enrobes the nanocapsules interacting with their surface layer of chitosan. This suggests that mucoadhesion mechanism is driven by the electrostatic interaction of the positively charged amine groups of D-glucosamine molecules of chitosan with the negatively charged sialic acid residues of mucin [72].

The SVT-loaded lipid core nanocapsules formulation was able to control drug release, due to the two diffusional barriers: the PCL polymer wall and the lipid dispersion present in the nanocapsule core. The nanoencapsulation reduced the diffusion rate of SVT across a dialysis membrane, confirming data that is frequently described in the literature as a property of polymeric nanoparticles [33]. Regarding the comparison between the two formulations, $LNC_{SVT\text{-}HMWchit}$ afforded better control of drug release. In order to explain the different release profiles, we evaluated the differences in terms of their physicochemical properties. Firstly, this can be explained by the higher viscosity of the chitosan used to develop the $LNC_{SVT\text{-}HMWchit}$. Previous studies demonstrated that the viscosity of the chitosan is an important factor for modulating the release control [73]. Moreover, nanoparticle size can influence in the release profile, which increases with decreasing particle size. Indeed, $LNC_{SVT\text{-}LMWchit}$ had a lower mean particle diameter than $LNC_{SVT\text{-}HMWchit}$, which could contribute to explaining their different release profiles, because of the greater available surface area [74,75].

The permeation across the RPMI 2650 human nasal cell line showed that the SVT transported across the nasal cell model by $LNC_{SVT\text{-}LMWchit}$ and $LNC_{SVT\text{-}HMWchit}$ can enhance drug transport across a cell pseudo-monolayer that also secretes mucin on its apical surface. The increase of SVT permeation across the human nasal cell layer can be explained by different mechanisms. In literature, chitosan is associated with an opening of tight junctions that increase cell layer permeability. However, this mechanism generally favors the permeation of water-soluble drugs, and it has been evidenced that it is slightly less efficient for chitosan bound to nanoparticles, compared to simple polysaccharide solutions [76]. More recently, it has been demonstrated that the biodegradation of nanocapsules by enzymes in the mucus barrier or intracellularly could be pivotal in enhancing the transcellular transport of lipophilic drugs [77]. The results of the ex vivo permeation studies on rabbit nasal mucosa confirmed and further added evidence for the fact that the nanoencapsulation of SVT significantly increased its permeation across excised nasal mucosa. In this case, the higher permeation evidenced for $LNC_{SVT\text{-}LMWchit}$ could be explained by a combination of factors. The smaller particle sizes of nanocapsules coated with low molecular weight chitosan could have facilitated its absorption into the mucosal tissue as reported before [78]. Moreover, an important factor is the bioadhesion of the nanostructures, as previously explained, given by the particles shell of chitosan, which interacts with electrostatic forces at the anionic sites of the nasal mucus [65]. However, from the mucoadhesion data, a better interaction with mucus could be expected from nanocapsules coated with the high molecular weight chitosan. However, the slower release kinetics evidenced for these particles have probably contributed to limiting the amount of drug permeated, especially considering that drug accumulation into the tissue is superimposable for the two nanocapsule formulations.

Previous findings [79,80], agree that chitosan-coated nanoparticles increase drug permeation across the nasal mucosa, compared to the free drug control. This controlled SVT permeation, together with the mucoadhesion effects, may be an important strategy for prolonging the effects of the drug when it is administered via the nasal route.

5. Conclusions

In the present investigation, the coating process of lipid-core nanocapsules, using a one-pot technique approach, was presented. Furthermore, two chitosan-coated simvastatin-loaded lipid core nanocapsules suitable for nasal administration were successfully developed. Both the nanoparticles produced with different types of chitosan were designed to have adequate physicochemical and mucoadhesive properties for a potential nose-to-brain application. The formulations prepared combine a controlled release of simvastatin, and mucoadhesion properties that are able to increase drug permeation across the nasal mucosa, as demonstrated by using two different models of nasal epithelium. In summary, simvastatin-loaded chitosan-coated lipid core nanocapsules seem to be a promising mucoadhesive system for the nose-to-brain delivery of poorly soluble anticancer drugs. Follow up studies will focus on the investigation of the potential of these nanoparticles for the treatment of brain tumors, involving studies with glioma cells, and an orthotopic intracranial tumor model in mice.

Author Contributions: Conceptualization, A.R.P., S.S.G., and F.S.; Methodology, F.A.B., S.P., T.A., G.D.S., G.G.P., M.M., L.T.F.; Investigation, F.A.B., S.P.; Resources, A.R.P., S.S.G.; Writing—Original Draft Preparation, F.A.B., S.P.; Writing—Review & Editing, F.A.B., F.S.; Supervision, A.B., G.C., F.S.

References

1. Chiang, K.H.; Cheng, W.L.; Shih, C.M.; Lin, Y.W.; Tsao, N.W.; Kao, Y.T.; Lin, C.T.; Wu, S.C.; Huang, C.Y.; Lin, F.Y. Statins, HMG-CoA Reductase Inhibitors, Improve Neovascularization by Increasing the Expression Density of CXCR4 in Endothelial Progenitor Cells. *PLoS ONE* **2015**, *10*, e0136405. [CrossRef] [PubMed]
2. Liao, J.K.; Ulrich, L. Pleiotropic effects of statins. *Annu. Rev. Pharmacol. Toxicol.* **2005**, *45*, 89–118. [CrossRef] [PubMed]
3. Davies, J.T.; Delfino, S.F.; Feinberg, C.E.; Johnson, M.F.; Nappi, V.L.; Olinger, J.T.; Schwab, A.P.; Swanson, H.I. Current and Emerging Uses of Statins in Clinical Therapeutics: A Review. *Lipid Insights* **2016**, *9*, 13–29. [CrossRef] [PubMed]
4. Jain, M.K.; Ridker, P.M. Anti-inflammatory effects of statins: Clinical evidence and basic mechanisms. *Nat. Rev. Drug Discov.* **2005**, *4*, 977–987. [CrossRef] [PubMed]
5. Liao, K.J. Isoprenoids as mediators of the biological effects of statins. *J. Clin. Investig.* **2002**, *110*, 285–288. [CrossRef] [PubMed]
6. Tanaka, S.; Fukumoto, Y.; Nochioka, K.; Minami, T.; Kudo, S.; Shiba, N.; Shimokawa, H. Statins exert the pleiotropic effects through small GTP-binding protein dissociation stimulator upregulation with a resultant Rac1 degradation. *Arter. Thromb. Vasc. Biol.* **2013**, *33*, 1591–1600. [CrossRef] [PubMed]
7. Hindler, K.; Cleeland, C.S.; Rivera, E.; Collard, C.D. The role of statins in cancer therapy. *Oncologist* **2006**, *11*, 306–315. [CrossRef] [PubMed]
8. Altwairgi, A.K. Statins are potential anticancerous agents (Review). *Oncol. Rep.* **2015**, *33*, 1019–1039. [CrossRef] [PubMed]
9. Gazzerro, P.; Proto, M.C.; Gangemi, G.; Malfitano, A.M.; Ciaglia, E.; Pisanti, S.; Santoro, A.; Laezza, C.; Bifulco, M. Pharmacological actions of statins: a critical appraisal in the management of cancer. *Pharmacol. Rev.* **2012**, *64*, 102–146. [CrossRef] [PubMed]
10. Wejde, J.; Hjertman, M.; Carlberg, M.; Egestad, B.; Griffiths, W.J.; Sjövall, J.; Larsson, O. Dolichol-like lipids with stimulatory effect on DNA synthesis: substrates for protein dolichylation. *J. Cell Biochem.* **1998**, *71*, 502–514. [CrossRef]
11. Bifulco, M. Therapeutic potential of statins in thyroid proliferative disease. *Nat. Clin. Pract. Endocrinol. Metab.* **2008**, *4*, 242–243. [CrossRef] [PubMed]
12. Chan, K.K.; Oza, A.M.; Siu, L.L. The statins as anticancer agents. *Clin. Cancer Res.* **2003**, *9*, 10–19. [PubMed]
13. Frick, M.; Dulak, J.; Cisowski, J.; Jozkowicz, A.; Zwick, R.; Alber, H.; Dichtl, W.; Schwarzacher, S.P.;

Pachinger, O.; Weidinger, F. Statins differentially regulate vascular endothelial growth factor synthesis in endothelial and vascular smooth muscle cells. *Atherosclerosis* **2003**, *170*, 229–236. [CrossRef]

14. Denoyelle, C.; Vasse, M.; Körner, M.; Mishal, Z.; Ganné, F.; Vannier, J.P.; Soria, J.; Soria, C. Cerivastatin, an inhibitor of HMG-CoA reductase, inhibits the signaling pathways involved in the invasiveness and metastatic properties of highly invasive breast cancer cell lines: an in vitro study. *Carcinogenesis* **2001**, *22*, 1139–1148. [CrossRef] [PubMed]
15. Yanae, M.; Tsubaki, M.; Satou, T.; Itoh, T.; Imano, M.; Yamazoe, Y.; Nishida, S. Statin-induced apoptosis via the suppression of ERK1/2 and Akt activation by inhibition of the geranylgeranyl-pyrophosphate biosynthesis in glioblastoma. *J. Exp. Clin. Cancer Res.* **2011**, *30*, 74. [CrossRef] [PubMed]
16. Wu, H.; Jiang, H.; Lu, D.; Xiong, Y.; Qu, C.; Zhou, D.; Mahmood, A.; Chopp, M. Effect of simvastatin on glioma cell proliferation, migration, and apoptosis. *Neurosurgery* **2009**, *65*, 1087–1096. [CrossRef] [PubMed]
17. Bababeygy, S.R.; Polevaya, N.V.; Youssef, S.; Sun, A.; Xiong, A.; Prugpichailers, T.; Veeravagu, A.; Hou, L.C.; Steinman, L.; Tse, V. HMG-CoA Reductase Inhibition Causes Increased Necrosis and Apoptosis in an In Vivo Mouse Glioblastoma Multiforme Model. *Anticancer Res.* **2009**, *29*, 4901–4908. [PubMed]
18. Parrish, K.E.; Sarkaria, J.N.; Elmquist, W.F. Improving drug delivery to primary and metastatic brain tumors: strategies to overcome the blood-brain barrier. *Clin. Pharmacol. Ther.* **2015**, *97*, 336–346. [CrossRef] [PubMed]
19. Romana, B.; Batger, M.; Prestidge, C.A.; Colombo, G.; Sonvico, F. Expanding the therapeutic potential of statins by means of nanotechnology enabled drug delivery systems. *Curr. Top. Med. Chem.* **2014**, *14*, 1182–1193. [CrossRef] [PubMed]
20. Mittal, D.; Ali, A.; Md, S.; Baboota, S.; Sahni, J.K.; Ali, J. Insights into direct nose to brain delivery: current status and future perspective. *Drug Deliv.* **2014**, *21*, 75–86. [CrossRef] [PubMed]
21. Sonvico, F.; Clementino, A.; Buttini, F.; Colombo, G.; Pescina, S.; Guterres, S.S.; Pohlmann, A.R.; Nicoli, S. Surface-Modified Nanocarriers for Nose-to-Brain Delivery: From Bioadhesion to Targeting. *Pharmaceutics* **2018**, *10*, 34. [CrossRef] [PubMed]
22. Bernardi, A.; Braganhol, E.; Jäger, E.; Figueiró, F.; Edelweiss, M.I.; Pohlmann, A.R.; Guterres, S.S.; Battastini, A.M. Indomethacin-loaded nanocapsules treatment reduces in vivo glioblastoma growth in a rat glioma model. *Cancer Lett.* **2009**, *281*, 53–63. [CrossRef] [PubMed]
23. Patel, T.; Zhou, J.; Piepmeier, J.M.; Saltzman, W.M. Polymeric Nanoparticles for Drug Delivery to the Central Nervous System. *Adv. Drug Deliv. Rev.* **2012**, *64*, 701–705. [CrossRef] [PubMed]
24. Rodrigues, S.F.; Fiel, L.A.; Shimada, A.L.; Pereira, N.R.; Guterres, S.S.; Pohlmann, A.R.; Farsky, S.H. Lipid-Core Nanocapsules Act as a Drug Shuttle Through the Blood Brain Barrier and Reduce Glioblastoma After Intravenous or Oral Administration. *J. Biomed. Nanotechnol.* **2016**, *12*, 986–1000. [CrossRef] [PubMed]
25. Bahadur, S.; Pathak, K. Physicochemical and physiological considerations for efficient nose-to-brain targeting. *Expert Opin. Drug Deliv.* **2012**, *9*, 19–31. [CrossRef] [PubMed]
26. Comfort, C.; Garrastazu, G.; Pozzoli, M.; Sonvico, F. Opportunities and challenges for the nasal administration of nanoemulsions. *Curr. Top. Med. Chem.* **2015**, *15*, 356–368. [CrossRef] [PubMed]
27. Illum, L. Nasal drug delivery-possibilities, problems and solutions. *J. Control. Release* **2003**, *87*, 187–198. [CrossRef]
28. Prego, C.; Torres, D.; Alonso, M.J. Chitosan nanocapsules: a new carrier for nasal peptide delivery. *J. Nanosci. Nanotechnol.* **2006**, *6*, 2921–2928. [CrossRef] [PubMed]
29. Fonseca, F.N.; Betti, A.H.; Carvalho, F.C.; Gremião, M.P.; Dimer, F.A.; Guterres, S.S.; Tebaldi, M.L.; Rates, S.M.; Pohlmann, A.R. Mucoadhesive Amphiphilic Methacrylic Copolymer-Functionalized Poly(ε-caprolactone) Nanocapsules for Nose-to-Brain Delivery of Olanzapine. *Biomed. Nanotechnol.* **2015**, *11*, 1472–1481. [CrossRef]
30. Clementino, A.; Batger, M.; Garrastazu, G.; Pozzoli, M.; Del Favero, E.; Rondelli, V.; Gutfilen, B.; Barboza, T.; Sukkar, M.B.; Souza, S.A.; et al. The nasal delivery of nanoencapsulated statins—an approach for brain delivery. *Int. J. Nanomed.* **2016**, *11*, 6575–6590. [CrossRef] [PubMed]
31. Couvreur, P.; Barratt, G.; Fattal, E.; Vauthier, C. Nanocapsule Technology: A Review. *Crit. Rev. Ther. Drug Carrier Syst.* **2002**, *19*, 99–134. [CrossRef] [PubMed]
32. Mora-Huertas, C.E.; Fessi, H.; Elaissari, A. Polymer-based nanocapsules for drug delivery. *Int. J. Pharm.* **2010**, *385*, 113–142. [CrossRef] [PubMed]
33. Pohlmann, A.R.; Fonseca, F.N.; Paese, K.; Detoni, C.B.; Coradini, K.; Beck, R.C.; Guterres, S.S.

Poly(e-caprolactone) microcapsules and nanocapsules in drug delivery. *Expert Opin. Drug Deliv.* **2013**, *10*, 623–638. [CrossRef] [PubMed]

34. Jäger, E.; Venturini, C.G.; Poletto, F.S.; Colomé, L.M.; Pohlmann, J.P.; Bernardi, A.; Battastini, A.M.; Guterres, S.S.; Pohlmann, A.R. Sustained release from lipid-core nanocapsules by varying the core viscosity and the particle surface area. *J. Biomed. Nanotechnol.* **2009**, *5*, 130–140. [CrossRef] [PubMed]
35. Venturini, C.G.; Jäger, E.; Oliveira, C.P.; Bernardi, A.; Battastini, A.M.O.; Guterres, S.S.; Pohlmann, A.R. Formulation of lipid core nanocapsules. *Colloids Surf. A Physicochem. Eng. Asp.* **2011**, *375*, 200–208. [CrossRef]
36. Fiel, L.A.; Rebêlo, L.M.; Santiago, T.M.; Adorne, M.D.; Guterres, S.S.; Sousa, J.S.; Pohlmann, A.R. Diverse Deformation Properties of Polymeric Nanocapsules and Lipid-Core Nanocapsules. *Soft Matter* **2011**, *7*, 7240–7247. [CrossRef]
37. Frozza, R.L.; Bernardi, A.; Paese, K.; Hoppe, J.B.; da Silva, T.; Battastini, A.M.; Pohlmann, A.R.; Guterres, S.S.; Salbego, C. Characterization of trans-resveratrol-loaded lipid-core nanocapsules and tissue distribution studies in rats. *J. Biomed. Nanotechnol.* **2010**, *6*, 694–703. [CrossRef] [PubMed]
38. Zanotto-Filho, A.; Coradini, K.; Braganhol, E.; Schröder, R.; de Oliveira, C.M.; Simões-Pires, A.; Battastini, A.M.; Pohlmann, A.R.; Guterres, S.S.; Forcelini, C.M.; et al. Curcumin-loaded lipid-core nanocapsules as a strategy to improve pharmacological efficacy of curcumin in glioma treatment. *Eur. J. Pharm. Biopharm.* **2013**, *83*, 156–167. [CrossRef] [PubMed]
39. Dimer, F.A.; Ortiz, M.; Pase, C.S.; Roversi, K.; Friedrich, R.B.; Pohlmann, A.R.; Burger, M.E.; Guterres, S.S. Nanoencapsulation of Olanzapine Increases Its Efficacy in Antipsychotic Treatment and Reduces Adverse Effects. *J. Biomed. Nanotechnol.* **2014**, *10*, 1137–1145. [CrossRef] [PubMed]
40. Figueiró, F.; Bernardi, A.; Frozza, R.L.; Terroso, T.; Zanotto-Filho, A.; Jandrey, E.H.; Moreira, J.C.; Salbego, C.G.; Edelweiss, M.I.; Pohlmann, A.R.; et al. Resveratrol-loaded lipid-core nanocapsules treatment reduces in vitro and in vivo glioma growth. *J. Biomed. Nanotechnol.* **2013**, *9*, 516–526.
41. Figueiró, F.; de Oliveira, C.P.; Rockenbach, L.; Mendes, F.B.; Bergamin, L.S.; Jandrey, E.H.; Edelweiss, M.I.; Guterres, S.S.; Pohlmann, A.R.; Battastini, A.M. Pharmacological Improvement and Preclinical Evaluation of Methotrexate-Loaded Lipid-Core Nanocapsules in a Glioblastoma Model. *J. Biomed. Nanotechnol.* **2015**, *11*, 1808–1818. [CrossRef] [PubMed]
42. Drewes, C.C.; Fiel, L.A.; Bexiga, C.G.; Asbahr, A.C.; Uchiyama, M.K.; Cogliati, B.; Araki, K.; Guterres, S.S.; Pohlmann, A.R.; Farsky, S.P. Novel therapeutic mechanisms determine the effectiveness of lipid-core nanocapsules on melanoma models. *Int. J. Nanomed.* **2016**, *11*, 1261–1279. [PubMed]
43. Bender, E.A.; Adorne, M.D.; Colomé, L.M.; Abdalla, D.S.P.; Guterres, S.S.; Pohlmann, A.R. Hemocompatibility of poly(epsilon-caprolactone) lipid-core nanocapsules stabilized with polysorbate 80-lecithin and uncoated or coated with chitosan. *Int. J. Pharm.* **2012**, *426*, 271–279. [CrossRef] [PubMed]
44. Muxika, A.; Etxabide, A.; Uranga, J.; Guerrero, P.; De la Caba, K. Chitosan as a bioactive polymer: Processing, properties and applications. *Int. J. Biol. Macromol.* **2017**, *105*, 1358–1368. [CrossRef] [PubMed]
45. Kim, I.Y.; Seo, S.J.; Moon, H.S.; Yoo, M.K.; Park, I.Y.; Kim, B.C.; Cho, C.S. Chitosan and its derivatives for tissue engineering applications. *Biotechnol. Adv.* **2008**, *26*, 1–21. [CrossRef] [PubMed]
46. Rodrigues, S.; Dionísio, M.; López, C.R.; Grenha, A. Biocompatibility of Chitosan Carriers with Application in Drug Delivery. *J. Funct. Biomater.* **2012**, *3*, 615–641. [CrossRef] [PubMed]
47. Ways, T.M.M; Lau, W.M.; Khutoryanskiy, V.V. Chitosan and Its Derivatives for Application in Mucoadhesive Drug Delivery Systems. *Polymers* **2018**, *10*, 267. [CrossRef]
48. Ali, A.; Ahmed, S. A review on chitosan and its nanocomposites in drug delivery. *Int. J. Biol. Macromol.* **2018**, *109*, 273–286. [CrossRef] [PubMed]
49. Bernkop-Schnürch, A.; Dünnhaupt, S. Chitosan-based drug delivery systems. *Eur. J. Pharm. Biopharm.* **2012**, *81*, 463–469. [CrossRef] [PubMed]
50. Eliyahu, S.; Aharon, A.; Bianco-Peled, H. Acrylated Chitosan Nanoparticles with Enhanced Mucoadhesion. *Polymers* **2018**, *10*, 106. [CrossRef]
51. Castile, J.; Cheng, Y.H.; Simmons, B.; Perelman, M.; Smith, A.; Watts, P. Development of in vitro models to demonstrate the ability of PecSys®, an in situ nasal gelling technology, to reduce nasal run-off and drip. *Drug Dev. Ind. Pharm.* **2013**, *39*, 816–824. [CrossRef] [PubMed]
52. Pozzoli, M.; Ong, H.X.; Morgan, L.; Sukkar, M.; Traini, D.; Young, P.M.; Sonvico, F. Application of RPMI 2650 nasal cell model to a 3D printed apparatus for the testing of drug deposition and permeation of nasal products. *Eur. J. Pharm. Biopharm.* **2016**, *107*, 223–233. [CrossRef] [PubMed]

53. Bortolotti, F.; Balducci, A.G.; Sonvico, F.; Russo, P.; Colombo, G. In vitro permeation of desmopressin across rabbit nasal mucosa from liquid nasal sprays: the enhancing effect of potassium sorbate. *Eur. J. Pharm. Sci.* **2009**, *37*, 36–42. [PubMed]
54. Vaz, G.R.; Hädrich, G.; Bidone, J.; Rodrigues, J.L.; Falkembach, M.C.; Putaux, J.L.; Hort, M.A.; Monserrat, J.M.; Varela Junior, A.S.; Teixeira, H.F.; et al. Development of Nasal Lipid Nanocarriers Containing Curcumin for Brain Targeting. *J. Alzheimers Dis.* **2017**, *59*, 961–974. [CrossRef] [PubMed]
55. Oliveira, P.; Venturini, C.G.; Donida, B.; Poletto, F.S.; Guterres, S.S.; Pohlmann, A.R. An algorithm to determine the mechanism of drug distribution in lipid-core nanocapsule formulations. *Soft Matter* **2013**, *9*, 1141–1150. [CrossRef]
56. Bianchin, M.D.; Külkamp-Guerreiro, I.C.; Oliveira, C.P.; Contri, R.V.; Guterres, S.S.; Pohlmann, A.R. Radar charts based on particle sizing as an approach to establish the fingerprints of polymeric nanoparticles in aqueous formulations. *J. Drug Deliv. Sci. Technol.* **2016**, *30*, 180–189. [CrossRef]
57. Frank, L.A.; Chaves, P.S.; D'Amore, C.M.; Contri, R.V.; Frank, A.G.; Beck, R.C.; Pohlmann, A.R.; Buffon, A.; Guterres, S.S. The use of chitosan as cationic coating or gel vehicle for polymeric nanocapsules: Increasing penetration and adhesion of imiquimod in vaginal tissue. *Eur. J. Pharm. Biopharm.* **2017**, *114*, 202–212. [CrossRef] [PubMed]
58. Gouda, M.; Elayaan, U.; Youssef, M.M. Synthesis and Biological Activity of Drug Delivery System Based on Chitosan Nanocapsules. *Adv. Nanopart.* **2014**, *3*, 148–158. [CrossRef]
59. Mir, M.; Ishtiaq, S.; Rabia, S.; Khatoon, M.; Zeb, A.; Khan, G.M.; Ur Rehman, A.; Ud Din, F. Nanotechnology: from In Vivo Imaging System to Controlled Drug Delivery. *Nanoscale Res. Lett.* **2017**, *12*, 500. [CrossRef] [PubMed]
60. Komninou, E.R.; Remião, M.H.; Lucas, C.G.; Domingues, W.B.; Basso, A.C.; Jornada, D.S.; Deschamps, J.C.; Beck, R.C.; Pohlmann, A.R.; Bordignon, V.; et al. Effects of Two Types of Melatonin-Loaded Nanocapsules with Distinct Supramolecular Structures: Polymeric (NC) and Lipid-Core Nanocapsules (LNC) on Bovine Embryo Culture Model. *PLoS ONE* **2016**, *11*, e0157561. [CrossRef] [PubMed]
61. Haliza, K.; Alpar, H.O. Development and characterization of chitosan nanoparticles for siRNA delivery. *J. Control. Release* **2006**, *115*, 216–225.
62. Sonvico, F.; Cagnani, A.; Rossi, A.; Motta, S.; Di Bari, M.T.; Cavatorta, F.; Alonso, M.J.; Deriu, A.; Colombo, P. Formation of self-organized nanoparticles by lecithin/chitosan ionic interaction. *Int. J. Pharm.* **2006**, *324*, 67–73. [CrossRef] [PubMed]
63. Zaki, S.S.O.; Ibrahim, M.N.; Katas, H. Particle Size Affects Concentration-Dependent Cytotoxicity of Chitosan Nanoparticles towards Mouse Hematopoietic Stem Cells. *J. Nanotechnol.* **2015**, *15*, 1–5.
64. Huang, M.; Khor, E.; Lim, L.Y. Uptake and cytotoxicity of chitosan molecules and nanoparticles: Effects of molecular weight and degree of deacetylation. *Pharm. Res.* **2004**, *21*, 344–353. [CrossRef] [PubMed]
65. Casettari, L.; Illum, L. Chitosan in nasal delivery systems for therapeutic drugs. *J. Control. Release* **2014**, *190*, 189–200. [CrossRef] [PubMed]
66. Mazzarino, L.; Coche-Guérente, L.; Labbé, P.; Lemos-Senna, E.; Borsali, R. On the mucoadhesive properties of chitosan-coated polycaprolactone nanoparticles loaded with curcumin using quartz crystal microbalance with dissipation monitoring. *J. Biomed. Nanotechnol.* **2014**, *10*, 787–794. [CrossRef] [PubMed]
67. Mistry, A.; Stolnik, S.; Illum, L. Nanoparticles for direct nose-to-brain delivery of drugs. *Int. J. Pharm.* **2009**, *379*, 146–157. [CrossRef] [PubMed]
68. Sosnik, A.J.; Neves, J.; Sarmento, B. Mucoadhesive polymers in the design of nano-drug delivery systems for administration by non-parenteral routes: A review. *Prog. Polym. Sci.* **2014**, *39*, 2030–2075. [CrossRef]
69. Sigurdsson, H.H.; Kirch, J.; Lehr, C.M. Mucus as a barrier to lipophilic drugs. *Int. J. Pharm.* **2013**, *453*, 56–64. [CrossRef] [PubMed]
70. Menchicchi, B.; Fuenzalida, J.P.; Bobbili, K.B.; Hensel, A.; Swamy, M.J.; Goycoolea, F.M. Structure of chitosan determines its interactions with mucin. *Biomacromolecules* **2014**, *15*, 3550–3558. [CrossRef] [PubMed]
71. Chaves, P.D.; Ourique, A.F.; Frank, L.A.; Pohlmann, A.R.; Guterres, S.S.; Beck, R.C. Carvedilol-loaded nanocapsules: Mucoadhesive properties and permeability across the sublingual mucosa. *Eur. J. Pharm. Biopharm.* **2017**, *114*, 88–95. [CrossRef] [PubMed]
72. Singh, I.; Rana, V. Enhancement of Mucoadhesive Property of Polymers for Drug Delivery Applications: A Critical Review. *Rev. Adhesion Adhesives* **2013**, *1*, 271–290. [CrossRef]

73. Chiou, S.H.; Wu, W.T.; Huang, Y.Y.; Chung, T.W. Effects of the characteristics of chitosan on controlling drug release of chitosan coated PLLA microspheres. *J. Microencapsul.* **2001**, *18*, 613–625. [PubMed]
74. Trotta, M.; Cavalli, R.; Chirio, D. Griseofulvin nanosuspension from triacetin-in-water emulsions. *S.T.P. Pharma Sci.* **2003**, *13*, 423–426.
75. Zili, Z.; Sfar, S.; Fessi, H. Preparation and characterization of poly-e-caprolactone nanoparticles containing griseofulvin. *Int. J. Pharm.* **2005**, *294*, 261–267. [CrossRef] [PubMed]
76. Vllasaliu, D.; Exposito-Harris, R.; Heras, A.; Casettari, L.; Garnett, M.; Illum, L.; Stolnik, S. Tight junction modulation by chitosan nanoparticles: comparison with chitosan solution. *Int. J. Pharm.* **2010**, *15*, 183–193. [CrossRef] [PubMed]
77. Barbieri, S.; Sonvico, F.; Como, C.; Colombo, G.; Zani, F.; Buttini, F.; Bettini, R.; Rossi, A.; Colombo, P. Lecithin/chitosan controlled release nanopreparations of tamoxifen citrate: loading, enzyme-trigger release and cell uptake. *J. Control. Release* **2013**, *167*, 276–283. [CrossRef] [PubMed]
78. Ahmad, J.; Singhal, M.; Amin, S.; Rizwanullah, M.; Akhter, S.; Kamal, M.A.; Haider, N.; Midoux, P.; Pichon, C. Bile salt stabilized vesicles (Bilosomes): a novel nano-pharmaceutical design for oral delivery of proteins and peptides. *Curr. Pharm. Des.* **2017**, *23*, 1575–1588. [CrossRef] [PubMed]
79. Colombo, M.; Figueiró, F.; de Fraga Dias, A.; Teixeira, H.F.; Battastini, A.M.O.; Koester, L.S. Kaempferol-loaded mucoadhesive nanoemulsion for intranasal administration reduces glioma growth in vitro. *Int. J. Pharm.* **2018**, *543*, 214–223. [CrossRef] [PubMed]
80. Khan, A.; Aqil, M.; Imam, S.S.; Ahad, A.; Sultana, Y.; Ali, A.; Khan, K. Temozolomide loaded nano lipid based chitosan hydrogel for nose to brain delivery: Characterization, nasal absorption, histopathology and cell line study. *Int. J. Biol. Macromol.* **2018**, *116*, 1260–1267. [CrossRef] [PubMed]

13

Nasal Administration and Plasma Pharmacokinetics of Parathyroid Hormone Peptide PTH 1-34 for the Treatment of Osteoporosis

Richard G. Pearson [1,*], Tahir Masud [2], Elaine Blackshaw [3], Andrew Naylor [4], Michael Hinchcliffe [5], Kirk Jeffery [4], Faron Jordan [4], Anjumn Shabir-Ahmed [4], Gareth King [4], Andrew L. Lewis [4], Lisbeth Illum [6] and Alan C. Perkins [3]

1 Division of Rheumatology, Orthopaedics and Dermatology, School of Medicine, Queen's Medical Centre, University of Nottingham, Nottingham NG7 2UH, UK
2 Nottingham University Hospitals NHS Trust, Queen's Med Centre, University of Nottingham, Nottingham NG7 2UH, UK; tahir.masud@nuh.nhs.uk
3 Radiological Sciences, School of Medicine, Queen's Medical Centre, University of Nottingham, Nottingham NG7 2UH, UK; elaine.blackshaw@nottingham.ac.uk (E.B.); alan.perkins@nottingham.ac.uk (A.C.P.)
4 Critical Pharmaceuticals Ltd., Bio City, Pennyfoot Street, Nottingham NG1 1GF, UK; anaylor@upperton.com (A.N.); kjeffery@upperton.com (K.J.); faron.jordan@hotmail.co.uk (F.J.); anjumnshabir@yahoo.com (A.S.-A.); gareth.king@catapult-ventures.com (G.K.); andrew.lewis@quotientsciences.com (A.L.L.)
5 Paracelsis Ltd., BioCity Nottingham, Pennyfoot Street, Nottingham NG1 1GF, UK; mh@paracelsis.com
6 Identity, 19 Cavendish Crescent North, The Park, Nottingham NG71BA, UK; lisbeth.illum@illumdavis.com
* Correspondence: richard.pearson@nottingham.ac.uk

Abstract: Nasal delivery of large peptides such as parathyroid 1-34 (PTH 1-34) can benefit from a permeation enhancer to promote absorption across the nasal mucosa into the bloodstream. Previously, we have published an encouraging bioavailability (78%), relative to subcutaneous injection in a small animal preclinical model, for a liquid nasal spray formulation containing the permeation enhancer polyethylene glycol (15)-hydroxystearate (Solutol® HS15). We report here the plasma pharmacokinetics of PTH 1-34 in healthy human volunteers receiving the liquid nasal spray formulation containing Solutol® HS15. For comparison, data for a commercially manufactured teriparatide formulation delivered via subcutaneous injection pen are also presented. Tc-99m-DTPA gamma scintigraphy monitored the deposition of the nasal spray in the nasal cavity and clearance via the inferior meatus and nasopharynx. The 50% clearance time was 17.8 min (minimum 10.9, maximum 74.3 min). For PTH 1-34, mean plasma C_{max} of 5 pg/mL and 253 pg/mL were obtained for the nasal spray and subcutaneous injection respectively; relative bioavailability of the nasal spray was ≤1%. Subsequently, we investigated the pharmacokinetics of the liquid nasal spray formulation as well as a dry powder nasal formulation also containing Solutol® HS15 in a crossover study in an established ovine model. In this preclinical model, the relative bioavailability of liquid and powder nasal formulations was 1.4% and 1.0% respectively. The absolute bioavailability of subcutaneously administered PTH 1-34 (mean 77%, range 55–108%) in sheep was in agreement with published human data for teriparatide (up to 95%). These findings have important implications in the search for alternative routes of administration of peptides for the treatment of osteoporosis, and in terms of improving translation from animal models to humans.

Keywords: PTH 1-34; teriparatide; nasal delivery; pharmacokinetics; osteoporosis; man; sheep; clinical trial; preclinical

1. Introduction

Fragility fractures are associated with osteoporosis, a skeletal disease that occurs mainly in the older population, and are associated with a reduced bone mineral density (BMD), with alterations in bone microarchitecture such that the bone exhibits a reduced capacity to resist fracture [1,2]. Osteoporosis is a significant contributor to non-traumatic hip fractures and vertebral fractures worldwide. In 2017, there were 66,668 hip fractures in those aged 60 years or over in the UK alone. The human cost in this patient group is high, with a mortality rate of 6.7%. A 30 day survival for patients with hip fracture can be accurately estimated using the Nottingham Hip Fracture Score [3,4]. This is mirrored by a huge health economic burden, and costs for the NHS and social care of £1 billion per year in the UK [5].

PTH 1-34 injections (teriparatide) are currently the only anabolic therapy specifically designed for the treatment of osteoporosis by promoting the deposition of bone to increase bone density as opposed to preventing bone loss. Poor compliance of between 25–30% at 12 months is widely reported in patient populations prescribed teriparatide treatment [6,7]. When this patient group is questioned, there is a reluctance to be prescribed teriparatide due to the need for repeated injection [8]. Therefore, we are researching nasal spray formulations as an alternative to daily injection, as a strategy for improving patient compliance which could afford improved patient outcomes and reduced economic healthcare/social care burden. In addition, there could be economic benefits due to reduced manufacturing costs.

Nasal spray delivery systems can facilitate easy, painless administration of a drug, and are convenient for patients to self-administer. However, large hydrophilic molecules such as peptides and proteins are poorly transported across the nasal membrane, and hence require the use of a permeation enhancer to achieve a therapeutically relevant bioavailability. Furthermore, it can be a challenge to develop a suitable nasal formulation since many permeation enhancers are poorly tolerated by the nasal membrane [9–11]. Enabling technologies in the form of both nasal delivery devices and nasal mucosal permeation enhancers are presently being developed for effective nasal delivery of peptides/proteins. Such technologies are being pursued in clinical trials [12,13]. The nasal delivery system investigated here contains a permeation enhancer aimed at promoting absorption of the PTH 1-34 (4.1 kDa 34 N-terminal amino acid peptide) across the nasal mucosa in a safe manner [9]. The selected permeation enhancer is a pharmaceutical excipient, polyethylene glycol (15)-hydroxystearate, also known as Macrogol (15)-hydroxystearate, polyoxyethylated 12-hydroxystearic acid, Solutol® HS 15, Kolliphor® HS 15 or CriticalSorb™ [10].

The therapeutic efficacy of the intranasal spray formulation of PTH 1-34 is dependent upon pharmacokinetics. To investigate this, the rat preclinical model was previously utilised, and showed that serum levels of PTH 1-34 were significantly greater when delivered in nasal formulations containing Solutol® HS15, compared to a simple PTH 1-34 formulation [14]. We have also previously demonstrated that Solutol® HS15 is an essential excipient for the enhancement of human growth hormone delivery via the intranasal route [10]. Solutol® HS15, a mixture of mono- and diesters of 12-hydroxystearate (macrogol 15-hydroxystearate), is a non-ionic surfactant with a hydrophilic–lipophilic balance value of 14–16. Due to its amphiphilic nature, Solutol® HS15 in solution forms micelles approximately 13 nm in diameter. Importantly, when peptides or proteins are dissolved in an aqueous solution comprising Solutol® HS15, they retain their tertiary structure [15]. The mechanism of action of Solutol® HS15 is considered to arise primarily from a combination of effects on the cell membrane (transcellular enhancement mechanism), and from an impact on the organization of the actin in the cell cytoskeleton resulting in tight junction opening (paracellular enhancement mechanism). Solutol® HS15 enhances the transport of drugs across the mucosal membrane without demonstrating toxicity to mucosal tissue [9]. The formulation is compliant with the European Medicines Agency guidelines on pharmaceutical quality of inhalation and nasal products (EMEA/CHMP/QWP/49313/2005).

Our previously published preclinical data in rats for a liquid nasal spray formation were encouraging, showing that the nasal systemic absorption of PTH 1-34 was increased considerably when administered in a formulation containing Solutol® HS15. The mean C_{max} obtained for the nasal spray (13.7 ng/mL after administering 100 μg/kg PTH 1-34) was comparable to that after subcutaneous injection (14.8 ng/mL after a 80 μg/kg dose), and the relative bioavailability was 78% [14]. These data led to the initiation of the clinical study assessing the liquid nasal spray formulation. This was carried out to assess nasal deposition, clearance and pharmacokinetics in human subjects [16]. In addition, on review of the clinical data obtained, we followed up this research using a large animal (ovine) model reported to be reliable and predictive of human intranasal drug delivery [17]. This replicated the evaluation of the liquid nasal spray formulation that was given to healthy human volunteers, in addition to piloting an intranasal dry powder formulation containing the same absorption enhancer excipient [18].

2. Materials

The PTH 1-34 acetate used for the nasal formulation was chemically synthesised (Polypeptide Inc., Torrance, CA, USA), and recombinant PTH 1-34 known as teriparatide was the active formulation ingredient (API) in the commercially available subcutaneous injection pen, Forsteo®, obtained from Lilly France S.A.S, Fegersheim, France. HyPure WFI Quality Water (Ph.Eur.) (Thermo Fisher Scientific, Loughborough, UK), Solutol® HS15 (BASF, Ludwigshafen, Germany). All other materials were supplied by Sigma Aldrich, Gillingham, UK: glacial acetic acid USP, sodium acetate USP, D-mannitol (Ph.Eur.) and L-methionine (Ph.Eur.). Gellan gum, Gelzan™ CM (CP Kelco), and trehalose USP Tc-99m-DTPA (Diethylenetriamine pentaacetate) supplied by the radiopharmacy unit of Queen's Medical Centre, University of Nottingham.

3. Methods

3.1. Preparation of Nasal Formulations for Clinical Study

The nasal formulation comprised 0.1% *w/v* PTH 1-34 (Polypeptide Inc., Torrance, CA, USA), 7.5% *w/v* polyethylene glycol (15)-hydroxystearate (Ph.Eur.), 5% *w/v* D-mannitol (Ph.Eur.), 3% *w/v* L-methionine (Ph.Eur.), 0.15% sodium acetate (Ph.Eur.), and 0.8% *w/v* acetic acid (Ph.Eur.) in water for injection (Ph.Eur.) containing the radiolabel (Tc-99m-DTPA). To achieve a 90 μg dose of PTH 1-34, 90 μL of the formulation was atomised in each actuation using a Standard Rexam 3959 winged spray actuator, SP270-90 pump (Rexam Healthcare, London, UK). In brief, for manufacture of the radiolabel (Tc-99m-DTPA) containing formulation, Solutol® HS15 was rendered molten by raising the temperature to 60 ± 10 °C. Molten Solutol® HS15 was then dissolved in 0.2 M acetate buffer (pH 4.0) containing the D-mannitol and L-Methionine at 50 ± 5 °C. The resulting 11% *w/v* Solutol HS15 was allowed to cool and was used to prepare the 1 mg/mL PTH 1–34, Tc-99m-DTPA (3–5 MBq activity), 7.5% Solutol® HS15 formulation in 0.1 M acetate buffer pH4 using water for injection (Ph.Eur.) as the diluent. Preparation of the formulations was performed at the GMP facility at the Queen's Medical Centre, Nottingham, UK.

The droplet size from the nasal spray was assayed for a 45 μL dose volume by Rexam (Suresnes, France) using a Spraytec (Malvern Panalytical, Malvern, UK) instrument, activation speed: 60 mm/s, acceleration: 2500 mm/s^2, with a symmetric profile. All parameters were analysed during the stabilization phase of the spray, with actuator positioned 6 cm from the laser. D10: Droplet diameter such that 10% of the total liquid volume consist of droplets of smaller diameter (in μm), similarly for D50 and D90. SPAN is a measure of the droplet size distribution and is defined by SPAN = (D90 − D10)/D50. D10 = 29.2 (26.8–33.5) μm, D50 = 59.7 (51.4–75.3) μm, D90 = 127.3 (102.7–155.6) μm, SPAN 1.64 (1.48–1.76).

A HPLC based analytical method was used to determine stability of the nasal formulation and was defined as 97.0–103.0 percent ($n = 4$) of the initial drug concentration in the formulation following storage (2–8 °C) over a period of 48 h, the maximum time elapsed between manufacture and dosing of the patients. Column: Discovery Bio wide pore C18 (25 mm × 4.6 mm i.d., 5 μm); Mobile Phase: Phase A: 0.1 M Sodium Perchlorate, pH 2.7, Phase B: Acetonitrile; Flow Rate: 1.0 mL/min; Run Time 50 min;

Injection Volume: 15 µL; Column Temperature: 60 °C; Auto Sampler Temperature: 2–8 °C; Detection: 210 nm.

3.2. Preparation of Nasal Formulations for Ovine Study

The liquid nasal formulation used in the sheep was prepared identically to that for the human study, with the exception that it was manufactured in the Critical Pharmaceutical Laboratories (CPL) and did not contain the Tc-99m-DTPA label. The dry powder formulation was also prepared at CPL as 1% *w/w* PTH (1-34) with 39% Gellan gum, 40% Solutol® HS15, 20% Trehalose. In brief, 97.5 mg Gellan gum was dissolved in 50 mL ultra-pure water overnight. Solutol® HS15 was rendered molten (60 ± 10 °C), and 100 mg was added to the Gellan gum solution and mixed for 30–45 min at 60 °C. 50 mg of trehalose was added and mixed for a further 10 min. A total 5 mg of PTH 1-34 was dissolved in 5 mL of ultra-pure water, and 2.5 mL was added to the formulation. Particles were prepared using a spray dryer Mini Spray Dryer B-290 (Buchi UK Ltd., Oldham, UK) with the inlet set at 85 °C (outlet modified by inlet temperature), the aspirator 100%, the pump set at 006 equivalent to 2 mL/ min, the spray pressure at 4 bar. Particle size of the dry powder formulation manufactured for use in the sheep was not measured, due to limited availability of material due to batch size. However, the particle size of similar formulations when prepared for loading into the delivery devices was monitored using Helos/BF (Sympatec GmbH, Clausthal-Zellerfeld, Germany) during formulation development, where the VMD was 73.7–91.8 µm (×10 = 10.6–23.7 µm, ×50 = 51.5–98.1 µm, ×90 = 142–153 µm). A total 2.4–2.8% of particles were below 10 µm. As the vast majority of particles were >10 µm, the formulations would be expected to be nasally deposited. The integrity of the spray dried PTH 1-34 was monitored during formulation development by HPLC analysis, which consistently revealed a purity of >82.5% PTH 1-34.

3.3. Healthy Human Volunteer Pharmacokinetic/Gamma Scintigraphy Study

The study was conducted in accordance with the Declaration of Helsinki, and the protocol for the clinical study was given a favourable opinion (12 September 2013) by the NRES committee London Westminster (ref 13/LO/1037, IRAS ID 126447). All participants gave their informed consent before they participated in the study. This included regulatory approvals from the Medicines and Healthcare products Regulatory Agency (MHRA), Nottingham University Hospitals NHS Trust Research & Innovation (NUH NHS Trust R&I) and certification from the Administration of Radioactive Substances Advisory Committee (ARSAC). The study was registered at https://clinicaltrials.gov/ website and with the Trent Comprehensive Local Research Network (Trent CLRN). A dose escalation component was included within the approved study using a developmental delivery device, however, the data are not reported here due to commercial sensitivities.

The focus of the study was to investigate the plasma pharmacokinetics of parathyroid hormone PTH 1-34 delivered in a liquid nasal spray formulation containing the excipient polyethylene glycol (15)-hydroxystearate (Solutol® HS15). Furthermore, the nasal deposition and clearance of the formulation was investigated using gamma scintigraphy. The pharmacokinetics and the deposition and clearance of the nasal spray by gamma scintigraphy were investigated in the same clinical study.

3.3.1. Pharmacokinetics

An open cross-over clinical IMP (investigative medicinal product) study was conducted in seven healthy female subjects aged over 55 years (mean age 67.7, range 58 to 81 years). Each participant provided informed consent in accordance with ethical committee requirements and good clinical practice. Pre-study screening assessments were carried out within 21 days of the participants receiving their first dose (Supplementary Materials: Section S1). Inclusion and exclusion criteria were applied (Supplementary Materials: Section S2). Participants were admitted to the study centre on the morning of dosing, having abstained from alcohol and smoking for at least 24 h previously and fasted from midnight. Participants were given a light meal on arrival. A cannula was then positioned in the participant's arm or hand to facilitate the collection of blood samples. The pre-dose sample was taken.

Participants received a single subcutaneous injection of 20 μg teriparatide into the abdomen at their first trial visit. Following a seven day wash out period, each participant self-administered 90 μg PTH 1-34 from the nasal spray formulation using the Rexam SP270 nasal spray device; the patients had previously been trained in operation of the Rexam device. Any episodes of sneezing after administration of the nasal formulation were recorded. The nasal spray formulation contained Tc-99m-DTPA, 3–5 MBq per Rexam SP270 nasal spray dose, resulting in an effective radiation dose of less than 0.14 mSv to each participant.

Following either subcutaneous or intranasal dosing, 10 mL blood samples (Becton Dickinson sodium heparin) were taken at 5, 15, 30, 60 120, 180, 240, 300 and 360 min. After each sample was taken, the cannula was flushed with 10 mL 0.9% saline. Blood was stored on ice and centrifuged within 30 min to prepare plasma (4 °C, 1100–1300 g, 10 min). These samples were stored at −20 °C before dispatching to Simbec Research Ltd. (Merthyr Tydfil, UK) for quantification by validated ELISA, in compliance with The UK Good Laboratory Practice Regulations 1999 (Statutory Instrument No. 310 6) and subsequent amendment, OECD Principles of Good Laboratory Practice (Paris 1998) and EC Commission Directive 2004/10/EC of February 2004.

Pharmacokinetic data were analysed using Phoenix® WinNonlin® 5.1 (Certara USA, Inc., Princeton, NJ, USA) from quantified PTH 1-34 in the plasma, using recorded sampling times. Summary statistics (mean, median, SD, coefficient of variation [CV%], minimum, maximum, *n*) and the following plasma pharmacokinetic parameters were calculated:

- C_{max}
- T_{max}
- Terminal half-life ($t_{1/2}$)
- AUC to 2 h (AUC_{0-2h})
- AUC to last measured time point (AUC_{last}) and corresponding F_{rel} for nasal formulation

3.3.2. Gamma Scintigraphy

For the gamma scintigraphy part of the study, a custom designed, rigid frame was attached to a single head X ring gamma camera (Mediso Ltd., Budapest, Hungary) and used to support the chin of the participant. This maintained a fixed position of the nose in a sagittal view relative to the camera, and negated the need to register the longitudinal image series. From immediately post-dose, a 20 min continuous (dynamic) image acquisition was recorded comprising 40 × 30 s frames. In addition, 30 min post administration, a 30 s frame was acquired which was repeated every 30 min thereafter, terminating at 2 h post-dose. Participants returned for a safety follow-up between 1 and 14 days after their final study procedure.

All seven participants attended the University of Nottingham MRI clinical facility (Sir Peter Mansfield Imaging Centre, School of Medicine) prior to the clinical study to generate a sagittal view of the head and neck to provide an anatomical image of the nasal cavity. The acquisition sequence protocol was: 3 plane localiser, Asset Calibration, Coronal STIR, Sagittal T_2 and Sagittal T_1 using a GE 750 3T MRI fitted with a 32 channel head coil.

Using a HERMES image workstation (Hermes Medical Solutions, Gravesend, UK) the scintigraphic images were superimposed upon the DICOM MRI images to enable reference of the nasal spray deposition site and to define formulation clearance relative to anatomical position within the nasal cavity. Using the sagittal MRI anatomical view, four regions of interest (ROI) were defined: one around the anterior site of deposition in the nasal cavity, the second covering the nasal cavity and nasopharynx to the level of the oropharynx, a third covering the entire region and a fourth distal region to obtain the background counts. The counts obtained from the ROIs were subject to various corrections to account for image time, background activity and radioactive decay. The time for 50% clearance of the total amount of radioactivity deposited in the nasal region ($T_{50\%}$) was calculated for each subject. $T_{50\%}$ was calculated from corresponding activity–time profiles by fitting 4 parameter logistic regression

(GraphPad Prism 6). For data where this program was unable to make a satisfactory curve fit, the $T_{50\%}$ was obtained by straight line interpolation.

3.3.3. Ovine Study

Research was conducted in accordance with the requirements of the Animals (Scientific Procedures) Act 1986 (ASPA) under Procedural Project Licence (PPL) number 40/3552 (Protocol 19b/1), between 26 April 2016 and 24 May 2016, at the University of Nottingham, Nottingham, UK (Procedural Establishment Licence (PEL) number PCD 40/2406). The overarching protocol (as detailed in the PPL) was subject to full review by the Animal Welfare and Ethical Review Board (AWERB), and the study-specific protocol received a more localised review by the Named Animal Care and Welfare Officer (NACWO) and Named Veterinary Surgeon (NVS). This research governance is compliant with recommended ethical review processes. In view of the clinical data obtained in the present study, the pharmacokinetics of the Solutol® HS15-based formulation of PTH 1-34 were further investigated in sheep. The sheep study replicated the clinical trial in that it tested the nasal solution formulation of PTH 1-34 as well as a subcutaneous injection, but also evaluated pharmacokinetics of PTH 1-34 following intravenous injection and an intranasal PTH1-34 dry powder formulation.

The study was conducted according to a four-way randomised cross-over study in four (Mule crossbred) female sheep (obtained from a reputable commercial supplier). The sheep were group housed in a heat and ventilation air conditioned (HVAC) facility for the duration of the study, and were uniquely identified by a combination of ear tag and electronic transponder. On arrival, the animals were also randomly assigned a unique identifier by the facilities Research Animal Facility Management system (LabTracks, Locus Technology Inc., Manchester, MD, USA) and an abbreviated study number (1, 2, 3 and 4). To aid identification during the study, the fleece of each animal was marked with the abbreviated study number by spraying with a commercial stockmarker (dye). The animals were acclimatised for 17 days prior to initiation of treatments. The animals were subject to a health inspection by the NVS prior to and after use in the study, and were monitored during the study by the PPL holder and facility personnel supported by the NACWO, NVS and University of Nottingham personnel. Animals were weighed weekly during the study (Supplementary Materials: Section S3).

The sheep were housed in a temperature and humidity controlled facility (14.2–22.2 °C and humidity from 42–70%) for the duration of the study. On the four study legs, temperature and humidity during the experimental period ranged from 17.6–19.8 °C and 51–61%, respectively. Sheep were routinely fed twice daily with hay and standard grower diet (pellets), with water ad libitum. The sheep were provided with food (approximately double rations of hay) to last overnight on the day prior to each study leg; remaining food was removed approximately 60 min before the start of dosing on each leg. Water was available throughout. Sheep were fed as normal following collection of the last blood sample on each study leg. At the end of the study, the animals were euthanised by overdose of anaesthetic.

Administration of the PTH 1-34 was either as an intranasal liquid, intranasal dry powder, subcutaneous injection or intravenous injection. The treatments were randomised according to a Latin Square design using an online randomisation programme (Experimental Design Generator and Randomiser (Edgar) accessed from: http://www.edgarweb.org.uk/) with a minimum of a two day washout period between study legs. Immediately prior to dosing, the four sheep were sedated by an intravenous injection of ketamine hydrochloride (100 mg/mL solution administered at 2.25 mg/kg). This provided approximately 3 min sedation, during which period the sheep were dosed.

The formulations were prepared at Critical Pharmaceuticals' Laboratories and transported, refrigerated, to the study facility. The intranasal liquid was administered via the right nostril using a LMA™ MAD110 Nasal™ Intranasal mucosal atomization device (MAD110) (Wolfe-Tory Medical, Inc., Salt Lake City, UT, USA) customised for use in sheep (to allow circumvention of the nostril and delivery of the dose to the respiratory mucosa of the nasal cavity). The intranasal powder formulation was also administered via the right nostril using a 5 mm oral/nasal tracheal tube Portex® Blueline 100/111/050,

(Smiths Medical, Ashford, UK) and one-way bellows. The amount of powder administered to each animal, and thus the nominal dose of PTH 1-34, was determined by weighing the devices before and after the nasal administrations. The subcutaneous and intravenous bolus injections of PTH 1-34 were administered into the flank and a jugular vein, respectively. Further details relating to dose administration are provided in Table 1. It has been reported in the literature that injections into the thigh as opposed to the abdomen have been estimated to result in a 21% slower rate of absorption, resulting in an 18% reduction in maximum plasma teriparatide concentrations (C_{max}) and 1.5 min prolongation in the time to reach peak concentration (T_{max}) [19]. Therefore, care was taken to mirror the subcutaneous injection site (flank) in the sheep model.

Table 1. Dosing of four female sheep (Mule crossbred) with PTH 1-34.

Formulation	Route	Nominal PTH Concentration (µg/mL)	Dose Volume (mL)	Dose Weight (mg)	Nominal PTH Dose (µg)
Solution #	intranasal	1000	0.2 †	not applicable	200
Powder	intranasal	10 **	not applicable	20 † (13 ± 1.5) §	200 (130 ± 15) §
Solution *	subcutaneous	40	0.5	not applicable	20
Solution *	Intravenous	40	0.5 ‡	not applicable	20

nasal spray formulation as described for clinical study; * injection formulations did not contain 7.5% *w/v* polyethylene glycol (15)-hydroxystearate (Ph.Eur.); ** µg/mg; † nasal doses administered via single (right) nostril; ‡ intravenous doses given as a bolus injection; § Mean (± SE) powder and PTH 1-34 dose weights in parentheses calculated by weighing devices before and after dosing.

A qualitative assessment of local tolerability to the administered intranasal formulations (animals dosed by injection served as controls) was made by recording the incidences of sneezing/snorting in the first 60 min following dosing and any evidence of nasal discharge prior to dosing, at 15 min intervals in the first 60 min, and then at subsequent blood sampling time points thereafter. As part of the monitoring procedure, any other 'remarkable' observation was noted.

For pharmacokinetic evaluation, blood samples (3 mL) were collected by direct venepuncture of a cephalic vein (both veins used interchangeably) under local anaesthesia (topical application of EMLA™ Cream 5%, Astra Zeneca). For intranasal and subcutaneous treatments, blood samples were collected at time 0 (prior to dosing), 5, 10, 15, 30, 45, 60, 120, 180 and 240 min post-dose administrations. For the intravenous treatment, blood samples were collected at time 0 (prior to dosing), and at 2, 5, 15, 30, 45, 60, 120, 180 and 240 min post-dose administration. Each blood sample was dispensed into a BD Vacutainer and stored on crushed ice prior to centrifugation at 2000× *g* (3135 rpm) for 10 min at 4 °C (Sorvall™ legend RV refrigerated centrifuge). The samples were stored at −20 °C prior to PTH 1-34 quantification by ELISA kit (Immunotopic, San Clemente, CA USA) as directed by the manufacturer; optical densities were measured using an LT-4000 Microplate Reader (Labtech International Ltd, Heathfield, UK).

Pharmacokinetic analysis of the plasma PTH 1-34 concentration–time data was performed using Phoenix® WinNonlin® 6.4 (Certara USA, Inc., Princeton, NJ, USA) and Excel 2016 (Microsoft, Redmond, WA, USA). The following were used as the principal measures to evaluate intranasal and subcutaneous absorption of PTH 1-34 in the sheep compared to intravenous injection: C_{max}; T_{max}; $t_{1/2}$; AUC_{last}; and AUC_{INF} (definitions as before); C_0 (initial plasma concentration estimated by back-extrapolating from the first two concentration values) was also estimated after intravenous administration only. F_{rel} (bioavailability of intranasal (IN) or intravenous (IV) PTH 1-34, relative to subcutaneous (SC) injection) and F_{ab} (absolute bioavailability of IN or SC PTH 1-34, relative to IV) were estimated as follows:

$$F_{rel}\,(\%) = (AUC_{INF(IN\ or\ IV)} \times Dose_{(SC)}) \div (AUC_{INF(SC)} \times Dose_{(IN\ or\ IV)}) \times 100$$

$$F_{ab}\ (\%) = (AUC_{INF(IN\ or\ SC)} \times Dose_{(IV)}) \div (AUC_{INF(IV)} \times Dose_{(IN\ or\ SC)}) \times 100$$

4. Results

4.1. Clinical Study

All seven healthy volunteers completed the clinical study and all pre- and post-clinical assessments were acceptable. There were no serious adverse events during this study and no participant sneezed after nasal dosing.

4.1.1. Pharmacokinetics

The mean pharmacokinetic profiles of PTH 1-34 when delivered as a liquid nasal spray formulation or as a subcutaneous injection to healthy volunteers and corresponding summary pharmacokinetic data are presented in Figure 1 and Table 2, respectively. The mean profile obtained following subcutaneous administration (20 μg dose) of teriparatide was consistent with those obtained in individual subjects (not shown) and showed rapid absorption (mean C_{max} 253 pg/mL with range in C_{max} values of 141.8 to 406.5 pg/mL and mean T_{max} of 21 min) and elimination (mean $t_{1/2}$ approximately 1 h). Teriparatide concentrations returned to zero by 6 h. This was in contrast to PTH 1-34 delivered by liquid nasal spray (90 μg dose) with plasma concentrations only being measured above baseline in two of the seven subjects at 15 and 30 min (14.0–18.9 pg/mL) or 30 and 60 min (17.7–15.4 pg/mL) post-dose administration (for all seven subjects mean C_{max} 5 pg/mL with T_{max} 9 min; $t_{1/2}$ could not be calculated as PTH 1-34 was only measured in the plasma at two time points in these participants, where the concentration was observed to increase with time). The bioavailability of PTH 1-34 after intranasal dosing was approximately 1% (for the subjects with measurable plasma concentrations, but 0.26% if all seven subjects were included in the calculations) compared to the subcutaneous injection of Forsteo®. The pharmacokinetic parameters—C_{max}, T_{max}, $AUC_{0–2h}$ and $AUC_{0–last}$—for the two delivery routes differed markedly (Table 2).

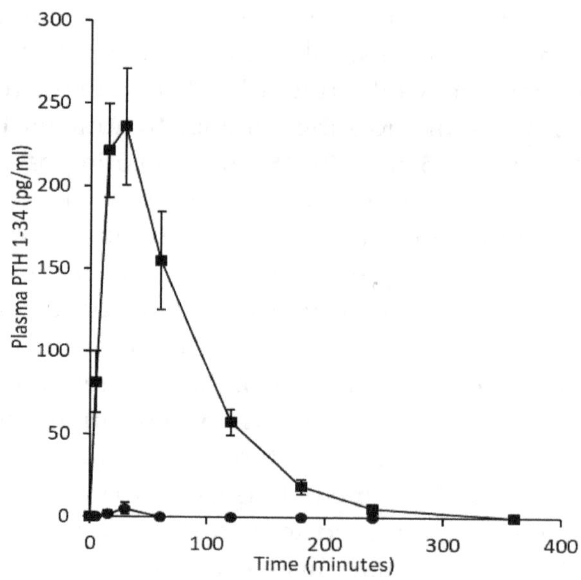

Figure 1. Pharmacokinetics of a single dose of either a liquid intranasal spray formulation containing the excipient Solutol® HS15 or a subcutaneous injection of teriparatide by a pen to healthy female subjects aged over 55 years (mean age 67.7, range 58 to 81 years). Circles represent the mean ± SE of the PTH 1-34 plasma concentration delivered from a Rexam SP270 nasal spray device (n = 7). Squares depict the PTH 1-34 plasma concentration in participants following subcutaneous injection using a commercially available formulation and injection pen (Eli Lilly).

Table 2. Pharmacokinetics of a single dose of an intranasal liquid spray formulation containing the excipient Solutol® HS15 or of a commercially available subcutaneous teriparatide injection formulation.

	Subcutaneous Injection (20 μg Teriparatide) *	**Intranasal Spray (90 μg PTH 1-34) ‡**
C_{max} (pg/mL)	252.5	5.2
t_{max} (min)	21.4	8.6
$t_{1/2}$ (min)	64.8	NC
AUC_{0-2h} (pg·min/mL)	17,381.9	242.3
AUC_{0-last} (pg·min/mL)	20,725.6	242.3

* $n = 7$ volunteers, each dose was given within a cross-over study with a one week washout between doses. ‡ $n = 7$, values were not detectable in 5 of the 7 volunteers. NC: not calculable.

4.1.2. Gamma Scintigraphy

An overview of the deposition and clearance of the nasal spray formulation delivered using a Rexam SP270 device is presented as a time series of scintigraphy images (Figure 2 and Supplementary Materials: Section S4). This represents the anatomical location of the Tc-99m-DTPA containing formulation, plotted as a density plot superimposed upon the sagittal view MRI of the participant. These data are a typical example and depicts Subject 2 in this study. The time series of images, 3, 15, 30, 60, 90 and 120 min, illustrates that the formulation was deposited in the anterior of the nasal cavity, extending to the mid-part of the nasal cavity in the region corresponding to the inferior meatus/turbinate, and was subsequently cleared from the inferior turbinates to the nasopharynx. The mean clearance curve obtained for the nasal spray formulation is shown in Figure 3. This depicts the amount of radioactivity (Tc^{99m}) that was present in the nasal cavity at each image timepoint. To adjust for variation between subjects in terms of the precise dose of Tc-99m-DTPA deposited, the counts obtained after analysis of the first frame (i.e., after 30 s) were taken as the total counts (100%) for each subject. The scintigraphy clearance data identified that the administered formulation underwent a rapid initial clearance phase (0–20 min) from the nasal cavity. The second phase demonstrated clearance at a slower rate (30–120 min). There was some variability in the clearance data between participants, graphically represented using 95% CI (Figure 3). These data can be summarised as having a median value for $T_{50\%}$ of 17.8 min (minimum 10.9, maximum 74.3 min).

4.1.3. Ovine Study

The mean pharmacokinetic profiles of PTH 1-34 in sheep when delivered nasally, as a liquid nasal spray formulation or dry powder, or by subcutaneous injection is shown in Figure 4. Corresponding summary pharmacokinetic data are presented in Table 3. The ovine study data replicate the clinical study regarding the liquid nasal spray formulation containing Solutol® HS15 making comparison to the subcutaneous injection. As in humans, the subcutaneous profile obtained in sheep showed rapid absorption and elimination of PTH 1-34; C_{max} for the 20 μg subcutaneous injection was 121 ± 47 pg/mL (mean, SE), with a median T_{max} of 10 min (range 5–15 min) and an elimination half-life of 54 ± 8 min (range 43–71 min, $n = 3$). A 200 μg intranasal dose of the PTH 1-34 liquid formulation produced a C_{max} of 47 ± 21 pg/mL and T_{max} of 10 min (range 10–15 min), and concentrations had returned to near baseline values by 30 min post-dose. The dry powder formulation was introduced to the experimental design in an attempt to improve upon the pharmacokinetic profile obtained for the liquid nasal spray. However, this formulation resulted in poor absorption of PTH 1-34 across the nasal mucosa following administration of a nominal 200 μg dose (actual dose based on weighing devices before and after administration ranged from 100–170 μg): C_{max} 8 ± 3 pg/mL. The intravenous injection provided reference pharmacokinetic data and facilitated calculation of absolute bioavailability (Figure 5). The intravenous pharmacokinetic profile of the PTH 1-34 plasma concentration demonstrated rapid elimination of PTH 1-34. The observed C_{max} for a 20 μg dose was 1142 ± 198 pg/mL at 2 min post-injection, returning to near baseline at 30–45 min. The bioavailabilities (F_{rel}) of PTH 1-34 from the liquid nasal formulation containing Solutol® HS15 and dry powder formulation, relative to subcutaneous injection, were 1.4 ± 0.3% and 1.0 ± 0.1%, respectively. The absolute bioavailability of subcutaneous injection of PTH 1-34 was 77.0 ± 13.7%.

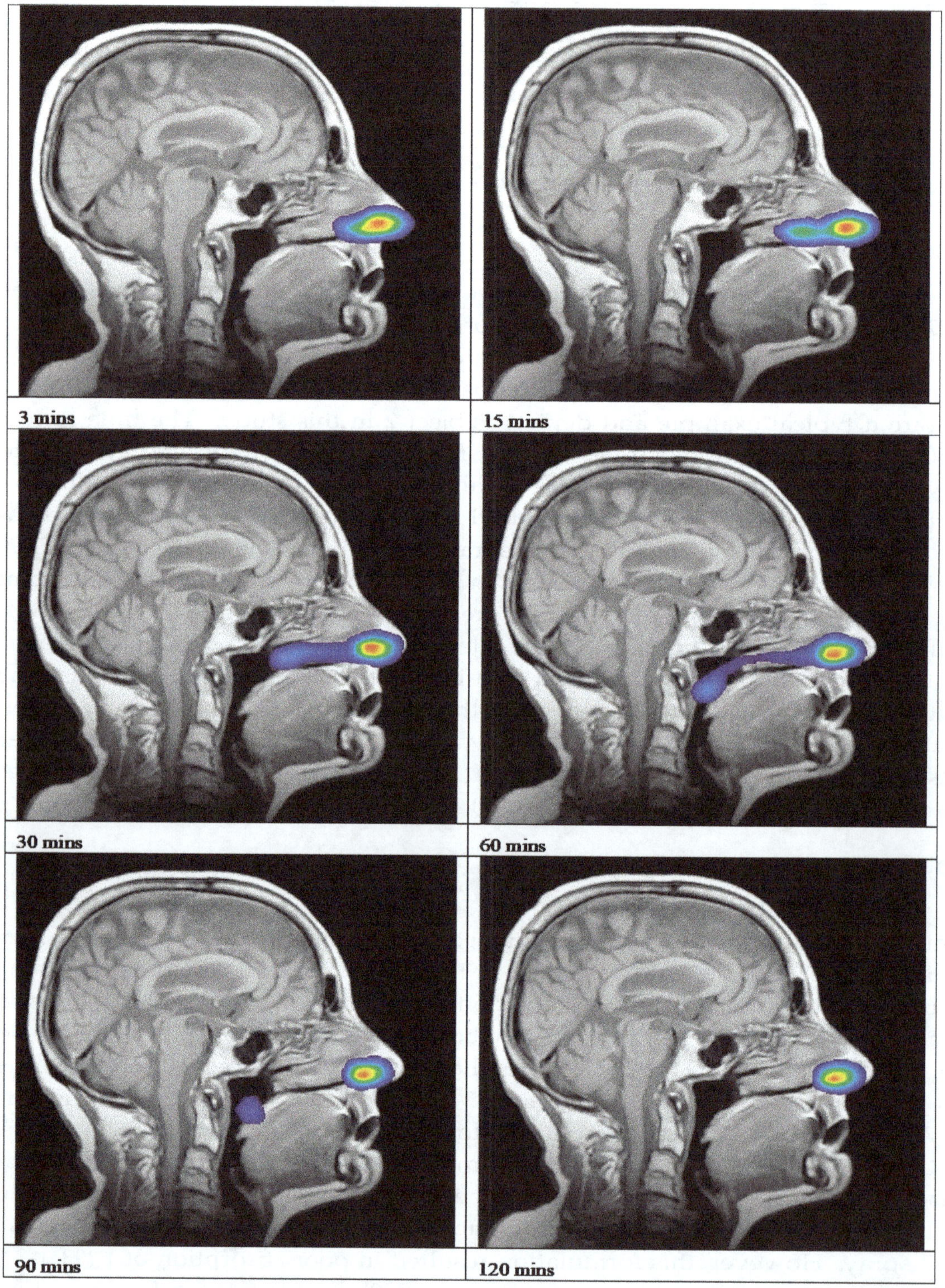

Figure 2. Deposition and clearance of nasal spray formulations delivered using a Rexam SP270 device. Scintigraphic images superimposed upon the MRI sagittal image of Subject 2, showing the clearance of the Tc^{99m}-DTPA nasal spray formulation. (The highest levels of activity are shown in red and yellow.).

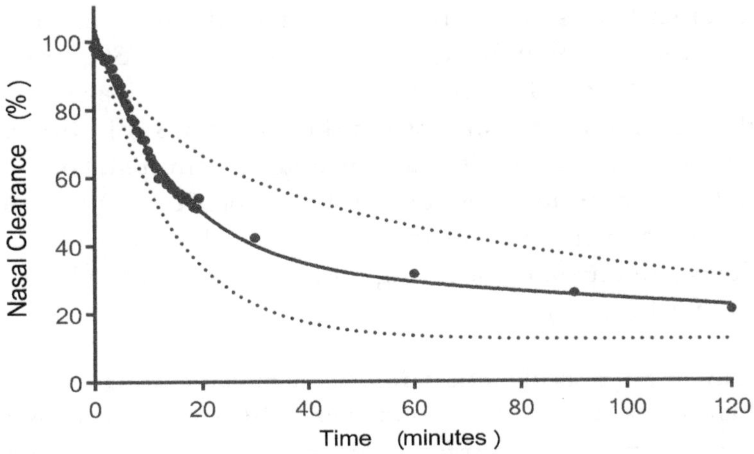

Figure 3. The clearance of Tc-99m-DTPA PTH 1-34 liquid formulation, delivered from a Rexam SP270 nasal spray device fitted with a Rexam 3959 standard winged applicator to healthy female subjects aged over 55 years (two phase decay clearance curve (Prism 7.03) fitted to mean values = solid line, ±95% CI = dotted line, n = 7).

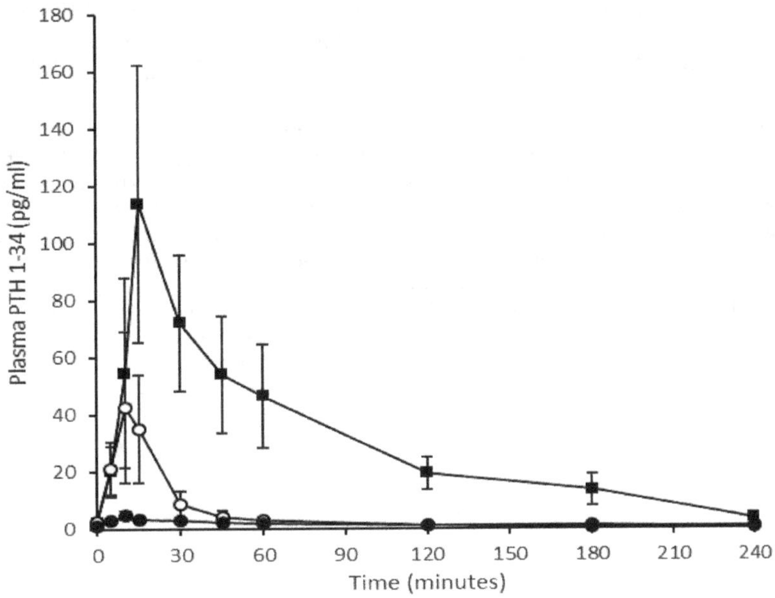

Figure 4. Pharmacokinetic profile of change of plasma PTH (1-34) concentration with time when delivered to an ovine model. Quantification of PTH (1-34) in plasma prepared from blood sampled at 5, 10, 15, 30, 45, 60, 120, 180, 240 min. Squares represent subcutaneous injection (20 μg), open circles represent intranasal liquid formulation (200 μg) and solid circles represent Gellan gum dry powder formulation (130 μg). (Mean values ± SE, n = 4 with the exception of the subcutaneous injection where n = 3.).

Monitoring of body weight (Supplementary Materials: Section S3) and adverse effects was conducted during the sheep study. One animal, Sheep 1, was withdrawn from the study prior to dosing on study leg 4 due to the animal suffering what appeared to be a seizure, further details are provided in Supplementary Materials, Section S3. All other general observations with regards to adverse effects monitoring were considered unremarkable.

In terms of monitoring for local tolerability, one incidence of sneezing/snorting was recorded across the four sheep that received the intravenous injection of PTH 1-34, and one incidence across the three sheep that received the subcutaneous injection. After administration of the PTH 1-34 liquid nasal spray formulation, there were six incidences of sneezing/snorting across three of four study animals, compared to ten incidences across three of four study animals after administration of the dry powder formulation. However, 9 of these 16 incidences were in Sheep 1, which, as stated above, was subsequently withdrawn due to ill health. Slight nasal discharge was noted on a single occasion in each of the two sheep that received subcutaneous and intravenous injections. Slight nasal discharge was observed in three of four study animals after intranasal administration of solution (one, two or four incidences observed) and powder (one, two or three incidences) formulations. Similarly, 7 of the 13 incidences of sneezing/snorting in nasally dosed animals were observed in Sheep 1. (Further details relating to incidences of sneezing/snorting and nasal discharge in sheep are summarised in Supplementary Materials, Section S5.)

Table 3. Summary of ovine pharmacokinetic parameters obtained for PTH 1-34 following intranasal (200 μg dose), subcutaneous (20 μg dose) and intravenous (20 μg dose) administration of PTH 1-34.

	Intranasal Liquid (200 μg)	Intranasal Powder (200 μg [1])	Subcutaneous Injection (20 μg)	Intravenous Injection (20 μg)
C_{max} (pg/mL)	47 ± 21	8 ± 3	121 ± 47	1142 ± 198 [2]
T_{max} (min)	10 ± 2.0 (10)	11 ± 6.6 (8)	12 ± 1.5 (10)	2 ± 0 (2)
$t_{1/2}$ (min)	109 ± 43.7 (77)	96 ± 29.8 (71)	54 ± 8.7 (47)	75 ± 18.1 (78)
$AUC_{0\text{-}last}$ (pg·min/mL)	1094 ± 410	317 ± 49	7197 ± 2204	10,660 ± 1888
AUC_{INF} (pg·min/mL)	1222 ± 370	442 ± 41	7460 ± 2220	10,799 ± 1900 [3]
F_{rel} (%) [4]	1.4 ± 0.31	1.0 ± 0.12	100	155.8 ± 24.0
F_{ab} (%) [5]	1.1 ± 0.26	0.7 ± 0.03	77.0 ± 13.71	100

Data presented as mean ± SE (median values presented in parentheses where applicable); n = 4 except in the subcutaneous injection group, where n = 3. Except in the case of F_{rel}/F_{ab} values, no correction has been made to the data to account for the dose of PTH 1-34 administered. [1] For the powder formulation, this represents the nominal dose; the estimated dose, based on emitted dose weight of powder, was 100 μg Sheep 1, 170 μg Sheep 2, 130 μg Sheep 3 and 120 μg Sheep 4 (mean ± SE 130 ± 15μg); [2] C_0 was 2182 ± 696 pg/mL following extrapolation to t = 0; [3] Since the subcutaneous injection group only comprised data from three animals (Sheep 2, 3, and 4) the corresponding mean AUC_{INF} ± SE value from these three animals was 9361 ± 1758 pg/mL·min; [4] relative to subcutaneous injection for each individual animal, where subcutaneous data were missing (Sheep 1), the average AUC_{INF} (n = 3) was used in the calculation (in the case of the intravenous injection, the calculated F_{rel} for n = 4 was approximately 156% compared to 140% for n = 3, the nominal PTH 1-34 was used throughout except for the powder formulation, where the estimated dose, as given above, was used; [5] relative to intravenous injection, the nominal PTH 1-34 dose was used throughout except for the powder formulation, where the estimated dose, as given above, was used.

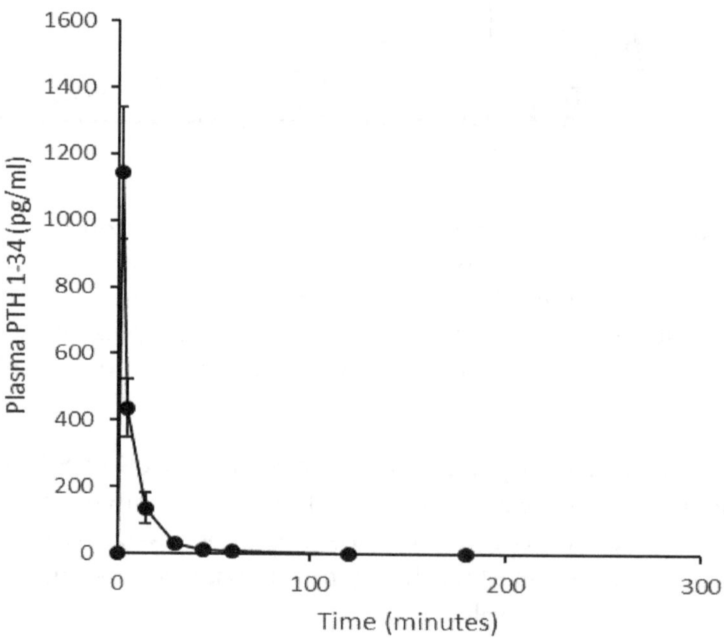

Figure 5. Plasma pharmacokinetic profile of an intravenous injection (20 μg) of PTH (1-34) in an ovine model. Quantification of PTH (1-34) in plasma prepared from blood sampled at 2, 5, 15, 30, 45, 60, 120, 180, 240 min. (Mean ± SE, n = 4.).

5. Discussion

Currently, in the UK and also globally, bisphosphonates are the first line of drug treatment for osteoporosis in the majority of patients. Subcutaneous injection of teriparatide has received regulatory approval for the treatment of post-menopausal women with osteoporosis, men with hypogonadal or idiopathic osteoporosis, and men and women with glucocorticoid-induced osteoporosis at high risk for fracture. In the UK, this is a second-line treatment in the National Health Service (NHS). At present, the course of treatment is up to 24 months [20]. Teriparatide has an imminent patent expiry date, which is of commercial interest [21]. Greater costs are incurred in the manufacture of injectable formulations compared to those for nasal delivery. An economic consideration regarding teriparatide prescription exists, as it is considerably more expensive than a course of bisphosphonate treatment [22]. Research indicates that patients poorly adhere to the long course of injections prescribed, and therefore a therapeutically efficient simple nasal spray, while cheaper to produce, would also be welcomed by patients being treated with PTH 1-34 [6–8].

An absolute bioavailability of 95% (i.e., intravenous injection 100%) has previously been reported for PTH 1-34 in human subjects when administered by subcutaneous injection into the abdominal wall [23]. Our clinical study did not attempt to replicate an assessment of absolute bioavailability, but instead focused on the current clinical route of administration of PTH 1-34 as a comparator for the nasal formulation under investigation, and therefore relative bioavailability to this delivery route. Our study data showed a plasma PTH 1-34 $t_{1/2}$ of 65 min post subcutaneous injection, which is similar to previously published values [19]. C_{max} for this delivery route was 253 pg/mL which is also comparable to those reported [24]. The pharmacokinetics we report for subcutaneous injection represent the consensus option in the literature [25–27]. As detailed above, the relative bioavailability of the intranasally dosed liquid nasal spray was approximately 0.26–1% of the subcutaneous injection of Forsteo® (Lilly France S.A.S, France) [28]. Published literature regarding nasal spray formulations are sparse, and those that are available tend to lack formulation and or pharmacokinetic data, making comparison difficult [28,29].

We consider the scintigraphy data to be an important aspect of our study, which demonstrated that the liquid nasal spray was deposited predominantly anteriorly in the nasal cavity. There is sparse literature regarding how the anatomical site of the deposition of the nasal spray formulation within the nasal regions influences transmucosal entry of peptides into the blood [30]. Deposition of the formulation is reported to be required posterior to the nasal valve, possibly within a larger and supra region of the turbinates than we achieved in order to attain optimal absorption of teriparatide [31–34]. The liquid formulation delivered to the nasal cavity in humans was rapidly cleared, and, hence, the time available for absorption was limited. It is not possible from the scintigraphic images obtained in the study to determine the percentage of formulation that did not reach (and deposit) past the nasal valve. Hence, suboptimal deposition could have contributed to the low bioavailability obtained. Similarly, we do not have data regarding how the excipient polyethylene glycol (15)-hydroxystearate, included in the formulation to promote absorption of PTH 1-34 into the plasma, interacted with the nasal mucosal surface. Perhaps a longer residency could improve drug plasma concentration, and this warrants further research. However, the $T_{50\%}$ median clearance time of 17.8 min (minimum 10.9, maximum 74.3 min) is comparable to published data on nasal clearance of liquid formulation [35].

The present clinical study showed disappointing relative bioavailability following delivery in a liquid formulation via the nasal route. This was not consistent with the previous data from our small animal preclinical studies [14]. In the preceding preclinical conscious rat model, we reported the pharmacokinetic performance of an intranasally administered PTH 1-34 subcutaneous formulation, an intranasal liquid formulation with no enhancer and an intranasal solution containing Solutol® HS15. PTH 1-34 doses of 80 μg/kg by subcutaneous injection and 100 μg/kg intranasally were given to rats. The C_{max} and T_{max} were approximately 14 ng/mL at 10 min, with 78% relative bioavailability for intranasally administered PTH 1-34 for the Solutol® HS15-based formulation, compared to 2 ng/mL,

13 min and 8% for the intranasal delivery without enhancer. We therefore expected that a relative bioavailability of at least 10% in humans should have been achievable.

Our sheep pharmacokinetic data for the SC and IV injections of PTH 1-34 are comparable with published values in human subjects. A 20 μg PTH 1-34 subcutaneous dose delivered to post-menopausal women with osteoporosis has been reported in a peer reviewed manuscript by the manufacturers of the commercial formulation to have a C_{max} in the region of 150 pg/mL and an elimination half-life of approximately 1 h. As previously stated, the absolute bioavailability of PTH SC injection in human subjects is approximately 95%. F_{ab} obtained in sheep herein was 77 ± 14% (range 55–108%). The relative bioavailability (F_{rel}) of the liquid intranasal formulation in the sheep was 1.4% ± 0.43%, close to that calculated for humans in the clinical study of approximately 1%. The mean C_{max} value in sheep of 47 ± 21 pg/mL can be put in context against reported values for the typical basal endogenous PTH concentration for post-menopausal women (28 pg/mL) and the 65 pg/mL upper limit in premenopausal women for endogenous PTH, yet at the dose given, were below the therapeutic concentrations currently used in treatment of osteoporosis [19,23].

With the aim of improving upon the pharmacokinetics of the liquid nasal spray in humans, our continued research evaluated a bioadhesive powder formulation within a large animal (ovine) model. This is a model known to be highly representative of intranasal drug delivery that closely replicates the clinical findings [17,36]. When using the ovine model to assess the dry powder formulation containing the same absorption enhancer, excipient delivered via the intranasal dry powder formulation did not improve upon the pharmacokinetics of the liquid nasal formulation. Likewise, we have published on the nasal administration in conscious rats of human growth hormone (hGH) (MW 22kDa), a molecular mass approximately five times that of PTH 1-34, with the permeation enhancer Solutol® HS15 (10%) added to the liquid formulation. For the first 2 h after administration, there was a relative bioavailability of 49% [11]. Powder formulations of the hGH with Solutol® HS15 were subsequently administered to human volunteers and compared to a subcutaneous injection of hGH. The relative bioavailability was found to be about 3%, although clinically relevant plasma concentrations could be reached with a twice daily hGF intranasal dose [18].

Observations made during the clinical study with healthy human subjects did not concur with the indicated mild irritation caused to the nasal cavities of the sheep (Supplementary Materials: Section S5) after administration of the nasal formulations [37]. However, the dose of PTH 1-34 in sheep was increased to 200 μg from the 90 μg delivered in the clinical study. A previously published clinical study reported in the literature, where 250, 500 and 1000 μg doses were delivered, reported some symptoms indicative of nasal irritation [28].

6. Conclusions

In conclusion, our study shows that PTH 1-34 was poorly absorbed from a liquid nasal spray containing the permeation enhancer Solutol® HS15 in healthy individuals with a 1% relative bioavailability. The scintigraphy imaging confirmed the anatomical site of deposition and rapid clearance of the administered dose in humans. The $T_{50\%}$ median was 17.8 min (minimum 10.9, maximum 74.3 min). When increasing the dose in the liquid nasal spray to 200 μg of PTH 1-34, this dose then resulted in a mean C_{max} value of 47 pg/mL in sheep. This value is between one third and one fifth of the C_{max} values for the drug administered at the prescribed dose of 20 μg as a subcutaneous injection for the treatment of osteoporosis in men and women.

The results discussed here for PTH 1-34 in two animal models, rats and sheep, and in humans, together with the results previously reported for hGH in rat and humans, highlights the issue of translation from animal models to humans, not only for the therapeutic effects of drugs but also for the effect of specific drug delivery systems, such as the Solutol® HS15 permeation enhancer. Many nasal delivery systems that include permeation enhancers for peptide drugs have been tested in various animal models, such as rats, rabbits and dogs, where they have been shown to effectively promote the uptake of peptide drugs, only to fail in clinical trials. The translation of effects seen in animal models to humans may depend on many factors, such as the type of intervention, study protocol, animal model and case specific factors. There are opposing opinions in the research community about the relevance of animal models [38]. However from our data, we consider that for peptide nasal delivery, the sheep model provides a better indication of the potential of translation to humans than the rat. Translational research has recently been made a priority both in the US by NIH (budget $500 million per year), in the EU (budget €6 billion) and in the UK (budget £500 million over five years) in order to assess the likelihood of successful cross-species translation [39].

Author Contributions: Conceptualization, A.L.L., L.I., T.M., A.C.P. and R.G.P.; methodology, R.G.P., A.N., M.H., K.J., F.J., A.S.-A., A.C.P.; formal analysis, R.G.P, M.H., F.J., G.K., A.C.P.; investigation, R.G.P., E.B., A.N., M.H., K.J., F.J., G.K., A.C.P.; resources, R.G.P., T.M., M.H., G.K., A.C.P.; data curation, R.G.P., F.J., G.K., M.H., A.C.P.; writing—original draft preparation, R.G.P.; writing—review and editing, R.G.P., T.M., A.N, M.H., G.K., A.L.L., L.I., A.C.P.; visualization, R.G.P., M.H., A.C.P.; supervision, R.G.P., T.M., G.K., A.C.P.; project administration, R.G.P., T.M., G.K., A.C.P.; funding acquisition, R.G.P., T.M., A.L.L., L.I., A.C.P.

Acknowledgments: The authors would like to acknowledge the support of Robin Spiller for holding the ARSAC licence for the human administration of the radiolabelled formulation.

References

1. Baron, R.; Hesse, E. Update on Bone Anabolics in Osteoporosis Treatment: Rationale, Current Status, and Perspectives. *J. Clin. Endocrinol. Metab.* **2012**, *97*, 311–325. [CrossRef] [PubMed]
2. Dhiman, P.; Andersen, S.; Vestergaard, P.; Masud, T.; Qureshi, N. Does bone mineral density improve the predictive accuracy of fracture risk assessment? A prospective cohort study in Northern Denmark. *BMJ Open* **2018**, *8*, 018898. [CrossRef] [PubMed]
3. Moppett, I.K.; Wiles, M.D.; Moran, C.G.; Sahota, O. The Nottingham Hip Fracture Score as a predictor of early discharge following fractured neck of femur. *Age Ageing* **2012**, *41*, 322–326. [CrossRef] [PubMed]
4. Maxwell, M.J.; Moran, C.G.; Moppett, I.K. Development and validation of a preoperative scoring system to predict 30 day mortality in patients undergoing hip fracture surgery. *Br. J. Anaesth.* **2008**, *101*, 511–517. [CrossRef] [PubMed]
5. Bunning, T.; Dickinson, R.; Fagan, E.; Inman, D.; Johansen, A.; Judge, A.; Hannaford, J.; Liddicoat, M.; Wakeman, R. *National Hip Fracture Database (NHFD) Annual Report 2018*; Royal College of Physicians: London, UK, 2017.
6. Modi, A.; Sajjan, S.; Insinga, R.; Weaver, J.; Lewiecki, E.M.; Harris, S.T. Frequency of discontinuation of injectable osteoporosis therapies in US patients over 2 years. *Osteoporos. Int.* **2017**, *28*, 1355–1363. [CrossRef] [PubMed]
7. Chan, D.C.; Chang, C.H.C.; Lim, L.C.; Brnabic, A.J.M.; Tsauo, J.Y.; Burge, R.; Hsiao, F.Y.; Jin, L.; Gurbuz, S.; Yang, R.S. Association between teriparatide treatment persistence and adherence, and fracture incidence in Taiwan: Analysis using the National Health Insurance Research Database. *Osteoporos. Int.* **2016**, *27*, 2855–2865. [CrossRef] [PubMed]
8. Fraenkel, L.; Gulanski, B.; Wittink, D. Patient treatment preferences for osteoporosis. *Arthritis Care Res. Off. J. Am. Coll. Rheumatol.* **2006**, *55*, 729–735. [CrossRef] [PubMed]
9. Brayden, D.J.; Bzik, V.A.; Lewis, A.L.; Illum, L. CriticalSorb promotes permeation of flux markers across isolated rat intestinal mucosae and Caco-2 monolayers. *Pharm. Res.* **2012**, *29*, 2543–2554. [CrossRef] [PubMed]
10. Illum, L. Nasal drug delivery—Recent developments and future prospects. *J. Control. Release* **2012**, *161*, 254–263. [CrossRef] [PubMed]
11. Illum, L.; Jordan, F.; Lewis, A.L. CriticalSorb (TM): A novel efficient nasal delivery system for human growth hormone based on Solutol HS15. *J. Control. Release* **2012**, *162*, 194–200. [CrossRef] [PubMed]
12. Rohrer, J.; Lupo, N.; Bernkop-Schnurch, A. Advanced formulations for intranasal delivery of biologics. *Int. J. Pharm.* **2018**, *553*, 8–20. [CrossRef] [PubMed]
13. Maggio, E.T. Intravail™: Highly effective intranasal delivery of peptide and protein drugs AU-Maggio. *Expert Opin. Drug Deliv.* **2006**, *3*, 529–539. [CrossRef] [PubMed]

14. Williams, A.J.; Jordan, F.; King, G.; Lewis, A.L.; Illum, L.; Masud, T.; Perkins, A.C.; Pearson, R.G. In vitro and preclinical assessment of an intranasal spray formulation of parathyroid hormone PTH 1-34 for the treatment of osteoporosis. *Int. J. Pharm.* **2018**, *535*, 113–119. [CrossRef] [PubMed]
15. Shubber, S.; Vllasaliu, D.; Rauch, C.; Jordan, F.; Illum, L.; Stolnik, S. Mechanism of Mucosal Permeability Enhancement of CriticalSorb (R) (Solutol (R) HS15) Investigated In Vitro in Cell Cultures. *Pharm. Res.* **2015**, *32*, 516–527. [CrossRef] [PubMed]
16. Soane, R.J.; Frier, M.; Perkins, A.C.; Jones, N.S.; Davis, S.S.; Illum, L. Evaluation of the clearance characteristics of bioadhesive systems in humans. *Int. J. Pharm.* **1999**, *178*, 55–65. [CrossRef]
17. Illum, L. Nasal delivery. The use of animal models to predict performance in man. *J. Drug Target.* **1996**, *3*, 427–442. [CrossRef]
18. Lewis, A.L.; Jordan, F.; Patel, T.; Jeffery, K.; King, G.; Savage, M.; Shalet, S.; Illum, L. Intranasal Human Growth Hormone (hGH) Induces IGF-1 Levels Comparable With Subcutaneous Injection With Lower Systemic Exposure to hGH in Healthy Volunteers. *J. Clin. Endocrinol. Metab.* **2015**, *100*, 4364–4371. [CrossRef]
19. Satterwhite, J.; Heathman, M.; Miller, P.D.; Marin, F.; Glass, E.V.; Dobnig, H. Pharmacokinetics of Teriparatide (rhPTH 1–34) and Calcium Pharmacodynamics in Postmenopausal Women with Osteoporosis. *Calcif. Tissue Int.* **2010**, *87*, 485–492. [CrossRef]
20. Joint Formulary Committee. *British National Formulary*, 72th ed.; BMJ Group and Pharmaceutical Press: London, UK, 2018.
21. Takacs, I.; Jokai, E.; Kovats, D.E.; Aradi, I. The first biosimilar approved for the treatment of osteoporosis: Results of a comparative pharmacokinetic/pharmacodynamic study. *Osteoporos. Int.* **2019**, *30*, 675–683. [CrossRef]
22. Basu, P.; Joglekar, G.; Rai, S.; Suresh, P.; Vernon, J. Analysis of Manufacturing Costs in Pharmaceutical Companies. *J. Pharm. Innov.* **2008**, *3*, 30–40. [CrossRef]
23. Eli_Lilly. *Highlights of Prescribing Information*; AbbVie Inc.: North Chicago, IL, USA, 2014; Available online: https://pi.lilly.com/us/forteo-pi.pf (accessed on 20 November 2018).
24. Haemmerle, S.P.; Mindeholm, L.; Launonen, A.; Kiese, B.; Loeffler, R.; Harfst, E.; Azria, M.; Arnold, M.; John, M.R. The single dose pharmacokinetic profile of a novel oral human parathyroid hormone formulation in healthy postmenopausal women. *Bone* **2012**, *50*, 965–973. [CrossRef] [PubMed]
25. Forssmann, W.-G.; Tillmann, H.-C.; Hock, D.; Forssmann, K.; Bernasconi, C.; Forssmann, U.; Richter, R.; Hocher, B.; Pfuetzner, A. Pharmacokinetic and Pharmacodynamic Characteristics of Subcutaneously Applied PTH-1-37. *Kidney Blood Press. Res.* **2016**, *41*, 507–518. [CrossRef]
26. Henriksen, K.; Andersen, J.R.; Riis, B.J.; Mehta, N.; Tavakkol, R.; Alexandersen, P.; Byrjalsen, I.; Valter, I.; Nedergaard, B.S.; Teglbjaerg, C.S.; et al. Evaluation of the efficacy, safety and pharmacokinetic profile of oral recombinant human parathyroid hormone rhPTH(1-31)NH_2 in postmenopausal women with osteoporosis. *Bone* **2013**, *53*, 160–166. [CrossRef] [PubMed]
27. Liu, Y.; Shi, S.; Wu, J.; Li, Z.; Zhou, X.; Zeng, F. Safety, Tolerability, Pharmacokinetics and Pharmacodynamics of Recombinant Human Parathyroid Hormone after Single- and Multiple-Dose Subcutaneous Administration in Healthy Chinese Volunteers. *Basic Clin. Pharmacol. Toxicol.* **2012**, *110*, 154–161. [CrossRef] [PubMed]
28. Matsumoto, T.; Shiraki, M.; Hagino, H.; Iinuma, H.; Nakamura, T. Daily nasal spray of hPTH(1–34) for 3 months increases bone mass in osteoporotic subjects: A pilot study. *Osteoporos. Int.* **2006**, *17*, 1532–1538. [CrossRef] [PubMed]
29. Brandt, G.C.; Spann, B.M.; Sileno, A.P.; Costantino, H.R.; Li, C.; Quay, S.C. Teriparatide nasal spray: Pharmacokinetics and safety versus subcutaneous teriparatide in healthy volunteers. *Calcif. Tissue Int.* **2006**, *78*, S45.
30. Djupesland, P.G. Nasal drug delivery devices: Characteristics and performance in a clinical perspective—A review. *Drug Deliv. Transl. Res.* **2013**, *3*, 42–62. [CrossRef] [PubMed]
31. McInnes, F.J.; O'Mahony, B.; Lindsay, B.; Band, J.; Wilson, C.G.; Hodges, L.A.; Stevens, H.N.E. Nasal residence of insulin containing lyophilised nasal insert formulations, using gamma scintigraphy. *Eur. J. Pharm. Sci.* **2007**, *31*, 25–31. [CrossRef]
32. Takala, A.; Kaasalainen, V.; Seppala, T.; Kalso, E.; Olkkola, K.T. Pharmacokinetic comparison of intravenous and intranasal administration of oxycodone. *Acta Anaesthesiol. Scand.* **1997**, *41*, 309–312. [CrossRef]

33. Djupesland, P.G.; Skretting, A. Nasal Deposition and Clearance in Man: Comparison of a Bidirectional Powder Device and a Traditional Liquid Spray Pump. *J. Aerosol Med. Pulm. Drug Deliv.* **2012**, *25*, 280–289. [CrossRef]
34. Charlton, S.; Jones, N.S.; Davis, S.S.; Illum, L. Distribution and clearance of bioadhesive formulations from the olfactory region in man: Effect of polymer type and nasal delivery device. *Eur. J. Pharm. Sci.* **2007**, *30*, 295–302. [CrossRef] [PubMed]
35. Al-Ghananeem, A.; Sandefer, E.; Doll, W.; C Page, R.; Chang, Y.; A Digenis, G. Gamma scintigraphy for testing bioequivalence: A case study on two cromolyn sodium nasal spray preparations. *Int. J. Pharm.* **2008**, *357*, 70–76. [CrossRef] [PubMed]
36. Soane, R.J.; Hinchcliffe, M.; Davis, S.S.; Illum, L. Clearance characteristics of chitosan based formulations in the sheep nasal cavity. *Int. J. Pharm.* **2001**, *217*, 183–191. [CrossRef]
37. Masud, T.; Pearson, R.G. Nasally and sc Administered Teriparatide in Healthy Volunteers (NINTTO). Available online: https://clinicaltrials.gov/ct2/show/NCT01913834 (accessed on 5 June 2019).
38. Ioannidis, J.P.A. Extrapolating from Animals to Humans. *Sci. Transl. Med.* **2012**, *4*, 15. [CrossRef] [PubMed]
39. Woolf, S.H. The meaning of translational research and why it matters. *JAMA J. Am. Med. Assoc.* **2008**, *299*, 211–213. [CrossRef]

Permissions

All chapters in this book were first published by MDPI; hereby published with permission under the Creative Commons Attribution License or equivalent. Every chapter published in this book has been scrutinized by our experts. Their significance has been extensively debated. The topics covered herein carry significant findings which will fuel the growth of the discipline. They may even be implemented as practical applications or may be referred to as a beginning point for another development.

The contributors of this book come from diverse backgrounds, making this book a truly international effort. This book will bring forth new frontiers with its revolutionizing research information and detailed analysis of the nascent developments around the world.

We would like to thank all the contributing authors for lending their expertise to make the book truly unique. They have played a crucial role in the development of this book. Without their invaluable contributions this book wouldn't have been possible. They have made vital efforts to compile up to date information on the varied aspects of this subject to make this book a valuable addition to the collection of many professionals and students.

This book was conceptualized with the vision of imparting up-to-date information and advanced data in this field. To ensure the same, a matchless editorial board was set up. Every individual on the board went through rigorous rounds of assessment to prove their worth. After which they invested a large part of their time researching and compiling the most relevant data for our readers.

The editorial board has been involved in producing this book since its inception. They have spent rigorous hours researching and exploring the diverse topics which have resulted in the successful publishing of this book. They have passed on their knowledge of decades through this book. To expedite this challenging task, the publisher supported the team at every step. A small team of assistant editors was also appointed to further simplify the editing procedure and attain best results for the readers.

Apart from the editorial board, the designing team has also invested a significant amount of their time in understanding the subject and creating the most relevant covers. They scrutinized every image to scout for the most suitable representation of the subject and create an appropriate cover for the book.

The publishing team has been an ardent support to the editorial, designing and production team. Their endless efforts to recruit the best for this project, has resulted in the accomplishment of this book. They are a veteran in the field of academics and their pool of knowledge is as vast as their experience in printing. Their expertise and guidance has proved useful at every step. Their uncompromising quality standards have made this book an exceptional effort. Their encouragement from time to time has been an inspiration for everyone.

The publisher and the editorial board hope that this book will prove to be a valuable piece of knowledge for researchers, students, practitioners and scholars across the globe.

List of Contributors

Giovanna Rassu, Paolo Giunchedi and Elisabetta Gavini
Department of Chemistry and Pharmacy, University of Sassari, via Muroni 23/a, 07100 Sassari, Italy

Luca Ferraro
Department of Life Sciences and Biotechnology, University of Ferrara, via Borsari 46, 44121 Ferrara, Italy

Barbara Pavan
Department of Biomedical and Specialist Surgical Sciences, University of Ferrara, via Borsari 46, 44121 Ferrara, Italy

Alessandro Dalpiaz
Department of Chemical and Pharmaceutical Sciences, University of Ferrara, via Fossato di Mortara 19, 44121 Ferrara, Italy

Hsiu-Chao Lin, Chih-Chi Cheng, Kuan-Lin Ku and I-Ming Chu
Department of Chemical Engineering, National Tsing Hua University, Hsinchu 300, Taiwan

Cheng-Hung Lin and Madonna Rica Anggelia
Center for Vascularized Composite Allotransplantation, Department of Plastic and Reconstructive Surgery, Chang Gung Memorial Hospital, Chang Gung Medical College and Chang Gung University, Taoyuan 333, Taiwan
Graduate Institute of Biomedical Sciences, College of Medicine, Chang Gung University, Taoyuan 333, Taiwan

Hui-Yun Cheng, Chih-Jen Wen and Aline Yen Ling Wang
Center for Vascularized Composite Allotransplantation, Department of Plastic and Reconstructive Surgery, Chang Gung Memorial Hospital, Chang Gung Medical College and Chang Gung University, Taoyuan 333, Taiwan

Ju Hyang Park, Da In Kim, Ji Hyun Choi, Jin Ho Son and Dong Choon Hyun
Department of Polymer Science and Engineering, Kyungpook National University, Daegu 41566, Korea

Hojun Seo and Geon Dae Moon
Dongnam Regional Division, Korea Institute of Industrial Technology, Busan 46938, Korea

Jongbok Kim
Department of Materials Science and Engineering, Kumoh National Institute of Technology, Gumi, Gyeongbuk 39177, Korea

Anja Haasbroek, Clarissa Willers, Lissinda du Plessis and Josias Hamman
Centre of Excellence for Pharmaceutical Sciences (Pharmacen™), Potchefstroom Campus, North West University, Potchefstroom 2520, South Africa

Matthew Glyn
Preclinical Drug Development Platform (PCDDP), Potchefstroom Campus, North West University, Potchefstroom 2520, South Africa

Narsimha Mamidi and Aldo González-Ortiz
Tecnologico de Monterrey, Department of Chemistry and Nanotechnology, School of Engineering and Science, Monterrey 64849, Nuevo Leon, Mexico

Irasema Lopez Romo
Tecnologico de Monterrey, Department of Biotechnology, School of Engineering and Science, Monterrey 64849, Nuevo Leon, Mexico

Enrique V. Barrera
Department of Materials Science and Nano Engineering, Rice University, Houston, TX 77005, USA
Department of Chemistry, Rice University, Houston, TX 77005, USA

Fuat Topuz and Tamer Uyar
Institute of Materials Science & Nanotechnology, UNAM-National Nanotechnology Research Center, Bilkent University, 06800 Ankara, Turkey

Ghada M. El-Zaafarany, Mahmoud E. Soliman and Gehanne A. S. Awad
Department of Pharmaceutics and Industrial Pharmacy, Faculty of Pharmacy, Ain Shams University, Monazzamet Elwehda Elafrikeya Street, Abbaseyya, Cairo 11566, Egypt

Samar Mansour
Department of Pharmaceutics and Industrial Pharmacy, Faculty of Pharmacy, Ain Shams University, Monazzamet Elwehda Elafrikeya Street, Abbaseyya, Cairo 11566, Egypt
Department of Pharmaceutical Technology, Faculty of Pharmacy and Biotechnology, German University in Cairo, Al-Tagmoaa Alkhames, Cairo 11835, Egypt

Marco Cespi and Giovanni Filippo Palmieri
School of Pharmacy, University of Camerino, Via S. Agostino 1, 62032 Camerino (MC), Italy

Luca Casettari
Department of Biomolecular Sciences, School of Pharmacy, University of Urbino, Piazza del Rinascimento 6, 61029 Urbino (PU), Italy

Laura Modica de Mohac
DIBIMIS Department, University of Study of Palermo, 90128 Palermo, Italy
Drug Delivery Group, Institute of Pharmaceutical Science Faculty of Life Sciences and Medicine, King's College London, London SE1 9NH, UK

Alison Veronica Keating and Bahijja Tolulope Raimi-Abraham
Drug Delivery Group, Institute of Pharmaceutical Science Faculty of Life Sciences and Medicine, King's College London, London SE1 9NH, UK

Maria de Fátima Pina
Department of Pharmaceutics, University College London School of Pharmacy, London WC1N 1AX, UK

Maliheh Ghadiri, Paul M. Young and Daniela Traini
Respiratory Technology, Woolcock Institute of Medical Research and Discipline of Pharmacology, Faculty of Medicine and Health, The University of Sydney, Camperdown, NSW 2006, Australia

Weidong Huang
School of Chemistry and Chemical Engineering, Hubei Polytechnic University, Huangshi 435003, China
Hubei Key Laboratory of Mine Environmental Pollution Control and Remediation, Hubei Polytechnic University, Huangshi 435003, China

Xian-Li Liu
Hubei Key Laboratory of Mine Environmental Pollution Control and Remediation, Hubei Polytechnic University, Huangshi 435003, China

Yaoyao Yang, Biwei Zhao, Gangqiang Liang, Shiwei Liu and Deng-Guang Yu
School of Materials Science and Engineering, University of Shanghai for Science and Technology, Shanghai 200093, China

Sam Maher
School of Pharmacy, Royal College of Surgeons in Ireland, St. Stephens Green, Dublin 2, Ireland

David J. Brayden
School of Veterinary Medicine and UCD Conway Institute, University College Dublin, Belfield, Dublin 4, Ireland

Franciele Aline Bruinsmann
Programa de Pós-Graduação emCiências Farmacêuticas, Universidade Federal do Rio Grande do Sul, Porto Alegre 90610-000, Brazil
Food and Drug Department, University of Parma, Parco Area delle Scienze 27/a, 43124 Parma, Italy

Gabriele Dadalt Souto, Gabriela Garrastazu Pereira and Silvia Stanisçuaski Guterres
Programa de Pós-Graduação emCiências Farmacêuticas, Universidade Federal do Rio Grande do Sul, Porto Alegre 90610-000, Brazil

Stefania Pigana, Annalisa Bianchera and Fabio Sonvico
Food and Drug Department, University of Parma, Parco Area delle Scienze 27/a, 43124 Parma, Italy

Tanira Aguirre
Programa de Pós-Graduação em Biociências, Universidade Federal de Ciências da Saúde de Porto Alegre, Porto Alegre RS 900500-170, Brazil

Laura Tiozzo Fasiolo
Department of Life Sciences and Biotechnology, University of Ferrara, Via Fossato di Mortara 17/19, 44121 Ferrara, Italy
Food and Drug Department, University of Parma, Parco Area delle Scienze 27/a, 43124 Parma, Italy

Gaia Colombo
Department of Life Sciences and Biotechnology, University of Ferrara, Via Fossato di Mortara 17/19, 44121 Ferrara, Italy

Magno Marques
Programa de Pós-Graduação emCiências Fisiológicas, Universidade Federal do Rio Grande, Rio Grande RS 96203-000, Brazil

Adriana Raffin Pohlmann
Programa de Pós-Graduação emCiências Farmacêuticas, Universidade Federal do Rio Grande do Sul, Porto Alegre 90610-000, Brazil
Departamento de Química Orgânica, Instituto de Química, Universidade Federal do Rio Grande do Sul, Porto Alegre 91501-970, Brazil

Richard G. Pearson
Division of Rheumatology, Orthopaedics and Dermatology, School of Medicine, Queen's Medical Centre, University of Nottingham, Nottingham NG72UH, UK

Tahir Masud
Nottingham University Hospitals NHS Trust, Queen's Med Centre, University of Nottingham, Nottingham NG7 2UH, UK

Elaine Blackshaw and Alan C. Perkins
Radiological Sciences, School of Medicine, Queen's Medical Centre, University of Nottingham, Nottingham NG7 2UH, UK

Andrew Naylor, Kirk Jeffery, Faron Jordan, Anjumn Shabir-Ahmed, Gareth King and Andrew L. Lewis
Critical Pharmaceuticals Ltd., Bio City, Pennyfoot Street, Nottingham NG1 1GF, UK

Michael Hinchcliffe
Paracelsis Ltd., BioCity Nottingham, Pennyfoot Street, Nottingham NG1 1GF, UK

Lisbeth Illum
IDentity, 19 Cavendish Crescent North, The Park, Nottingham NG7 1BA, UK

Index